Managing Dismounted Complex Blast Injuries in Military & Civilian Settings

Joseph M. Galante • Matthew J. Martin
Carlos J. Rodriguez • Wade Travis Gordon
Editors

Managing Dismounted Complex Blast Injuries in Military & Civilian Settings

Guidelines and Principles

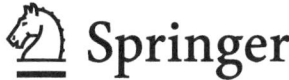

Editors
Joseph M. Galante
Division of Trauma and Acute
Care Surgery
University of California
Davis Medical Center
Sacramento, CA, USA

Carlos J. Rodriguez
Department of Surgery
Walter Reed National Military
Medical Center
Bethesda, MD, USA

Matthew J. Martin
Madigan Army Medical Center
Tacoma, WA, USA

Wade Travis Gordon
Department of Orthopaedics
Walter Reed National Military
Medical Center
Bethesda, MD, USA

ISBN 978-3-319-74671-5   ISBN 978-3-319-74672-2   (eBook)
https://doi.org/10.1007/978-3-319-74672-2

Library of Congress Control Number: 2018937082

© Springer International Publishing AG, part of Springer Nature 2018
This work is subject to copyright. All rights are reserved by the Publisher, whether the whole or part of the material is concerned, specifically the rights of translation, reprinting, reuse of illustrations, recitation, broadcasting, reproduction on microfilms or in any other physical way, and transmission or information storage and retrieval, electronic adaptation, computer software, or by similar or dissimilar methodology now known or hereafter developed.
The use of general descriptive names, registered names, trademarks, service marks, etc. in this publication does not imply, even in the absence of a specific statement, that such names are exempt from the relevant protective laws and regulations and therefore free for general use.
The publisher, the authors and the editors are safe to assume that the advice and information in this book are believed to be true and accurate at the date of publication. Neither the publisher nor the authors or the editors give a warranty, express or implied, with respect to the material contained herein or for any errors or omissions that may have been made. The publisher remains neutral with regard to jurisdictional claims in published maps and institutional affiliations.

Printed on acid-free paper

This Springer imprint is published by the registered company Springer International Publishing AG part of Springer Nature.
The registered company address is: Gewerbestrasse 11, 6330 Cham, Switzerland

Contents

1. **Introduction: Why We Do What We Do** 1
   Carlos J. Rodriguez and Joseph M. Galante

2. **Explosive Blasts: A Primer on a Multidimensional Mechanism of Injury** 7
   Raymond Fang

3. **Initial Care of Blast Injury: TCCC and TECC** 15
   Babak Sarani, Geoffrey L. Shapiro, James J. Geracci, and E. Reed Smith

4. **MASCAL** 29
   Jayson Aydelotte

5. **Resuscitation** 43
   Phillip Kemp Bohan and Martin A. Schreiber

6. **Damage Control Surgery in the Blast-Injured Patient** 57
   Travis M. Polk, Matthew J. Martin, and Ronald R. Barbosa

7. **Hemorrhage Control** 77
   Rachel M. Russo and Joseph J. DuBose

8. **Blast-Related Pelvic Fractures** 99
   George C. Balazs and Jean-Claude G. D'Alleyrand

9. **Thoracic Injuries** 111
   Ryan P. Dumas and Jeremy W. Cannon

10. **Abdominal Trauma** 121
    Luke R. Johnston, Elliot M. Jessie, and Matthew J. Bradley

11. **Vascular Injuries** 135
    Timothy K. Williams and W. Darrin Clouse

12. **Genitourinary Trauma** 151
    Matthew Banti and Jack Ryan Walter

13. **Soft Tissue Injuries and Amputations** 159
    Gabriel J. Pavey and Benjamin K. Potter

14. **Soft Tissue Infection** 181
    Jason Scott Radowsky and Debra L. Malone

15	**The Rational Care of Burns**........................... 197 Gary Vercruysse	
16	**Soft Tissue Reconstruction of Complex Blast Injuries in Military and Civilian Settings: Guidelines and Principles**.. Corinne E. Wee, Jason M. Souza, Terri A. Zomerlei, and Ian L. Valerio	209
17	**Rehabilitation of the Blast Injury Casualty with Amputation**....................................... Keith P. Myers, Tirzah VanDamme, and Paul F. Pasquina	225
18	**Mild Traumatic Brain Injury Rehabilitation**............... Bruno S. Subbarao, Rebecca N. Tapia, and Blessen C. Eapen	241
19	**Moderate and Severe Traumatic Brain Injury Rehabilitation**.. William Robbins and Ajit B. Pai	251
20	**Management of Dismounted Complex Blast Injury Patients at a Role V Military Treatment Facility: Special Considerations**................................ John S. Oh and Ashley E. Humphries	259
21	**Infection Control and Prevention After Dismounted Complex Blast Injury**............................... Heather C. Yun, Dana M. Blyth, and Clinton K. Murray	269
22	**Organizing the Trauma Team in the Military and Civilian Settings**.................................. Michael B. Yaffe, Alok Gupta, Allison Weisbrod, and James R. Dunne	285

Index... 293

Contributors

Jayson Aydelotte Trauma and Surgical Critical Care, Dell Seton Medical Center, University of Texas, Austin, TX, USA

Dell Medical School, University of Texas at Austin, Austin, TX, USA

George C. Balazs Department of Orthopaedic Surgery, Walter Reed National Military Medical Center, Bethesda, MD, USA

Norman M. Rich Department of Surgery, Uniformed Services University of Health Sciences, Bethesda, MD, USA

Matthew Banti Urology Service, Madigan Army Medical Center, Tacoma, WA, USA

Ronald R. Barbosa Trauma and Emergency Surgery Service, Legacy Emanuel Medical Center, Portland, OR, USA

Dana M. Blyth San Antonio Military Medical Center, JBSA-Fort Sam Houston, TX, USA

Uniformed Services University of the Health Sciences, Bethesda, MD, USA

Matthew J. Bradley Uniformed Services University of the Health Sciences and Walter Reed National Military Medical Center, Bethesda, MD, USA

Jeremy W. Cannon Division of Traumatology, Surgical Critical Care & Emergency Surgery, Perelman School of Medicine at the University of Pennsylvania, Philadelphia, PA, USA

W. Darrin Clouse Harvard Medical School, Massachusetts General Hospital, Division of Vascular and Endovascular Surgery, Boston, MA, USA

Jean-Claude G. D'Alleyrand Department of Orthopaedic Surgery, Walter Reed National Military Medical Center, Bethesda, MD, USA

Norman M. Rich Department of Surgery, Uniformed Services University of Health Sciences, Bethesda, MD, USA

Joseph J. DuBose Department of Vascular and Endovascular Surgery, David Grant USAF Medical Center, Travis Air Force Base, California, Fairfield, CA, USA

Ryan P. Dumas Division of Traumatology, Surgical Critical Care and Emergency Surgery, Perelman School of Medicine at the University of Pennsylvania, Philadelphia, PA, USA

James R. Dunne Department of Trauma/Surgical Critical Care, Memorial Health University Medical Center, Savannah, GA, USA

Blessen C. Eapen Polytrauma Rehabilitation Center, South Texas Veterans Health Care System, San Antonio, TX, USA

Department of Rehabilitation Medicine, University of Texas Health Science Center San Antonio, San Antonio, TX, USA

Raymond Fang Johns Hopkins University School of Medicine, Department of Surgery, Baltimore, MD, USA

Joseph M. Galante Division of Trauma and Acute Care Surgery, University of California, Davis Medical Center, Sacramento, CA, USA

James J. Geracci US Army III Corps (Armored), Fort Hood, Killeen, TX, USA

Alok Gupta Division of Acute Care Surgery, Trauma, and Critical Care, Beth Israel Deaconess Medical Center, Harvard Medical School, Boston, MA, USA

Ashley E. Humphries Department of General Surgery, Walter Reed National Military Medical Center, Bethesda, MD, USA

Elliot M. Jessie Uniformed Services University of the Health Sciences and, Walter Reed National Military Medical Center, Bethesda, MD, USA

Luke R. Johnston Uniformed Services University of the Health Sciences and, Walter Reed National Military Medical Center, Bethesda, MD, USA

Phillip Kemp Bohan San Antonio Military Medical Center, Ft. Sam Houston, TX, USA

Debra L. Malone Department of Surgery, Walter Reed National Military Medical Center, Bethesda, MD, USA

Matthew J. Martin Madigan Army Medical Center, Tacoma, WA, USA

Clinton K. Murray San Antonio Military Medical Center, JBSA-Fort Sam Houston, TX, USA

Uniformed Services University of the Health Sciences, Bethesda, MD, USA

Keith P. Myers Department of Rehabilitation, Walter Reed National Military Medical Center, Bethesda, MD, USA

Department of Physical Medicine and Rehabilitation, Uniformed Services University of the Health Sciences, Bethesda, MD, USA

John S. Oh Department of Surgery, Division of Trauma, Milton S. Hershey Medical Center, Hershey, PA, USA

Ajit B. Pai Physical Medicine & Rehabilitation, Polytrauma Rehabilitation Center, Hunter Holmes McGuire VA Medical Center, Richmond, VA, USA

Paul F. Pasquina Department of Rehabilitation, Walter Reed National Military Medical Center, Bethesda, MD, USA

Department of Physical Medicine and Rehabilitation, Uniformed Services University of the Health Sciences, Bethesda, MD, USA

Gabriel J. Pavey Uniformed Services University-Walter Reed Department of Surgery, Walter Reed National Military Medical Center, Bethesda, MD, USA

Travis M. Polk Department of General Surgery, Naval Medical Center Portsmouth, Portsmouth, VA, USA

Benjamin K. Potter Uniformed Services University-Walter Reed Department of Surgery, Walter Reed National Military Medical Center, Bethesda, MD, USA

Jason Scott Radowsky Blanchfield Army Community Hospital, Fort Campbell, TN, USA

William Robbins Polytrauma Transitional Residential Program, Hunter Holmes McGuire VA Medical Center, Richmond, VA, USA

Carlos J. Rodriguez Department of Surgery, Walter Reed National Military Medical Center, Bethesda, MD, USA

Rachel M. Russo Department of General Surgery, University of California Davis Medical Center, Sacramento, CA, USA

Babak Sarani Center for Trauma and Critical Care, George Washington University, Washington, DC, USA

Martin A. Schreiber Division of Trauma, Critical Care, and Acute Care Surgery, Oregon Health and Science University, Portland, OR, USA

Geoffrey L. Shapiro Emergency Medical Services Program, George Washington University, Washington, DC, USA

E. Reed Smith George Washington University, Arlington County Emergency Medical Services, Arlington, VA, USA

Jason M. Souza Department of Plastic and Reconstructive Surgery, Walter Reed National Military Medical Center, Bethesda, MD, USA

Bruno S. Subbarao Polytrauma/Transition and Care Management Programs, Phoenix VA Health Care System, Phoenix, AZ, USA

Rebecca N. Tapia Polytrauma Network Site, South Texas Veterans Health Care System, San Antonio, TX, USA

Department of Rehabilitation Medicine, University of Texas Health Science Center San Antonio, San Antonio, TX, USA

Ian L. Valerio Department of Plastic & Reconstructive Surgery, The Ohio State University Wexner Medical Center, Columbus, OH, USA

Department of Plastic & Reconstructive Surgery, Walter Reed National Military Medical Center, Bethesda, MD, USA

Tirzah VanDamme Department of Rehabilitation, Walter Reed National Military Medical Center, Bethesda, MD, USA

Department of Physical Medicine & Rehabilitation, Uniformed Services University of the Health Sciences, Bethesda, MD, USA

Gary Vercruysse University of Michigan School of Medicine, Ann Arbor, MI, USA

Jack Ryan Walter Urology Service, Madigan Army Medical Center, Tacoma, WA, USA

Corinne E. Wee Department of Plastic and Reconstructive Surgery, The Ohio State University Wexner Medical Center, Columbus, OH, USA

Allison Weisbrod Department of Surgery, Naval Hospital Camp Lejeune, Camp Lejeune, NC, USA

Timothy K. Williams Wake Forest Baptist Health, Winston-Salem, NC, USA

Michael B. Yaffe Acute Care Surgery, Trauma and Surgical Critical Care, Beth Israel Deaconess Medical Center, Boston, MA, USA

Heather C. Yun San Antonio Military Medical Center, JBSA-Fort Sam Houston, TX, USA

Uniformed Services University of the Health Sciences, Bethesda, MD, USA

Terri A. Zomerlei Department of Plastic & Reconstructive Surgery, The Ohio State University Wexner Medical Center, Columbus, OH, USA

Introduction: Why We Do What We Do

Carlos J. Rodriguez and Joseph M. Galante

Injury

This is a story of a 34-year-old active duty warrior who was on dismounted patrol during the fall of 2010 in Southern Helmand Province, Afghanistan, as part of the 2009–2010 surge in support of Operation Enduring Freedom. The morning was just like the previous 35 for this warrior—hot, dirty, and full of the unknown. The patrol he was leading had just finished night operations, and his team was heading back to the Forward Operating Base which he called home, when his lead foot stepped on a buried pressure plate improvised explosive device (IED). That step changed his life forever.

The pressure wave, heat, and debris associated with the blast had ready access to his lead left leg, exposed perineum, trailing right leg, and both upper extremities. The team's medic arrived quickly to assess the situation as the Wounded Warrior's team members secured the area. The medic's initial exam revealed an awake, but confused victim in severe pain who had sustained a very proximal left lower extremity traumatic amputation with active bleeding, destructive perineum wounds, a right lower extremity below-knee amputation with active bleeding, and bilateral open hand/forearm fractures. Removal of his flak jacket revealed a peppering pattern below the umbilicus without immediate ability to determine if any of these wounds penetrated abdominal fascia.

The medic quickly placed Combat Action Tourniquets (CATs) to both lower extremities. While the right-sided CAT effectively stopped the bleeding, the left side did not due to the junctional nature of the amputation. There was no room to place a second left lower extremity CAT, so direct pressure was held, but the pressure only slowed the hemorrhage. While the medic was tending the injured Wounded Warrior, the unit had radioed for casualty evacuation helicopter. By the time CATs were applied, the help had arrived.

In the air, an interosseous catheter was placed into the right humeral head. While total flight time to the closest Role 2 facility was only 8 min, blood loss could not be controlled and pulses were lost in the air. Chest compressions began as the casualty evacuation helicopter touched down at the Role 2. From the Role 2 flight line, the Wounded Warrior was placed on a rickshaw litter and brought to the ED at a full sprint.

C. J. Rodriguez
Department of Surgery, Walter Reed National Military Medical Center, Bethesda, MD, USA
e-mail: Carlos.J.Rodriguez4.mil@mail.mil

J. M. Galante (✉)
Division of Trauma and Acute Care Surgery, University of California, Davis Medical Center, Sacramento, CA, USA
e-mail: jmgalante@ucdavis.edu

© Springer International Publishing AG, part of Springer Nature 2018
J. M. Galante et al. (eds.), *Managing Dismounted Complex Blast Injuries in Military & Civilian Settings*, https://doi.org/10.1007/978-3-319-74672-2_1

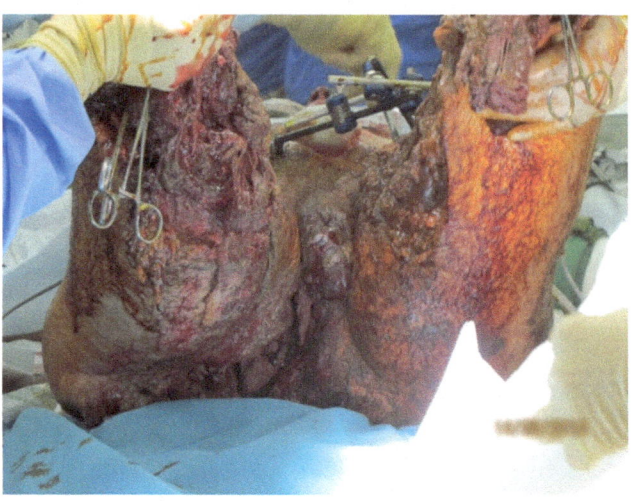

Fig. 1.1 Devastating bilateral lower extremity and perineal wounds are demonstrated

Role 2 Care

Upon arrival to the Role 2, surgeons immediately worked to gain proximal control of the left lower extremity junctional hemorrhage, while a team of anesthesiologists secured the airway and began uncrossmatched massive transfusion. Given the extent of proximal left lower extremity injury, it was relatively straightforward to make an incision cephalad to the left common femoral artery, dividing the inguinal ligament, thereby exposing his external iliac artery, suitable for clamping. With the artery clamped and initiation of blood transfusion, his pulse returned. He was then taken emergently to the operating room.

Given the extent of abdominal wall injury, perineal injuries, and proximal nature of his junctional hemorrhage, surgeons began with a laparotomy where they found significant stool soilage and intra-abdominal hemorrhage from the sigmoid mesocolon. The Sigmoid colon was mobilized and quickly resected. There were no other significant intra-abdominal injuries noted.

The left lower extremity amputation was so proximal; it was almost a complete hip disarticulation. The surgeons performed suture ligation of the left femoral vessels prior to taking down the iliac artery clamp. As he regained blood volume and blood pressure improved, bleeding from deep within the pelvis became evident. This prompted abdominal aortic cross-clamping and pre-peritoneal pelvic packing with external pelvic fixator placement. The cross-clamp was removed.

However, hypotension returned, indicating continued bleeding. The aorta was again cross-clamped, while the surgeons followed the external iliac artery proximally into the pelvis to ligate both internal and external iliac arteriovenous systems. The aortic cross-clamp was finally able to be successfully removed (Fig. 1.1).

From an orthopedic standpoint, he underwent a left above-knee amputation debridement; debridement, hemostasis, and conversion to a right above-knee amputation; and quick debridement/drip irrigation of his upper extremities.

On further examination, he was found to have a disrupted perineum, destructive right testicular injury, and injuries to the corpora cavernosa and urethra. This injury pattern prompted a completion right orchiectomy and placement of a suprapubic catheter.

His hemodynamics had stabilized. He was flown to the Role 3, expeditiously.

Role 3

A team of trauma, vascular, and orthopedic surgeons were waiting to evaluate the injured Wounded Warrior. Once acidosis was corrected, he did receive formal radiographic images to include CT scan of the head, chest, abdomen, and pelvis and plain films of all extremities. The team proceeded to the operating room where all dressings were taken down. Both the right and left lower extremity amputations were revised, with the left being revised one level higher—hip disarticulation on the left. The abdomen was explored and found to be hemostatic. The pelvic packing remained in place as it had been placed just 4 h prior. All wounds were sharply debrided to healthy appearing tissue. Wounds were dressed with gauze. He was made ready for an 8-h Critical Care Air Transport Team (CCATT) flight in the back of an Air Force C-17.

In total, 16 h had elapsed since the time of injury. In that time span, he had gone to the operating room twice and had received 41 u prbc, 38 u FFP, 8 u whole blood, 11 u platelets, 4 u cryoprecipitate, 1.5 gm TXA, and 7.2 mg FVIIa.

Role 4

The long flight to Germany was without incident. He arrived to the intensive care unit, where he and all his accompanying data (operative reports, progress notes, radiographic images, etc.) were evaluated by a team of physicians. Operative plans were made, and the Wounded Warrior was taken to the operating room for the third time in 24 h.

All dressings were taken down. On his lower extremities, what had been healthy tissue appeared to be somewhat necrotic in nature. While there was some thought that this necrosis was just secondary to blast effect and its penumbra, cultures and histopathology were sent to the lab for evaluation. His abdomen was noted to be clean and hemostatic. His abdominal fascia was closed, and a sigmoid colostomy was matured. External fixators were placed on his forearms. This time, instead of gauze dressings, negative pressure wound vacuums were placed on all extremities. Rigid proctoscopy revealed distal rectal injury.

Gastroenterology came to the operating room and placed a long naso-jejunal (i.e., beyond the ligament of Treitz) feeding tube to allow for feedings to occur, while non-abdominal surgical procedures were being performed.

Postoperatively, sedation was weaned. He was found to be following commands and was extubated. Intermittently, his temperature would spike to 103 F and leukocytosis was developing. Given these markers of infection and the recurrently necrotic wounds, he was started on meropenem and vancomycin.

He would remain in Germany for 60 h. During his stay, he made two trips to the operating room. Each time, recurrent wound necrosis was noted. He was extubated after his second trip. He left Germany for the United States 96 h after injury.

Role 5

The injured Wounded Warrior arrived late in the evening on post-injury day number 5—his temperature was 99.5 F with a leukocytosis of 24.3 k. He was taken to the operating room where his wounds were found to once again be necrotic (Fig. 1.2).

Histopathological specimen and wound cultures were taken from the border of necrotic and healthy tissue, wounds were debrided sharply, and liposomal amphotericin B and voriconazole were empirically started. Additionally, Dakin's (0.025%) solution was instilled through a negative pressure wound vacuum which was applied to wounds.

Over the next 12 h, fever curve spiked, leukocytosis increased (now 29.5 k), and fungal elements were seen on histopathological slides. He was taken back to the OR on Role 5 hospital day 2 for a second look. Again, necrotic tissue was found. He returned to the OR on days 4 and 6–11 (daily). On hospital day 7, with cultures now showing both *Mucor* spp. and *Fusarium* spp., he underwent bilateral nephrostomy tube placement as cystectomy was anticipated due to the extensive necrosis of the bladder wall. Ultimately, the bladder was spared. However, the zone necrosis became so proximal that, on hospital day 10, a left hemipelvectomy was required to finally surgically remove all invasive fungal elements (Fig. 1.3).

During his hospital stay, he was continually fed through the naso-jejunal feeding tube. Once he was re-liberated from the vent, he was able to undergo the standard blast consults of physical therapy, occupational therapy, dental examination, ophthalmologic examination, audiologic evaluation, and traumatic brain injury screening.

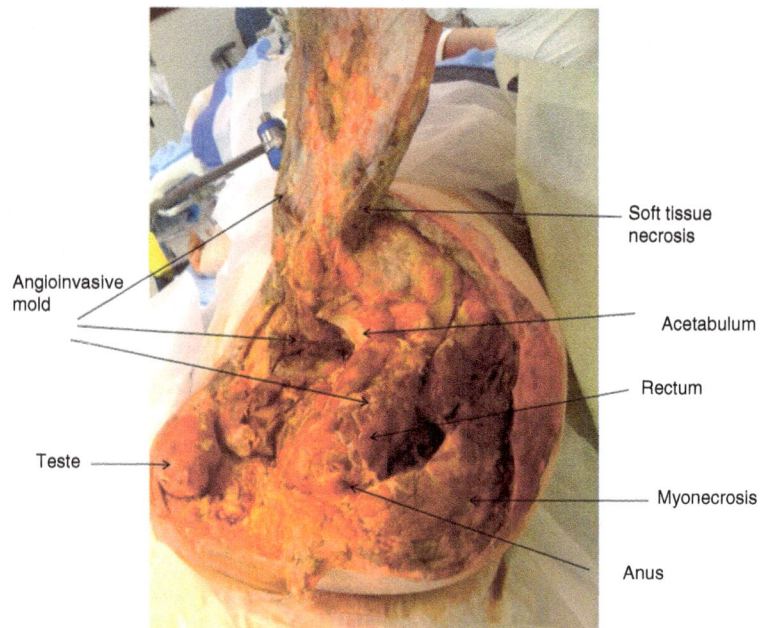

Fig. 1.2 Role 5 hospital day 1 reveals high-level lower extremity amputation with necrotic fibrinous material demonstrated on histopathology as a septate mold with angioinvasion (From Warkentien et al., *Invasive mold infections following combat-related injuries*, Clin Infect Dis. 2012 Dec;55(11):1441–9. doi: https://doi.org/10.1093/cid/cis749. Epub 2012 Oct 5, by permission of Oxford University Press)

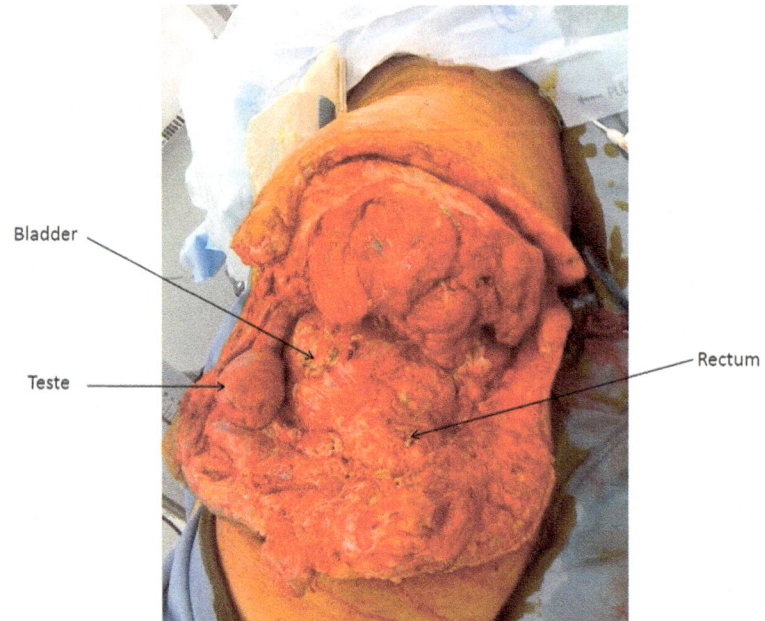

Fig. 1.3 Wound appearance after serial debridements, hemipelvectomy, and antifungal therapy (HD15) (From Warkentien et al., *Invasive mold infections following combat-related injuries*, Clin Infect Dis. 2012 Dec;55(11):1441–9. doi: https://doi.org/10.1093/cid/cis749. Epub 2012 Oct 5, by permission of Oxford University Press)

Outcome

In total, this Wounded Warrior spent 86 days in the hospital—23 of those days were spent in the ICU. He received a total of 113 u PRBC and 66 u of FFP. He underwent 26 trips to the operating room and was able to have all of his wounds closed with a combination of delayed primary closure and split thickness skin grafting. His injuries were reconstructed, and hospital course moved forward, albeit sometimes slowly, in a manner consistent with the chapters contained herein. He actually did retain rectal tone, but

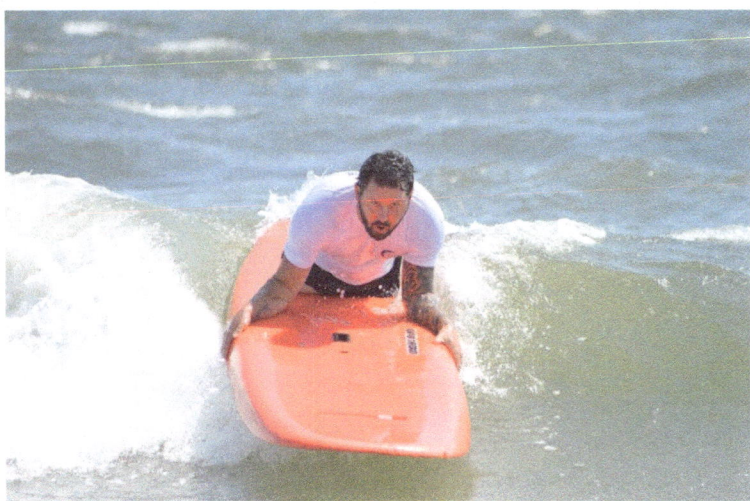

Fig. 1.4 Gunnery Sergeant John Hayes today, as determined as ever. He is living in Florida with his wife of 16 years and their four children

deferred anoplasty. He did not know how well he would have been able to conduct transfer from chair to a commode as he aged.

Today

The motivation of this text is rooted in each and every Wounded Warrior who came through the continuum of care from the battlefield to the states. Much has been written on combat trauma; our aim is a little different. In the chapters that follow, not only do we present acute combat trauma techniques and protocols, but we also focus on what occurs beginning day 1 following injury.

The Marine presented above is Gunnery Sergeant John Hayes. We reached out to him and asked permission for us to tell his story. We also requested personal insight into what he endured, "after the dust settled" (Fig. 1.4).

"Before the injury, I pushed life on all fronts," said Gunnery Sergeant Hayes in April 2017. "I hadn't acknowledged my PTSD symptoms or focused on my family enough. I tell people every day when they ask what happened that, 'It was the best thing that's happened to me', and their heads tilt. Yes, it does stink that it took this massive of an injury to slow me down, but it did just that. Even though the injury took my legs, I believe it made me a better person. I am so lucky to have made it Bethesda Naval Medical Center (WRNMMC). Having the most passionate and caring surgeons and nurses caring for me made me push harder when things were tough, and never give up."

Explosive Blasts: A Primer on a Multidimensional Mechanism of Injury

Raymond Fang

Explosive blasts caused 78% of US battle injuries sustained in support of Operations Iraqi Freedom and Enduring Freedom and recorded in the Joint Theater Trauma Registry from October 2001 through January 2005 [1]. Against most potential adversaries, the US military's significant technological advantages in weapons' precision and lethality preclude conventional military engagement. Foes increasingly rely upon asymmetrical warfare tactics in which less discriminate explosives devices are the weapon of choice. Terrorists similarly utilize explosive devices because they are inexpensive and easy to acquire, require minimal training to construct and to operate, and generate high casualty numbers and property damage without requiring the hazards of direct confrontation to deploy. Understanding basic blast physics and pathophysiology will assist clinicians caring for casualties injured by explosive blasts in not only military but also civilian settings.

ABCs of Explosives

A material capable of producing an explosion with release of its own potential energy is an explosive. An explosion results from the rapid exothermic chemical conversion of the solid or liquid explosive material to gas with the simultaneous release of energy. Explosives are classified as either low-order explosives or high-order explosives depending on whether they undergo deflagration or detonation as a chemical reaction.

Low-order explosives release energy relatively slowly in a process termed *deflagration* (from Latin *deflagrare*, "to burn down") in that they burn but do not explode. The first low explosive commonly used worldwide was black powder, also known as gun powder, which is a mixture of charcoal, sulfur, and potassium nitrate. Deflagration burns at subsonic speeds ranging from a few centimeters/second to 400 m/sec and generates large volumes of hot gas. When ignited in a confined space, the pressurized gas products lead to an effect similar to a detonation. Low-order explosives are used as propellants for bullet or rockets and in fireworks and theatrical special effects. Examples of low-order explosives include pipe bombs, the pressure-cooker bombs utilized in the 2013 "Boston Marathon" bombing, and petroleum-based bombs such Molotov cocktails.

High-order explosives react in a process termed *detonation* (from Latin *detonare*, "to expend thunder"). Detonation occurs similarly

R. Fang (✉)
Johns Hopkins University School of Medicine, Department of Surgery, Baltimore, MD, USA
e-mail: rfang2@jhmi.edu

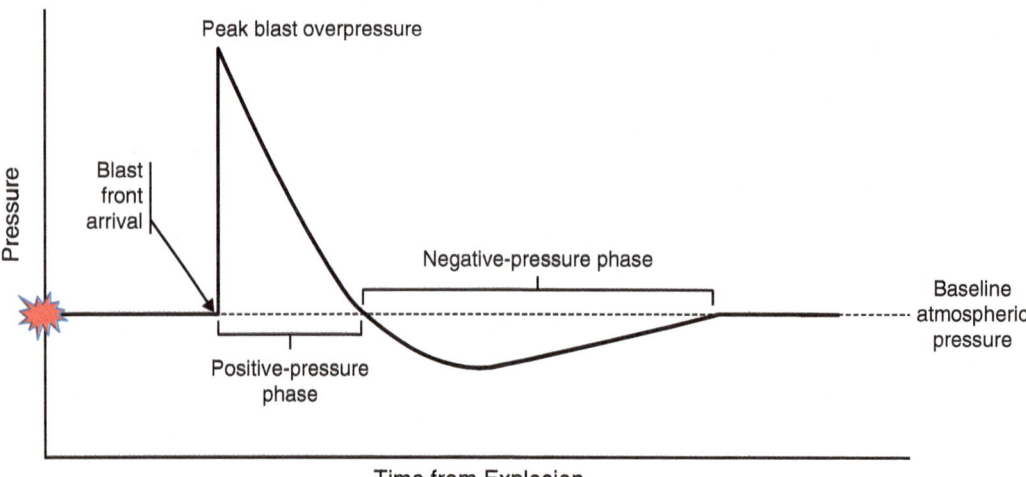

Fig. 2.1 The Friedlander curve, named after the British mathematician Frederick Friedlander (1917–2001) who studied blasts physics for civil defense purposes during World War II, describes the pressure-time relationship of an open-field explosion

with the near instantaneous transformation of the solid or liquid explosive material into extremely high-pressure gas with the simultaneous liberation of energy. The highly pressurized gas initially occupies the same physical volume as the original solid or liquid material and nearly instantaneously expands outward in all directions. The expanding gas compresses and heats the molecules of the surrounding medium into a few millimeters thick *blast wave* that travels at supersonic speeds of 3000–8000 m/sec. The leading edge of the blast wave, the *blast front*, possesses a shattering effect called *brisance* (from French *briser*, "to break or shatter") that exerts both stress and shear forces as it passes. In air, the blast force dissipates according to the cube of the distance so doubling one's distance from the epicenter reduces the blast effect experienced by a factor of eight. Because water is less compressible than air, an underwater blast retains its energy over a much farther distance than in air. As the blast front travels in air, the outward traveling gas creates an immediate peak positive-pressure region, a *blast wind*, flowing away from the detonation. A negative-pressure phase follows as air reverses flow to equilibrate back to the ambient pressure baseline (Fig. 2.1). Examples of high-order explosives include commercially manufactured compounds such as dynamite, trinitrotoluene (TNT), and Composition C-4. Several major terrorist attacks successfully utilized improvised high-order explosive devices that combined ammonium nitrate (fertilizer) with fuel oil, components that are inexpensive and easily acquired. TNT equivalent is a commonly used unit of measure to describe the energy released in an explosion. By convention, one gram of TNT releases 4.184 J of energy (equivalent of 1 kilocalorie).

High-order explosives are further subcategorized as primary and secondary related to the stimuli needed to initiate detonation. Primary explosives may detonate when stimulated by heat, impact, friction, or spark. Primary explosives are dangerous to handle, so they are used in small quantities to trigger an explosive reaction powered by a larger mass of secondary explosive. Secondary explosives are relatively insensitive to stimuli and explode only when triggered by the detonation of an adequate primary explosive (initiator) making secondary explosives relatively safe to store and handle.

Injuries Following Explosive Blasts

In civilian practice, most traumatic injuries are simplistically classified as either blunt or penetrating injuries. Falls, assaults, and motor vehicle crashes are typical blunt injury mechanisms, while gunshot wounds and stabbings are penetrating. As the mechanism influences the clinical suspicion for resulting anatomic injuries, it affects the patient's diagnostic evaluation and management. Explosive blasts are not easily categorized. Blast injuries not only combine features of both blunt and penetrating mechanisms but also include the additional effects of the blast wave. These *multidimensional injuries* can create multiple, complex injuries in the same patient, or a cohort of simultaneously injured patients, and oftentimes require multidisciplinary treatment.

Injuries incurred from explosive blasts are categorized by four mechanisms of injury:

- *Primary blast injuries* are those resulting from the casualty's exposure to the blast wave following a high-explosive detonation.
- *Secondary blast injuries* are caused by energized debris from the explosion striking the casualty and causing penetrating wounds and/or blunt injuries.
- *Tertiary blast injuries* result from the casualty being propelled by the force of the blast wind.
- *Quaternary blast injuries* include all other injuries, illnesses, or diseases related to the explosion and not included by the preceding three categories.

Many factors influence the injuries sustained following an explosion. The type, construction, and energy content of the explosive are key variables. The casualty's distance from the epicenter, body position in relation to the blast wave, and personal protective equipment worn also influence risk. Structures and objects in the surrounding environment can act as protective barriers or create additional flying debris. Explosions within enclosed spaces such as buildings and vehicles reflect the destructive blast energy back toward occupants repeating their blast exposure and magnifying the risks of injury. Structural collapse greatly increases the lethality of these events (e.g., US Marine barracks in Beirut, Lebanon [1983], Alfred P. Murrah Federal Building in Oklahoma City [1995], and the World Trade Center towers in New York City [2001]).

Primary Blast Injuries

Primary blast injuries are unique to high-order explosive detonations and the resulting supersonic, overpressure blast wave. Low explosives do not initiate a true blast wave and therefore do not cause primary blast injuries. As the blast wave passes through the casualty's body, potentially devastating effects occur primarily in air-containing structures and especially at air-tissue interfaces. Tissues exposed to stress beyond their tensile strength fail and are permanently disrupted in a concept termed "irreversible work." Rapid pressure change causes entrapped gases within the body to suddenly compress and then re-expand with release of kinetic energy causing injury termed implosion. Spalling takes place when the pressure wave passes through media of differing densities resulting in displacement and fragmentation of the denser tissue into the less dense air. In response to the pressure wave, tissues of differing densities also move at differing velocities causing shear injuries. Following passage of the blast wave, tissue damage may continue to evolve leading to delayed presentations of occult tissue necrosis and visceral perforation.

The tympanic membrane is the anatomic structure most frequently injured by primary blast injury. Tympanic membrane rupture may occur at pressures as low as 5 pounds per square inch (psi) above atmospheric pressure, so rupture is frequently used as a marker of significant blast exposure. Injury to other organs generally requires pressures greater than 40 psi above atmospheric pressure. (For reference, Composition C-4 detonation can create initial overpressure of greater than 4 million psi.) Casualties with tympanic membrane rupture may complain of hearing loss, tinnitus, otalgia, vertigo, or bleeding from the external auditory canal. Spontaneous healing occurs in most cases of tympanic membrane rupture, but extensive perforations may necessitate tympanoplasty. High-frequency hearing loss may be permanent. Since 2007, the Department of Defense (DoD) Joint Trauma System (JTS) has published a clinical practice guideline (CPG) for the management of "aural blast injury/acoustic trauma and hearing loss." [2] Despite its widespread use as a blast injury biomarker, tympanic membrane perforation has not proven to be a sensitive marker of serious primary blast injury during contemporary military practice. In a published report, Harrison et al. reported on 167 consecutive, blast-exposed casualties treated at a US military Role III facility in January 2006 [3]. In this cohort, 27 patients (16%) suffered tympanic membrane perforation. Twelve casualties (7%) sustained other serious primary blast injuries to include pneumothorax, pneumomediastinum, pulmonary contusion, facial sinus injury, or bowel perforation; 6 of these 12 casualties also suffered tympanic membrane perforation. The sensitivity and specificity of tympanic membrane perforation for the presence of other serious primary blast injuries were 50% and 87%, respectively.

Devastating primary blast injury to the lung is not only a common postmortem finding in patients killed at the scene of an explosive blast, but it is also a common cause of early death among casualties who survive the initial blast event. While individual body armor (IBA) protects soldiers from ballistic injuries to the chest, it does not prevent the barotrauma of primary blast injury. Clinical findings on presentation range from mild hypoxia to rapidly progressive respiratory failure accompanied by pink, frothy respiratory secretions. All casualties with suspected high-pressure blast exposure or blast exposure with pulmonary complaints should undergo a chest radiograph. A bihilar, central "butterfly" pattern of lung infiltrates is frequently associated with primary pulmonary blast injury. If symptomatic, but with a normal chest radiograph, chest CT imaging should be considered. Primary blast injuries to the lung include pulmonary contusions, pneumothorax, hemothorax, pneumomediastinum, and subcutaneous emphysema. Disruptions of the alveolar-venous interfaces predispose casualties to arterial air embolism especially with the initiation of positive-pressure mechanical ventilation. When massive, these emboli can cause stroke, myocardial infarction, spinal cord infarction, intestinal ischemia, and/or death. If a blast-injured casualty requires positive-pressure ventilation, low-pressure strategies including permissive hypercapnia should be employed. The long-term prognosis for survivors of primary pulmonary blast injury is excellent with near-complete physical and functional recovery anticipated at 1-year post-injury [4].

Gastrointestinal injuries to air-containing visceral structures likely occur in an analogous manner to the lung injuries with an anatomic incidence following the distribution of gastrointestinal air. Peritonitis on physical examination or free intraperitoneal air on diagnostic imaging are both straightforward indications for operative exploration. The ileocecal region is most commonly injured; rupture may occur acutely or even several days after the blast exposure. Delayed injuries occur when initially contused bowel, characterized by submucosal hemorrhage, progresses to full-thickness necrosis, and perforation. Solid organ lacerations are not common. Generally, blast forces sufficient to shear the spleen, liver, or kidneys will simultaneously result in lethal pulmonary lesions and immediate death.

Primary blast exposure is increasingly appreciated as a cause of traumatic brain injuries without a direct blow to the head. Military helmets are protective for ballistic fragments but not primary blast forces. These injuries are most frequently categorized as mild in severity (concussions) without diagnostic findings on standard neuroimaging. Traumatic axonal injury has been detected by advanced magnetic resonance imaging techniques such as diffusion tensor imaging [5]. Loss of consciousness, "seeing stars," and being "dazed and confused" may be described in the casualty's history. Post-injury symptoms include headache, tinnitus, noise intolerance, retrograde and anterograde amnesia, and irritability. These findings were historically attributed to psychoemotional disorders, "shell shock," and "combat fatigue." With overlapping symptomology, primary blast injury to the brain and post-traumatic stress disorder appear to be linked diagnoses. The DoD Instruction 6490.11, September 18, 2012, details the official policy for the management of deployed military personnel exposed to potential concussive events and is accessible as a JTS CPG [6]. All military patients who have suffered a potential concussive blast should have a standard trauma evaluation that includes administration of the Military Acute Concussion Evaluation (MACE). This test provides a rapid and objective score that measures the patient's current mental capacity, memory, and cognition. The combination of the trauma evaluation plus the MACE can then be used to help determine whether further testing or evaluations are indicated or if the service member can return to duty. Determining both the specific mechanisms of and identifying diagnostic biomarkers for primary blast-related brain injury remain foci of significant DoD-funded medical research.

Secondary Blast Injuries

Secondary blast injuries are caused by debris energized by the explosion striking the casualty and causing penetrating wounds and/or blunt injuries (Fig. 2.2). These projectiles originate from the explosive device itself or from the surrounding environment. Military explosive munitions are designed to maximize the number and velocity of shell casing fragments inflicting injury. Builders of improvised explosive devices pack nails, ball bearings, rocks, or other objects within the device to amplify their injury potential. Fragments leave the explosive at high velocity, but quickly decelerate similar to a shotgun blast. Commonly, all fragments are incorrectly described as shrapnel. Shrapnel specifically refers to an antipersonnel artillery shell devised in 1804 by Henry Shrapnel that contained lead balls which would rain down upon enemy forces at relatively low velocity following an aerial explosion. The shrapnel shell was rendered obsolete with the development of more effective, high-velocity explosive artillery shells early in World War I [7].

The injury radius for secondary blast injury from fragments is considerably farther than that from primary blast overpressure. In the absence of protective structures such as steel-reinforced concrete T-walls or bunkers, fragments derived from a 155-mm howitzer high-explosive artillery shell can cause penetrating injury at distances as far as 1800 feet. The lethal radius for primary blast injury is ~50 feet (Fig. 2.3) [8]. Small puncture wounds may be the only physical evidence of life-threatening internal injuries to the head, neck, and chest (Fig. 2.4). Fragmentation injuries caused the majority of injuries and deaths during combat operations in Iraq and Afghanistan. Unlike primary blast injury, individual body armor, helmets, ballistic eyewear, and other personal protective devices (e.g., "blast boxers") can reduce secondary blast injuries.

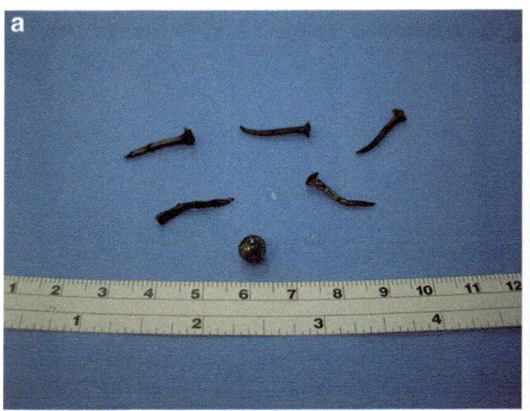
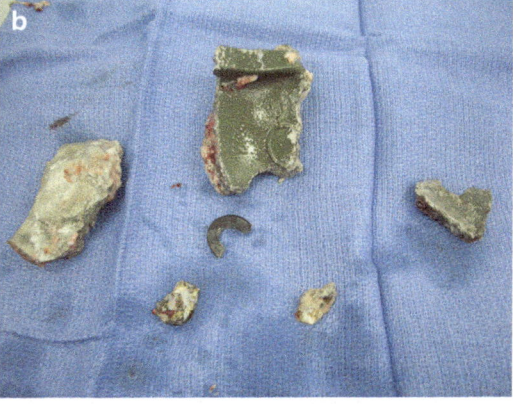

Fig. 2.2 Secondary blast injuries are caused by debris energized by the explosion. These fragments may include objects packed into the device such as nail, ball bearings, and rocks (**a**) as well as casing fragments of the explosive device (**b**)

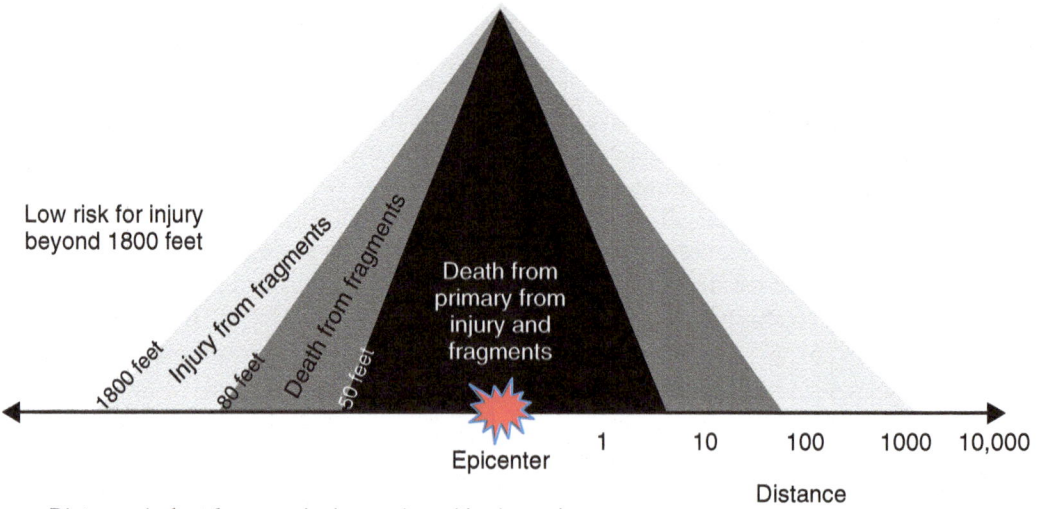

Fig. 2.3 Personal protective equipment can reduce injuries from blast fragments, but the extremities (**a**) and head (**b**) may remain vulnerable due to operational needs for mobility and sensory awareness. Small puncture wounds may be the only external evidence of significant internal injury such as this aortic laceration (**c**) and lumbar spinal cord transection (**d**)

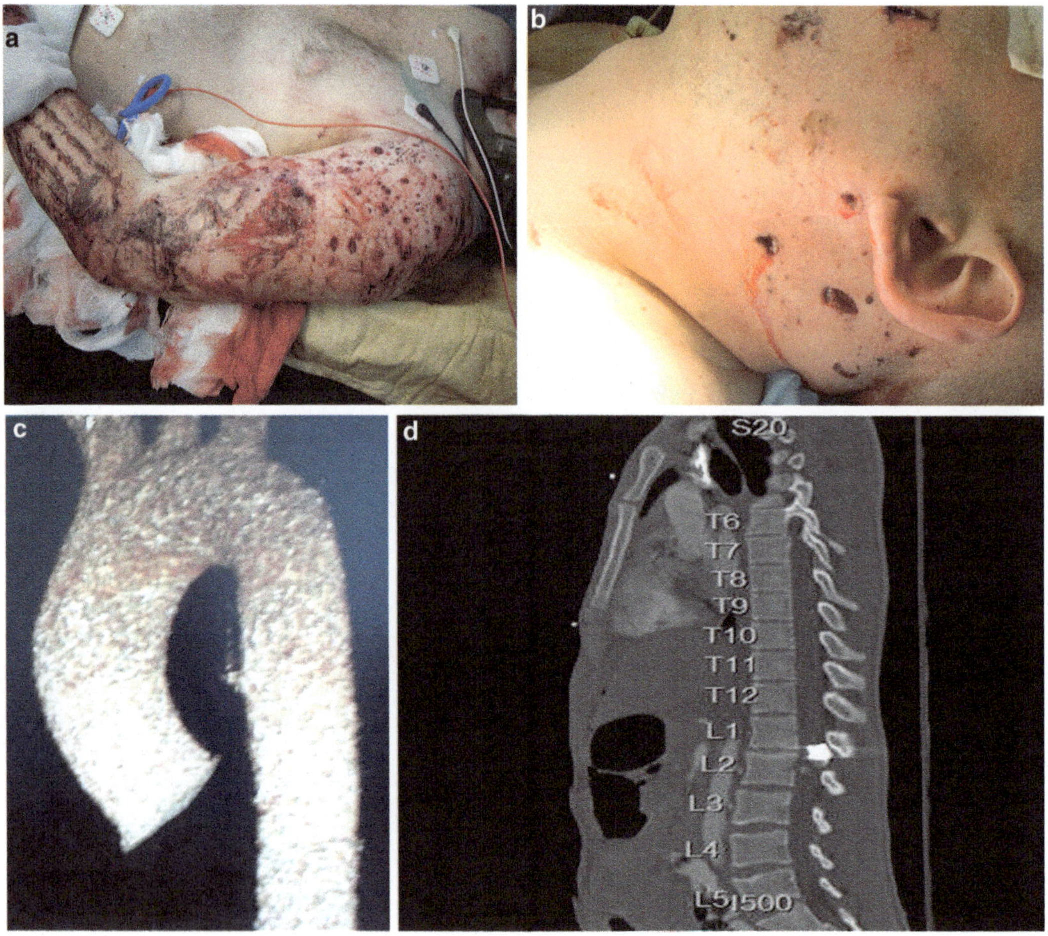

Fig. 2.4 Injury radius for the open-field detonation of a 155-mm artillery shell

In cases of suicide bombers, the bone, teeth, and other body tissues from the bombers themselves can become penetrating fragments. Some of these terrorist perpetrators are hepatitis and/or HIV positive with one reported case of hepatitis B virus transmission to a bombing victim in this manner. Thus, hepatitis B vaccination is recommended for survivors of suicide bombings [9].

Tertiary Blast Injuries

Tertiary blast injuries occur when the casualty is propelled by the blast wind and impacts the ground, wall, or other structures. The brief blast wind may exceed hurricane force and throw casualties considerable distances with great energy. These injuries are typical of a blunt trauma mechanism and include closed head injuries, blunt torso injuries, and extremity and spinal fractures. Rarely, casualties may suffer impalement injuries after being thrown in the air.

Quaternary Blast Injuries

Quaternary blast injuries include all other injuries, illnesses, or diseases related to the explosion and not included by the preceding three categories. These injuries may include thermal burns from the initial explosion or any resultant fire as well as crush injuries from falling debris or building collapse. "Dirty" bombs intentionally incorporate chemical, biological, or radiologic agents into the device. Exacerbations of underlying medical disease such as asthmas, chronic obstructive pulmonary disease, and angina are also considered in this category which may be especially significant when treating civilian casualties.

Dismounted Complex Blast Injury

Dismounted complex blast injury demonstrates the multidimensional nature of blast injuries requiring a multidisciplinary approach to care [10]. Low-energy blast events result from either small explosive devices or explosions distant from the casualty. Injuries incurred in these situations are generally from secondary blast fragments striking unprotected areas of the body. In contrast, high-energy events near dismounted personnel result in a pattern of devastating injuries: traumatic lower extremity amputations, upper extremity fractures and possible traumatic amputations, and perineal soft tissue injuries. Immediate mortality is extremely high with the initial blast event. A DoD JTS CPG for management of "high bilateral amputations and dismounted complex blast injuries" was released in 2011 [11]. Survival will be determined by the capabilities to rapidly diagnose and comprehensively manage the severe trauma sustained by the casualty from the four blast-induced mechanisms of injury.

Conclusions

Explosive blasts from improvised explosive devices and other weapons were the most common battlefield injury mechanism seen during the conflicts in Iraq and Afghanistan and are unfortunately also seen in the civilian trauma community. The number, type, severity, and anatomic distribution of resulting injuries depends on factors such as personal protective equipment, mounted or dismounted status, type and yield of the explosive device, distance from the blast, and associated factors such as building collapse or vehicle rollover. "Blast injury" is a catchall term, and patients are injured by multiple effects from primary to quaternary blast injury. These patients may sustain severe multisystem injuries unlike the vast majority of routine trauma seen in the civilian setting and that require a highly skilled and trained care team starting at the point of injury and proceeding through all phases of care to include reconstruction and rehabilitation. Further advances in understanding blast pathophysiology and treatment are needed in order to decrease the morbidity and mortality from blast injury. Additionally, preventive efforts aimed at improved vehicle design to dissipate blast forces away from occupants, detection and neutralization of explosive devices, and personal protective gear are as important or even more important to reducing the high level of lethality and disability associated with these events.

References

1. Owens BD, Kragh JF, Wenke JC, Macaitis J, Wade CE, Holcomb JB. Combat wounds in Operation Iraqi Freedom and Operation Enduring Freedom. J Trauma. 2008;64(2):295–9.
2. Parker M, Curtis K, Esquivel C, et al. Joint trauma system clinical practice guideline: aural blast injury/acoustic trauma and hearing loss. c2007. Updated 12 Aug 2016; cited 1 Jul 2017. Available from: http://www.usaisr.amedd.army.mil/cpgs.html.
3. Harrison CD, Bebarta VS, Grant GA. Tympanic membrane perforation after combat blast exposure in Iraq: a poor biomarker of primary blast injury. J Trauma. 2009;67(1):210–1.
4. Hirshberg B, Oppenheim-Eden A, Pizov R, et al. Recovery from blast lung injury: one-year follow-up. Chest. 1999;116(6):1683–8.
5. Mac Donald CL, Johnson AM, Cooper D, et al. Detection of blast-related traumatic brain injury in U.S. military personnel. N Engl J Med. 2011;364(22):2091–100.
6. Department of Defense. Department of Defense Instruction Number 6490.11: DoD Policy Guidance for Management of Mild Traumatic Brain Injury/Concussion in the Deployed Setting. c2012. Published 18 Sep 2012; cited 1 Jul 2017. Available from: http://www.usaisr.amedd.army.mil/cpgs.html.
7. Burris DG, Rich NM, Ryan JM. Shrapnel, the man, the missile and the myth. J R Army Med Corps. 2003;149(4):337–9.
8. Champion HR, Holcomb JB, Young LA. Injuries from explosions: physics, biophysics, pathology, and required research focus. J Trauma. 2009;66(5):1468–77.
9. Braverman I, Wexler D, Oren M. A novel mode of infection with hepatitis B: penetrating bone fragments due to the explosion of a suicide bomber. Isr Med Assoc J. 2002;4(7):528–9.
10. Cannon JW, Hofman LJ, Glasgow SC, et al. Dismounted complex blast injuries: a comprehensive review of the modern combat experience. J Am Coll Surg. 2016;223(4):652–64.
11. Gordon W, Talbot M, Fleming M, et al. Joint Trauma System Clinical Practice Guideline: High bilateral amputations and dismounted complex blast injury. c2011. Updated 26 Jul 2016; cited 1 Jul 2017. Available from: http://www.usaisr.amedd.army.mil/cpgs.html.

Initial Care of Blast Injury: TCCC and TECC

Babak Sarani, Geoffrey L. Shapiro, James J. Geracci, and E. Reed Smith

Tactical Combat Casualty Care (TCCC)

More than 15 years of continuous combat operations in Iraq and Afghanistan have resulted in many lessons and advancements in tactics, techniques, and procedures for saving lives on the battlefield. As compared to previous wars (World War II, Korea, Vietnam), a soldier wounded on the battlefield today has nearly twice the likelihood of surviving his wounds. Although this improvement in combat survivability is certainly multifactorial, numerous reports published in the medical literature document that Tactical Combat Casualty Care (TCCC) principles are saving lives and improving outcomes.

The concept of TCCC was first conceived in the mid-1990s in the US military's special operations community with the goal of improving combat trauma outcomes by optimizing the care rendered in the tactical prehospital environment. The TCCC principles, published first in August 1996 in *Military Medicine*, sought to avoid preventable deaths by combining good medicine with good tactics and redefining the prioritization of medical care under combat conditions to balance the competing priorities between achieving mission objectives and caring for the injured [1].

Prior to development and adoption of TCCC, the military followed essentially the same trauma guidelines used in the civilian sector. These guidelines, based upon the Emergency Medical Technicians Basic Course and the American College of Surgeon's Advanced Trauma Life Support (ATLS) curriculum, were initially developed in the 1970s and 1980s. Reflecting civilian trauma data, they recommend an "airway – breathing – circulation" approach to the evaluation and initial resuscitation of the injured. The assumptions upon which the standardized trauma management approach of ATLS is based – that the medical provider is in a safe, stable, resource-rich environment and that the most common cause of immediate death is related to loss of airway and respiratory failure – are often not valid in the combat setting (Table 3.1).

For decades, military wounding studies have reported significantly different wounding patterns in combat with a higher proportion of penetrating injuries as well as complex and

B. Sarani (✉)
Center for Trauma and Critical Care, George Washington University, Washington, DC, USA
e-mail: bsarani@mfa.gwu.edu

G. L. Shapiro
Emergency Medical Services Program, George Washington University, Washington, DC, USA

J. J. Geracci
US Army III Corps (Armored), Fort Hood, Killeen, TX, USA

E. R. Smith
George Washington University, Arlington County Emergency Medical Services, Arlington, VA, USA

Table 3.1 Differences between TCCC and ATLS

TCCC	ATLS
"CAB" – Circulation, airway, breathing	"ABC" – Airway, breathing, circulation
Factor tactical environment into medical decision making (see Table 3.2)	Assumes a safe environment for responders and patients
Support using hemostatic dressings and tranexamic acid	Does not mention hemostatic dressings or tranexamic acid
Urges tourniquets for severe hemorrhage	Teaches direct pressure only
Allows for permissive hypotension and limited fluid resuscitation	Calls for up to 2 liters of crystalloid to treat hypotension
Encourages the use of nasopharyngeal airway	Encourages the use of endotracheal intubation
Allows pain medications to be administered orally and encourages the use of nonnarcotic IV/IM pain medications	Only encourages the use of IV narcotics
Does not recommend spine immobilization for most mechanisms of injury depending on the tactical situation	Strongly supports the use of a rigid cervical collar and long spine board for many/most blunt mechanisms of injury
Recognizes the important need for early antibiotic administration for severe wounding	Does not address the role of antibiotics in initial trauma care

TCCC Tactical Combat Casualty Care, *ATLS* advanced trauma life support, *IM* intramuscular, *IV* intravenous

devastating injuries not typically seen in the civilian setting. The most complex of these are typically due to blast mechanisms from improvised explosive devices or other explosives, often creating devastating multi-system patterns of injury. Among battlefield deaths, hemorrhage from extremity or truncal wounds, rather than airway compromise, has been shown to be the most frequent etiology of potentially preventable combat deaths [1, 2]. Furthermore, 25% of battlefield fatalities have been noted to be potentially preventable with rapid application of simple stabilizing measures [3]. Over time, experience and the evidence documented in countless military studies have consistently concluded that, particularly in the prehospital setting where over 90% of combat deaths occur, civilian trauma care guidelines could not be wholly translated to combat casualty care. Although TCCC applies to any battlefield injury, it is most critical for patients injured by blast mechanisms and is likely responsible for the widely reported improvements in current battlefield survival statistics.

Tenets of TCCC

TCCC is prehospital combat casualty care rendered in a tactical environment and consists of a set of evidence-based guidelines customized for use on the battlefield and prioritizing the most common historical causes of preventable combat death [1]. Acknowledging that good medicine must be balanced with tactical considerations, the guiding premise of TCCC is performing the correct interventions at the correct time in the continuum of prehospital care in order to treat the casualty, prevent additional casualties, and complete the mission. Combat casualty care is divided into three phases characterized by distinct tactical considerations and limitations: Care Under Fire, Tactical Field Care, and Tactical Evacuation Care.

Care Under Fire

Care Under Fire refers to the immediate life-saving measures provided at the point of wounding, while both the casualty and the provider (nonmedic or medical first responder) are still under effective hostile fire. Risk of further injury is extremely high and available medical equipment and resources are low. Priorities are returning fire as necessary to suppress the enemy, moving the casualty to cover to prevent further wounding, and treating immediately life-threatening hemorrhage. Because the number one potentially preventable cause of death on the battlefield is hemorrhage from either an extremity or other compressible wound, medical interventions in this phase of care are focused on stopping bleeding as quickly as possible [3]. Direct pressure, pressure dressings, hemostatic dressings, and use of tourniquets are all recommended management. Airway compromise does not typically play as significant a role in preventable combat mortality. As the time, positioning, and equipment required to manage an airway expose both the casualty and first responder to increased risk, immediate airway management in the Care Under Fire phase is not recommended. Similarly, contrary to civilian standards, cervical spine immobilization is neither appropriate nor recommended except in cases of obvious and severe blunt trauma.

Tactical Field Care

Tactical Field Care refers to care rendered once the casualty is no longer under effective hostile fire or for an injury that has occurred on a mission without hostile fire. Risk of further injury is decreased, but evaluation and treatment are still dictated by the tactical situation, limitations in available medical equipment and resources, and time until evacuation (which may vary from minutes to hours). Priorities in this phase of care are completing the rapid trauma assessment and treatment focused on issues not addressed/fully addressed while under hostile fire. Compressible hemorrhage remains the focus. Any significant bleeding sites not previously noted should be treated, and all dressings and tourniquets should be reassessed. Use of junctional tourniquets is appropriate if wounds are amenable. Breathing problems (open chest wounds and suspected tension pneumothorax) are addressed with the use of chest seals and needle thoracentesis. Airway interventions, beginning with the least invasive (chin lift/jaw thrust, positioning, nasal pharyngeal airway, and cricothyroidotomy), should be considered for casualties that are not conscious or breathing well on their own. Contrary to civilian trauma guidelines, endotracheal intubation is not recommended during the tactical field care phase but remains as an option, along with subraglottic airways, in the tactical evacuation phase of care. Additional considerations in the Tactical Field Care phase of TCCC include management of the following:

- Shock. In the combat setting, signs of shock (altered mental status in the absence of obvious head trauma, weak/absent radial pulse) should be assumed to be due to hemorrhage. Fluid resuscitation should be reserved for those with signs of shock or traumatic brain injury (TBI). Sternal or other intraosseous (IO) access is the preferred route of fluid administration (speed of procedure, preservation of site by body armor) and blood/blood products (if available) are the preferred resuscitation fluids. Where blood products are not available, Hextend (6% hetastarch) rather than crystalloids (Lactated Ringers and Plasma-Lyte A) is preferred. Normal saline has been removed completely as an option, except in the case of burn-specific resuscitation, in the current TCCC guidelines. Continued resuscitation should be guided by signs and symptoms (mental status, radial pulse). Tranexamic acid (if available) should be considered if ongoing resuscitation/significant blood transfusion is anticipated.
- Hypothermia. Combat casualties are at extremely high risk of hypothermia regardless of ambient temperature (environmental exposure, blood loss, peripheral vasoconstriction), and its association with coagulopathy and high mortality has been well described in the literature. Every effort (minimize exposure, blankets, hypothermia prevention kits) must be made to prevent hypothermia.
- Pain. Analgesia should be considered for all combat casualties and is dependent on nature of injury, severity of pain, physiologic status of the casualty, and tactical situation. As further enemy contact is still possible in the Tactical Field Care phase, choice of analgesia will be dependent on the level of consciousness and whether the casualty is able to continue to fight or not. For casualties with mild to moderate pain that are conscious and able to continue as combatants, oral medications that will not alter level of consciousness (NSAIDs, acetaminophen) are recommended. For the more seriously injured and impaired who are unable to continue as combatants, IM/IV/IO/intranasal ketamine (where shock or respiratory distress is a concern) or opioid analgesic options such as oral

transmucosal fentanyl and IO/IV morphine are recommended.
- Infection. Infection is a significant cause of morbidity and mortality in combat casualties. All open wounds should be considered infected and treated as soon as all life-threatening injuries have been addressed. If the casualty is able to tolerate, oral moxifloxacin is recommended. Otherwise, IV/IM cefotetan or ertapenem is recommended.

Tactical Evacuation Care

Tactical Evacuation Care refers to care rendered after the casualty has been picked up by an aircraft or other form of transportation for transfer to a higher level of care. Risk of injury from hostile fire is further reduced, and additional medical personnel and equipment are typically available during this phase of care. Priority is reassessment and continuation of care initiated during Tactical Field Care. Treatment is focused on issues not addressed/fully addressed, and some additional care may be rendered based upon the increased medical capability (airway management, oxygen, monitoring, blood products, etc.) accompanying the evacuation team. Hypothermia management remains a priority during this phase of care and can be challenging depending on which mode of transport is utilized (helicopter, etc.).

TCCC Summary

In summary, TCCC was borne out of the need for an evidence-based and effective approach to prehospital care for the critically injured, including blast-injured patients, on the battlefield. Although primarily designed for military scenarios and use, the majority of the principles and practices of TCCC remain valid in the civilian environment and particularly for any blast or explosive scenario. However, it is also clear that TCCC cannot (and should not) be simply applied wholesale to the civilian environment, where the vast majority of patients will suffer markedly different injury patterns due to different wounding mechanisms. This recognition has led to the development of an alternative civilian-focused program of early trauma care, Tactical Emergency Casualty Care (TECC), which is discussed in the following sections. It is important to note that TCCC and TECC are not mutually exclusive or directly competing but should be thought of as complimentary approaches and programs with the unifying goal of improved care and survival after major traumatic injury.

Tactical Emergency Casualty Care (TECC)

The incidence of civilian active violence and complex coordinated terrorist attacks has increased over the last 15–20 years. These civilian attacks create unique operational environments which are somewhat akin to the military theater in which medical rescue must occur despite ongoing and active threats to the responders. The operational response to such events traditionally involved staging medical rescue assets off-scene until the tactical threat was completely eliminated by law enforcement personnel. Moreover, law enforcement personnel were not tasked with providing medical care to the wounded. However, this paradigm created a significant delay in care. Furthermore, the unique wounding patterns and medical needs fall outside the scope of traditional prehospital care. Thus, there is a knowledge gap in how medical responders train for and respond to operational scenarios in which there are known wounded yet there is ongoing threat. As such, given the proven success of TCCC, the civilian medical community began to integrate its key tenets into civilian trauma care as appropriate. Many civilian emergency medical system agencies simply integrated all TCCC guidelines into their operations, while others resisted the whole implementation, citing concerns about military language and operational processes, differences in patient populations, resource limitations, and legal constraints. Given these valid concerns, en bloc incorporation of TCCC guidelines in civilian protocols is as fundamentally flawed as the use of civilian ATLS principles was for battlefield trauma management.

An "all-hazards" approach to provision of care is needed in the civilian sector due to the wide variety of mechanisms of injury and age groups involved. Characteristics that distinguish civilian from military high-threat prehospital environments include, but are not limited to, the following:

- *Scope of practice and liability*: Civilian medical responders must practice under individual state and locally defined scopes of practice and protocols and are subject to liability concerns that the military provider is not.
- *Patient population to include geriatrics, pediatrics, pregnancy, and special needs*: Civilian medical responders must be equipped and trained to treat a wide range of age groups. Patients' body habitus also differ greatly in the civilian sector, making routine medical interventions more complicated and often requiring specialized equipment not needed in a homogenous, otherwise healthy, young cohort of patients. For example, needle thoracostomy using a standard-sized needle is less efficacious in the civilian sector [4], and tourniquets may be too big to be effective in the pediatric population.
- *Differences in barriers to evacuation and care*: Despite the threat of dynamic terrorist attacks, secondary attacks and armed resistance to evacuation are far less common in the civilian setting. Additionally, civilian operational scenarios typically involve greater resource for evacuation to definitive care, but these resources are not employed early following an event, as may occur in the military setting.
- *Baseline health of the population*: A significant number of civilian wounded persons have comorbid conditions that must be factored. Examples include the use of pharmacologic anticoagulants or renal failure, both of which impede clotting ability. Others may have chronic cardiac or pulmonary comorbidities which will blunt their ability to respond to injury and stress and also impede their ability to flee to safety.
- *Wounding patterns*: Although the weapons are similar between military and civilian active shooter scenarios, the wounding patterns differ given the paucity of protective ballistic gear in the civilian setting [5].
- *Budgetary constraints*: Civilian agencies must follow product and acquisition laws set by their individual jurisdictions. This limits their ability to acquire specific TCCC recommended products.

Tactical Emergency Casualty Care (TECC) was founded by a group of voluntary subject matter experts in emergency medicine, trauma surgery, critical care medicine, anesthesiology, pain management, EMS, law enforcement, tactical medicine, and medical education in 2011 to address the gap in civilian high-threat medical response. Based on TCCC guidelines, the medical literature, and expert opinion, TECC guidelines seek to balance the threat, varying scope of practice of responders, differences in patient population, limits on medical equipment and variable availability of resources that may be present in all high-threat atypical emergencies, and mass casualties in the civilian setting [6]. Additional goals of TECC include establishing a framework that balances risk-benefit ratios for all civilian operational medical response elements to minimize risk to the responder while optimizing patient care and accounting for differences in wounding pattern and patient cohort to provide guidance on medical management to mitigate preventable deaths. By emphasizing the importance of rapid stabilizing medical care at or near the point of wounding, the TECC guidelines are applicable to medical rescue operations for events such as active shooter/active violence and complex terror attacks, in addition to other mass casualty circumstances with ongoing risk to the rescuers such as industrial and hazardous materials events, structural collapse, and mass transportation accidents. Overall, the key tenets of TECC are similar to TCCC, but the developmental considerations and scope of application have been adapted to the civilian setting (Table 3.2). Additionally, the updates to the guidelines are firmly founded in civilian medical evidence. Since inception in 2011, TECC has been endorsed by a number of professional and governmental entities [7–9].

Table 3.2 Differences between TCCC and TECC

TCCC	TECC
Named categories in three phases of care 　Care under fire 　Tactical field care 　Tactical evacuation	Named categories in three phases of care 　Direct threat (hot zone) 　Indirect threat (warm zone) 　Evacuation care (cold zone)
Audience 　Soldier/sailor 　Medic 　Physician	Audience 　First care provider[a] 　First responder with a duty to act 　EMR/EMT 　Paramedic 　Physician
Designed for young, healthy cohort	Addresses pediatrics to geriatrics and accounts for comorbid conditions
Restricted to a uniform methodology and use of specific products/adjuncts	Allows for variability in practice and use of adjuncts based on jurisdiction and scope limitations

TCCC Tactical Combat Casualty Care, *TECC* Tactical Emergency Casualty Care
[a]Formerly called "civilian bystander"

Tenets of TECC

Decreasing the time from injury to initial stabilizing care is the most critical step in mitigating preventable trauma fatalities [10]. At most basic level, TECC balances the operational threat against the need for medical care for the wounded. As compared to a standard prehospital trauma scenario, which usually involves 1–2 patients with plentiful resources, there are significant differences when responding to a hostile scene where patients outnumber resources and/or scene security cannot be guaranteed. As such, TECC recommends organizing these tactical situations into phases of care defined by the threat itself: direct threat (hot zone), indirect threat (warm zone), and evacuation (cold zone) [11]. Within each phase, the feasibility and utility of medical interventions change based upon the risk of further injury to the patient or provider.

Throughout all phases of care, TECC stresses the importance of immediate hemorrhage control followed by simple airway management, hypothermia prevention, and damage control resuscitation based on one's scope of practice. Therefore, TECC strongly encourages the use of direct pressure, tourniquets, wound packing, and pressure and hemostatic dressings and the use of intravenous medications such as tranexamic acid based on the skill level and scope of practice of the responder. TECC also encourages the use of first care providers (formerly known as civilian bystanders) as well as first care responders (usually law enforcement personnel) to expedite delivery of care until specifically trained medical personnel arrive.

Direct Threat (Hot Zone)

A direct threat or hot zone is any area where the risk of harm to the patient or provider is imminent and may be greater than the risk of death posed by the injury itself. This may be a fixed, defined area such as seen in traditional hazardous materials or police response, but the hot zone may also be dynamic and shifting with fluid boundaries. Direct threat (hot zone) phase applies, but is not limited, to active shooter situations, hazardous materials spills, fire scene, unstable structural collapse, close proximity to unexploded improvised devices, and other technical rescue and mass casualty situations. The majority of effort during this phase is directed at mitigating the threat and extricating those in danger from the threat area. As such, very limited medical care is provided during this phase of care.

It is important to note, and is emphasized during this phase, that accessing and extricating the patient from an area of threat should be considered a medical intervention and prepared for by trained first responders. "It is no longer acceptable to stand and wait for casualties to be brought to the perimeter [because] external hemorrhage control is a core law enforcement skill" [12]. As such, joint training between police and fire/EMS units, often referred to as "rescue task force" units, prior to an actual event is pivotal as the EMS response paradigm has shifted, "from one of no risk entry to one of mitigated risk entry" [13]. Even with the use of rescue task force units, the persons most able to rapidly provide care will always be the uninjured, or minimally injured, civilian first care provider who is geographically close to the wounded followed by public safety personnel, usually law enforcement officers.

During direct threat (hot zone), external hemorrhage control is the only medical intervention that is recommended. Rapid application of tourniquets can be lifesaving if hemorrhage is so severe that it is likely the patient will exsanguinate prior to evacuation. Given the need to limit time spent in proximity to a threat, direct pressure should be applied immediately and followed quickly by tourniquet application as high up on the extremity as possible. These tourniquets should be placed over any clothing present to minimize time to application and control of bleeding. If tourniquets are not available and the injured person is capable, he or she should be instructed to apply direct pressure to his or her own wound during evacuation. Use of wound packing, pressure dressings, and hemostatic agents for hemorrhage control is deferred to later phases of care due to the amount of time and need for specialized equipment and training required to properly apply these interventions. All other medical interventions such as formal triage, spine immobilization, complex airway management, and shock management are deferred to later phases of care.

Indirect Threat (Warm Zone)

Indirect threat (warm zone) care begins once the patient and provider are in an area where there is still the potential for harm, or there is a chance that the dynamic situation may deteriorate back to a direct threat situation. Examples of indirect threat care include an active shooter event where a particular room/corridor has been cleared but the assailant has not yet been neutralized, the immediate aftermath of an exploded improvised explosive device where the risk of a secondary or delayed explosive device remains, or industrial accident where the possibility of further structural collapse or recurrent event is not likely but has not been definitively ruled out.

TECC recommends the establishment of casualty collection points depending on the geography and needs of the rescue operation. Traditional triage schemes such as START and SALT are not recommended. Instead, triage should be limited to defining patients only as ambulatory, non-ambulatory, and deceased.

Mitigation of the threat and safety considerations for responders remain paramount; however, in this phase, patient assessments and treatments are more comprehensive and methodical. The acronym, MARCHE, can be used to recall the correct order to address potentially preventable causes of death in this phase of care: major hemorrhage, airway, respirations/breathing, circulation, head injuries and hypothermia, and everything else (Table 3.3).

Table 3.3 MARCHE skills

Objective	Skill set/tasks
Major hemorrhage control	Direct pressure Wound packing Tourniquet Hemostatic dressing
Airway management	Sit up/lean forward or place on side Nasopharyngeal airway Supraglottic airway Surgical airway Endotracheal intubation (only in cold zone)
Respiration/breathing	Seal open chest wounds (release intermittently as needed) Needle thoracostomy Assist ventilation manually
Circulation	Use radial pulse and mental status as indices of shock Establish IV/IO access Minimize fluid/blood administration. Allow hypotensive resuscitation Administer TXA if appropriate
Traumatic brain injury	Use IV fluids to keep systolic blood pressure > 90 mmHg Avoid hypercapnia Provide analgesia/sedation Elevate head 30–45 degrees
Hypothermia prevention	Remove wet clothing, protect from cold surfaces, and cover patient
Multimodal pain control	Use combination of non-opioid and opioid medications
Smoke inhalation and burns	Invasive airway for airway edema/stridor Oxygen for carbon monoxide exposure Cyanide antidotes for smoke exposure with altered mental status

IV intravenous, *IO* intraosseous, *TXA* tranexamic acid

Major Hemorrhage

Major exsanguinating external hemorrhage remains the initial focus of care in this phase as well. This includes reassessing the efficacy of any tourniquets applied in a direct threat (hot zone) phase and immediately addressing any unrecognized or uncontrolled bleeding, such as junctional bleeding in the axilla, groin, or neck. The benefit of other hemorrhage control techniques instead of sole use of tourniquets can also be considered. Wound packing with mechanical pressure dressings and/or the use of topical hemostatic agents can be considered.

Tourniquets that are effectively controlling hemorrhage should be left in place. However, if these devices are found to be ineffective in controlling hemorrhage, additional tightening can be attempted or a second tourniquet may be placed. If operational conditions delay the evacuation of any patient with a tourniquet for more than 2 h, tourniquets may be downgraded through a methodical process of applying deep wound pack and pressure dressing directly to the wound, followed by gradual release of the tourniquet while assessing for the efficacy of hemorrhage control at the wound. Any downgraded tourniquet should be left loosely in place in case the need for reapplication arises.

Airway

Once all significant bleeding is controlled as best as possible, the next medical priority is airway maintenance. Clearing the oropharynx of obstruction, use of simple airway adjuncts, such as nasopharyngeal airways, and proper body positioning are emphasized over definitive airway techniques such as orotracheal intubation. These interventions can easily be incorporated into the skill set of the civilian first care responder and law enforcement personnel.

Emphasis is placed on allowing conscious patients to maintain whatever position they need in order to manage their own airway and improve breathing instead of forcing them to lay supine. Forcing patients to remain supine, especially to maintain cervical spine control, is ineffective, may be agitating, and may actually cause airway obstruction and aspiration or worsen respiratory mechanics.

Intubation in this phase is allowed and may be necessary depending on the operational situation and evacuation plan; however, supraglottic airways are recommended over traditional orotracheal intubation because the latter is time-consuming; requires advanced training, equipment, and supplies; and creates a patient with much higher requirements for medical maintenance. When needed, surgical techniques to obtain an airway are allowable if appropriately trained personnel are present.

Respiration

The primary focus of maintaining adequate respirations is through addressing and maintaining the integrity of the chest wall and pleural space. This includes covering open pneumothoraces ("sucking chest wounds") with an occlusive dressing and early recognition and treatment of tension pneumothoraces. Simple recognition of developing tension pneumothorax is accomplished through monitoring for increasing respiratory distress, hypoxia/air hunger, and hypotension. Tension pneumothorax should be treated through temporary removal ("burping") of an occlusive chest seal or through needle thoracostomy. Needle thoracostomy should be performed with a minimum 14-gauge, 3.25 inch device [4] and only by properly trained, appropriate scope providers. The decision to artificially ventilate any patient must be made with the consideration of the resources it will require as well as the feasibility of evacuating such a patient. As a whole, CPR is not recommended for any patient; however, consideration should be given to perform bilateral needle thoracostomies (if appropriately trained and authorized) in any patient with penetrating torso trauma prior to cessation of care to treat possible unrecognized tension pneumothorax.

Circulation

"Circulation" consists of early recognition of shock and implementation of damage control resuscitation. Limited administration of fluids is recommended only when it is determined that the patient is in profound shock [14]. Altered mental status in the absence of a head injury, skin condition and appearance, and absence of distal pulses can be used in lieu of an actual, measured blood pressure to assess for adequacy of perfusion and probability of shock. In general, if a patient is mentating appropriately, they are not in an immediately life-threatening state of shock irrespective of the vital signs. Similarly, the presence of a radial or pedal pulse connotes a sufficient blood pressure to maintain perfusion to the vital organs.

In addition to permissive hypotension, the use of tranexamic acid for patients in hemorrhagic shock from non-compressible hemorrhage is emphasized. A blood-based resuscitation using packed red blood cells, plasma, and platelets in a 1:1:1 ratio is preferred; however, the logistical requirements and advanced protocol and scope of practice required make this unlikely in most prehospital settings. As such, TECC recommends, if blood or blood products are not available, crystalloid should be administered in 500 mL boluses until a radial/pedal pulse is obtained or the patient's mental status improves.

Head Injury

Cerebral perfusion pressure is defined as the mean arterial pressure blood pressure minus the intracranial pressure and should be kept at 60 mm Hg or more at all times in any patient with suspected traumatic brain injury. Given that the intracranial pressure cannot be measured outside of the hospital setting, a systolic blood pressure of at least 90 mmHg should be maintained in all patients with suspected brain injury. Fluid resuscitation to achieve or support this blood pressure supersedes permissive hypotension that would otherwise be recommended under the tenets of damage control resuscitation. Positioning the patient in a semi-Fowler's position at 15–30 degrees, keeping the head midline, and loosening tight cervical collars may also allow for better venous drainage, thereby lowering intracranial pressure and increasing CPP. Pain relief can also lower intracranial pressure and help maintain CPP.

Hypothermia

Prevention of hypothermia is a key component of mitigating coagulopathy, hemorrhage, and death. In the prehospital, high-threat setting, it is easier to prevent hypothermia from occurring than it is to reverse it. TECC places emphasis on simple techniques such as removal of wet clothing, positioning the patient off of the ground, placing materials between the patient and whatever surface they are on, covering the patient, and utilizing reflective materials to prevent radiation heat loss.

Everything Else

TECC defers decontamination, treatment of burns, pain control, musculoskeletal injuries, and splinting until the final segment of indirect threat phase of care because these are least likely to be immediately fatal. This does not imply less significance to the management of these wounds but provides proper emphasis on the timing in resource-limited conditions.

Pain is best controlled using a multimodal strategy employing combinations of non-opioid and opioid analgesics in a strategy to maximize patient benefit without creating an additional medical burden as a result of over sedation. For situations involving smoke and fire, TECC addresses the potential for carbon monoxide and cyanide toxicity and provides recommendations for the use of specific antidotes.

Evacuation Care (Cold Zone)

The evacuation care phase describes actions taken to continue providing appropriate trauma care once the patient has been moved from an indirect threat (warm zone) area to any area where there is minimal, if any, further risk. A common casualty collection point should have already been identified during the indirect (warm) phase of care in order to concentrate medical transport resources and facilitate triage of injured to appropriate definitive care facilities. Evacuation care (cold zone) principles also apply during transport to definitive medical care and the initial phases of trauma bay resuscitation, especially in medical receiving facilities that are not designated trauma facilities.

Higher level of resources and additional personnel should be available during this phase of care. In addition to reassessing all previous interventions applied, it is in this phase that a traditional triage system should be applied to define both patient evacuation priority and to allow for proper destination distribution in order to avoid overwhelming any one receiving facility.

Care provided in the evacuation care (cold zone) more closely resembles that recommended by traditional trauma and emergency medicine manuals, such as the Prehospital Advanced Trauma Life Support or International Trauma Life Support. The difference in this phase of care as opposed to a routine trauma scenario is related to the number victims and nature of injuries present, need for resource and personnel allocation, and the ongoing operational scenario that create competing priorities for resources.

Decreased risk and increased resources allow for more definitive care. Definitive airways should be established as needed, spine immobilization protocols should be followed, oxygen should be administered as needed, fractures should be splinted, pain should be aggressively addressed, and damage control resuscitation with permissive hypotension, hemostatic resuscitation, and tranexamic acid should be considered if not already done. Tourniquets should be discontinued to be downgraded to other forms of hemostatic control as soon as practical. Communication between field providers and receiving facilities as well as proper medical treatment documentation is emphasized.

Implementation of TECC

Tactical Emergency Casualty Care is most effective when applied as an entire system of care for medical response to unexpected disasters. This TECC "chain of survival" links the continuity of care across all medical providers, from the civilian first care provider to the nonmedical law enforcement/first responder to the EMS first responder, lastly, to the trauma center first receiver (Fig. 3.1). Each link in the chain has an appropriate scope-limited set of TECC knowledge and procedures that are built upon and carried forward (Table 3.4).

TECC should be initiated at or near the point of wounding by non-injured bystanders/first care providers [12, 15]. Similar to the strategy utilized in teaching bystander CPR, to improve community resiliency and to improve immediate survival of the wounded in mass casualty and high-threat events, nonmedical individuals should be trained in the basic tenets of TECC as noted in Table 3.4. The US Army 75th Ranger Regiment's experience with TCCC [16] and the American Heart Association's experience with bystander CPR form the basis for this recom-

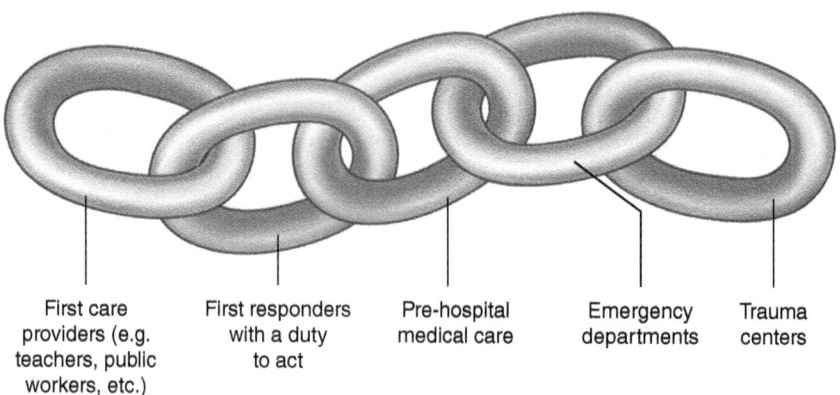

Fig. 3.1 TECC chain of survival

Table 3.4 TECC recommended skills by provider level of training [11]

Provider level	Direct pressure on wounds	Tourniquet for severe bleeding	Pack wound/ pressure dressing	Apply topical hemostatic agents	Body positioning	Nasopharyngeal airway	Supra/infraglottic airway	Cricothyroidotomy	Needle thoracostomy	Pain management
FCP	X	X	X	X	X					
FR	X	X	X	X	X	X				
EMR/EMT	X	X	X	X	X	X	X[a]			
EMT-P	X	X	X	X	X	X	X	X	X	X

FCP first care provider, *FCR* nonmedical first care responder with a duty to act, *EMT* emergency medical technician (basic/intermediate/advanced) *EMT-P* paramedic

[a]Supraglottic tube only

mendation. With sufficient funding and time, similar programs could be taught nationally for civilian initiation of TECC care in the immediate aftermath of a disaster [15]. There are multiple reports of civilian law enforcement officers applying tourniquets to successfully arrest hemorrhage. These reports clearly demonstrate that nonmedical first care providers can be trained in basic medical interventions and that they will apply these skills effectively when needed [13, 17, 18]. Current courses, such as Bleeding Control for the Injured (B-Con), and public awareness campaigns, such as the Stop the Bleed campaign, represent early efforts to promulgate this strategy to the lay public. Implementing TECC training for all law enforcement responders as a part of basic law enforcement training will solidify the next link in the chain of survival by allowing the first arriving law enforcement responders to both address the immediate tactical threat and also to begin or continue care for the wounded.

There is only one study on the cause of civilian mortality following public mass shooting events [5]. This study found that only 7% of patients had potentially survivable wounds. Moreover, these wounds consisted only of non-airway facial injuries and pneumo-/hemothoraces, not peripheral exsanguinating hemorrhage. It is possible that simply putting the patient on their side to mitigate aspiration may have allowed at least one victim to survive long enough for public safety first responders to arrive. Furthermore, it is also possible that a nonmedical first responder (e.g., law enforcement officer) may have been able to temporize some of these patients by simply inserting a nasopharyngeal airway and/or placing an occlusive chest seal to restore the integrity of the chest wall – similar to the strategies used by the soldiers of the 75th Ranger Regiment – until extrication of the wounded could be arranged.

There is no officially designated TECC course, and the Committee for Tactical Emergency Casualty Care does not endorse any specific training program in TECC. Instead, the Committee for TECC creates the specific guidelines, essentially the "what" and the "why," and allows the end user to create individualized training to implement them (the "how"). This approach allows for regional and agency-specific scope and culture.

Table 3.5 Sample of TECC pediatric guidelines

Use of pediatric-specific equipment/adjuncts
Communicating with the child during the event
Approach from eye level
Use non-threatening language and tone
Do not be too explicit
Have child repeat back what you said
Allow child to participate in his/her care as much as possible
Post-event care
Assign a single person to care for kids to establish trust
Do not separate siblings or repatriate as soon as possible
Reunify whole families as soon as possible

Special populations and the effect of age on trauma resuscitation are the current focus of TECC. Because civilian events often include pediatric patients, as best exemplified most recently in the Sandy Hook Elementary School public mass shooting event, TECC has a separate set of guidelines directed to care of these patients (Table 3.5) [19]. Physiologically, the approach to the injured child is the same as the adult: hemorrhage control first followed by airway management. However, TECC takes into account the unique psychosocial aspects that must be addressed in pediatric trauma. Kids cannot process complex events quickly making comprehension and communication difficult. This inability to understand and communicate can lead to lack of cooperation with first responders and exposes them to significant emotional distress with possible long-lasting effects. Simple strategies such as approaching them at eye level, softening one's tone and using non-threatening language, allowing the child to participate in their care as much as possible, keeping siblings (and ideally families) together, and assigning a single care taker for a number of children may significantly improve a child's well-being, both in the immediate and distant future. Additionally, equipment may have to be tailored specifically to a child, much as is the case with endotracheal tubes and other medical adjuncts.

Conclusion

In summary, prehospital trauma management has truly come full circle. TCCC in the US military evolved from civilian practices. More than 15 years of experience in continuous combat operations have driven revolutionary changes in TCCC techniques and equipment including the use of hemostatic dressings, tourniquets, tranexamic acid, point of wounding analgesia, etc. As TCCC continues to save lives on the battlefield, the principle continues to evolve through nearly real-time evidence-based process improvement. Well-documented clinical evidence and the increasing incidence of high-profile civilian active shooter incidents and mass casualty events resulting in casualties similar to those encountered in combat settings have, in turn, prompted recent efforts to translate TCCC lessons learned for use in the civilian sector. TECC is an adaptation of these proven military concepts to the civilian setting. It takes into account the various demographics and pre-existing comorbid conditions inherent in civilian mass casualty events. It provides guidelines for training of each specific level of provider, starting with civilian first care providers and ending with physicians working in dedicated trauma centers. Given the data available to date, the biggest opportunity to mitigate preventable death remains founded in the rapid evacuation of wounded to appropriate definitive care facilities; significantly more research is needed to guide and update TECC guidelines.

References

1. Butler FK Jr, Blackbourne LH. Battlefield trauma care then and now: a decade of Tactical Combat Casualty Care. J Trauma Acute Care Surg. 2012;73(6 Suppl 5):S395–402.
2. Eastridge BJ, Mabry RL, Seguin P, Cantrell J, Tops T, Uribe P, et al. Death on the battlefield (2001-2011): implications for the future of combat casualty care. J Trauma Acute Care Surg. 2012;73(6 Suppl 5):S431–7.
3. Champion HR, Bellamy RF, Roberts CP, Leppaniemi A. A profile of combat injury. J Trauma. 2003;54(5 Suppl):S13–9.
4. Schroeder E, Valdez C, Krauthamer A, Khati N, Rasmus J, Amdur R, et al. Average chest wall thickness at two anatomic locations in trauma patients. Injury. 2013;44(9):1183–5.
5. Smith ER, Shapiro G, Sarani B. The profile of wounding in civilian public mass shooting fatalities. J Trauma Acute Care Surg. 2016;81(1):86–92.
6. Smith R, Callaway DW. Tactical emergency casualty care. The need for & evolution of civilian high threat medical guidelines. JEMS. 2014;Suppl:10–5.
7. US Fire Administration. Fire/Emergency Medical Services Department operational considerations and guide for active shooter and mass casualty incidents. 2013 [cited 2015 2/9/2015]; Available from: https://www.usfa.fema.gov/downloads/pdf/publications/active_shooter_guide.pdf.
8. National tactical officers association. TEMS position statement. 2014 [cited 2015 2/9/2015]; Available from: https://ntoa.org/sections/tems/tems-position-statement/.
9. International association of firefighters. IAFF position statement: rescue task force training. 2014 [cited 2015 2/9/2015]; Available from: http://services.prod.iaff.org/ContentFile/Get/17073.
10. Jacobs LM, Wade DS, McSwain NE, Butler FK, Fabbri WP, Eastman AL, et al. The Hartford Consensus: THREAT, a medical disaster preparedness concept. J Am Coll Surg. 2013;217(5):947–53.
11. Sims K, Montgomery HR, Dituro P, Kheirabadi BS, Butler FK. Management of external hemorrhage in tactical combat casualty care: the adjunctive use of XStat compressed hemostatic sponges: TCCC guidelines change 15-03. J Spec Oper Med. 2016;16(1):19–28.
12. Jacobs LM, Rotondo M, McSwain N, Wade DS, Fabbri WP, Eastman A, et al. Joint committee to create a national policy to enhance survivability from mass casualty shooting events: Hartford Consensus II. Conn Med. 2014;78(1):5–8.
13. Pons PT, Jerome J, McMullen J, Manson J, Robinson J, Chapleau W. The Hartford Consensus on active shooters: implementing the continuum of prehospital trauma response. J Emerg Med. 2015;49(6):878–85.
14. Fisher AD, Miles EA, Cap AP, Strandenes G, Kane SF. Tactical damage control resuscitation. Mil Med. 2015;180(8):869–75.
15. Callaway D, Bobko J, Smith ER, Shapiro G, McKay S, Anderson K, et al. Building community resilience to dynamic mass casualty incidents: a multiagency white paper in support of the first care provider. J Trauma Acute Care Surg. 2016;80(4):665–9.
16. Fisher AD, Callaway DW, Robertson JN, Hardwick SA, Bobko JP, Kotwal RS. The ranger first responder program and tactical emergency casualty care implementation: a whole-community approach to reducing mortality from active violent incidents. J Spec Oper Med. 2015;15(3):46–53.
17. Callaway DW, Robertson J, Sztajnkrycer MD. Law enforcement-applied tourniquets: a case series of life-saving interventions. Prehosp Emerg Care. 2015;19(2):320–7.
18. Robertson J, McCahill P, Riddle A, Callaway D. Another civilian life saved by law enforcement-applied tourniquets. J Spec Oper Med. 2014;14(3):7–11.
19. Bobko JP, Callaway DW, Smith ER. Preparing for the unthinkable. Tactical emergency casualty care pediatric guidelines. JEMS. 2014;Suppl:28–32.

MASCAL

Jayson Aydelotte

Mass casualty incidents, also termed "MASCAL incidents" or simply "MASCALs," are common in wartime. In fact, managing frequent MASCAL incidents is one of the main differences in the practice of wartime surgery vs. civilian trauma surgery. One of the main instruments of creating immense numbers and severity of casualties is explosion/blast injuries. Although these are certainly more frequent in the military environment, and particularly during the recent wars in Iraq and Afghanistan, the civilian setting is not immune to blast events and should be familiar and prepared for these rare but challenging events. The responsible commander and clinical leadership team of any forward facility or civilian trauma center should always put together their MASCAL plan wall ahead of time, ensure it is widely disseminated and understood, and hold realistic drills and MASCAL practice sessions. The principles of developing a complete MASCAL plan involve:

1. Defining the mission
2. Making trauma simple
3. Understanding patient movement, space, and personnel
4. Understanding the biggest bang for the buck
5. Identifying the best triage officer
6. Understanding triage categories and where they can best be located
7. Understanding the roles of the command and leadership team
8. Understanding the rate-limiting step
9. Knowing and avoiding some pitfalls common to MASCALs

Different deployments at different echelons (roles) of care necessitate specific plans depending on the size of the medical unit and its capabilities. This chapter is written to describe a "typical" military role 3 deployment—essentially half of a combat support hospital with an appropriate complement of surgical, anesthesia, emergency physicians, nurses, and medics. However, these basic lessons and learning points will hold true in both the austere military and the civilian setting.

J. Aydelotte (✉)
Trauma and Surgical Critical Care, Dell Seton Medical Center, University of Texas, Austin, TX, USA

Dell Medical School, University of Texas at Austin, Austin, TX, USA

Defining the Mission

Under normal circumstances, "normal" meaning a routine day at a treatment facility in the modern world, the mission of a US Army Medical Department is to "conserve the fighting strength." But a wartime unit's mission must be more clearly defined so that everyone is on the same page. The mission of a deployed medical unit (any role) is *to mitigate death and suffering for all those that enter the facility*. It is important that everyone understands the mission as it helps facilitate everything that happens in the unit, everything from how the blood is given to what uniform is worn. But it especially affects the performance of the unit in a MASCAL as it helps define command structure, clinical behavior, and standards of care. For example, the usual standard of requiring a doctor's order to give a narcotic pain medicine is suspended to allow nurses to deliver necessary pain medicine (*mitigate suffering*) when they may be alone without medical supervision for an extended period of time. If everyone is focused on the mission of the unit, then problems are approached with one question in mind: *Does this course of action facilitate the mission?* This is an important step in establishing effective strategies/operations, and the command group must organize all the officers and NCOs to facilitate this line of thinking.

Making Trauma Simple

While some providers are skilled and experienced in the modern practice of caring for the injured, many deployed providers are not. It is not unusual to have a makeup of clinical personnel encompassing a wide range of backgrounds and common practice with only a small percentage of them with actual, real trauma experience. This is something the command group and the clinical leadership must assess before leaving the states. It is helpful to identify the most experienced surgeons, nurses, emergency medicine physicians, and NCOs and put them in positions to train the less experienced providers in a way the unit can function efficiently and effectively. It is a great mistake to lump all doctors, nurses, and NCOs into one group that "should" know how to care for the injured.

One way of delivering effective trauma care is to make the decision process as simple as possible. The American College of Surgeons Advanced Trauma Life Support (ATLS) course is a worldwide standard for the practice of trauma care. It is ideal to have all the members of the unit either take or audit the course prior to deployment. But if this is not possible or if the clinical leadership feels the unit needs different training, then it is incumbent on the officers to provide it. The best way to make providers who are uncomfortable or inefficient more effective in caring for the injured is to have simple training and repetitive practice.

Understanding Patient Movement, Treatment Personnel, and Space

It really all comes down to *moving* the patients through the *space* you have with the *personnel* available at the time. It is easiest to think about things in the reverse order presented above because special attention should be focused on the patient movement piece of the equation.

Space: In a standard half-CSH, there is going to be an EMT section, an ICU, an ICW, some operating rooms, and a PLX (pharmacy, lab, and X-ray) area. This is the space we have to work with. There is, essentially, a finite amount of bed space in each of the sections above. It is important for the leadership to recognize exactly what space is available and usable and keep tabs on what is being occupied at all times. In the modern US military system, the issue of moving patients *out* of the occupied space is a standard practice that has essentially been matured in the most recent conflicts in Iraq and Afghanistan. The key concept here is to keep a close eye on what space is used and when. The best way to do this is to have the triage officer, the chief medical officer (DCCS), and the chief nursing officer (DCN) keep redundant running lists with a pen or pencil of how many patients are in each area.

Personnel There are always variations in people's experience and comfort level in dealing with military or life-threatening trauma. Most deployed units are made up of a mix of people from various clinical backgrounds, some of which are brand-new to the concept of trauma care, especially the war-injured. This should be something the leadership recognizes and addresses, especially in regards to MASCAL management. A smart leader can put an experienced clinical provider in a position to force-multiply clinical care delivery in every area of the hospital. But *not* recognizing this variation can result in mismanagement of clinical personnel and lead to more confusion in an already confusing time. But the simpler way of approaching the personnel aspect of the equation is to recognize exactly who is available for treatment in each section at any given time. The easiest area to visualize is the operating rooms. If the Combat Support Hospital (CSH) has a total of four operating tables and four anesthesia providers; the math is very simple. There is one anesthesia provider per bed. Slightly more complicated is the EMT section. If there are five general surgeons (one of which is the triage officer), one urologist, one gynecologist, one orthopedic surgeon, and one emergency medicine doctor, then the CSH can staff eight beds in the EMT section or seven beds with the emergency medicine doctor "floating" to help the other seven providers perform procedures and helping to facilitate movement. The leadership team must assess the best tact to help accomplish the mission. This concept will be revisited in the *Triage Category* section below.

Patient Movement This is the most important aspect of MASCAL planning. The execution of patient movement has everything to do with changing the *culture* of patient movement. This requires the leadership to accept a few major changes in the way medicine is practiced in the US civilian or garrison healthcare world. This is best illustrated in a comparison between a traditional emergency department trauma admission to the ICU and a wartime admission to the ICU at the 28th CSH in Baghdad in 2007. In both cases the patient will have the same injuries: MVC rollover (HMMV rollover after explosion event), closed head injury requiring intubation, no abdominal injuries identified, and right closed femur fracture.

In the traditional/garrison model, the doctor taking care of the patient makes a decision to move to the ICU and articulates it to the bedside ED nurse (time zero). The nurse then tells the charge nurse that the patient needs to go to the ICU. The charge nurse then calls the bed coordinator (house supervisor) who takes notes on the patient and then calls the ICU after checking the bed status. The ICU and the bed coordinator have a conversation about when a bed will be available and when staffing will be ready for the patient. This is typically a 30-min time delay from initial phone call to another call when the ICU is now ready for the patient. The bed coordinator then calls the ED and lets the charge nurse know the ICU is ready for the patient. The charge nurse then alerts the bedside nurse, who is likely dealing with at least one other patient. The bedside nurse then gets on the phone and calls the ICU nurse who will take over care of the patient and gives a verbal report to him/her. The bedside ED nurse then assembles a team to help him/her package the patient for movement, and then they leave the ED. This is another 30-min delay at least. In total, if everything is moving just right, it's about an hour from decision to move to actually moving out of the ED. In the CSH, when the decision is made to move to the ICU, the patient was moved onto a transport stretcher with an oxygen tank, the brakes released, on their way to the ICU. This took approximately 3 min.

This is a major paradigm shift in thinking about traditional patient movement. It requires three things:

1. Recognizing (and coming to emotional terms with) the notion that an open ICU bed is going to be filled and everyone must help each other to overcome the adversity, the patients are *not* going to quit coming.
2. Eliminating communication with a bed coordinator. This is a necessary step because of the first item above.
3. Creating the expectation that bedside, face-to-face communication between the ED nurse and the ICU nurse is adequate and safe. This eliminates all the calling and, quite frankly, unnecessary preparation. The expectations for preparation for ICU admissions could be set well ahead of time: they will all likely be intubated and on the ventilator *and* likely requiring/continuing a big resuscitation or head injury management.

The leadership must be comfortable with all three elements of change and agree that those things *must* change in order to facilitate efficient movement in the hospital. This will be discussed more in depth in the *Biggest Bang for the Buck* section below but is illustrated with simple math in a traditional EMT area as outlined in the *Space* section above. With seven beds and one floater in the EMT section, with the traditional concept of patient movement, the CSH can see seven casualties per hour. But if the trauma workup is simple and the patient movement piece is outlined as above, each bed can be turned over in about 9 min (the average bed turnover time for another traditional CSH setup [47th CSH, Tikrit, Iraq 2009]), yielding an EMT section that can see nearly 50 patients per hour. Of course this description does not account for patients needing to go to the operating room and losing some of the surgeons from staffing the EMT section, but the point of the illustration is that a commitment to efficient patient movement can multiply the number of patients seen per hour by a factor of seven. This is a very important concept that must be acknowledged and incorporated into the MASCAL plan.

The Biggest Bang for the Buck

As much credit as surgeons get for heroically taking someone to the operating room and performing some lifesaving operation in one body cavity or another, they are actually the rate-limiting step in a MASCAL. Everything else in the hospital, if operating efficiently, moves way, way faster than they do. A *fast* surgeon can complete a damage control trauma case in about an hour skin to skin. But that would equate to a total of four patients per hour in the entire facility in a role 3 scenario described above.

The *biggest bang for the buck*, the way to help the most people with the resources available, is stopping external bleeding, securing an airway, giving some blood, and draining a pneumothorax the staples of ATLS. This is why movement through the EMT section is so important. Injuries that require a surgeon's hand are certainly going to come through the hospital, no question about it. But the vast majority of lifesaving interventions will come from the steady hand of someone caring for the patient in the EMT, putting pressure on a bleeding wound, placing a tourniquet, placing a chest tube, or intubating those that cannot control their airway. Knowing this will help guide the leadership team to best utilize their personnel in the space they have available and ensure efficient patient movement to make more open spots to treat more casualties. This is a major tenet of mass casualty management that must be recognized as it helps drive the culture of movement both in and out of the EMT section.

The Triage Officer

The triage officer is the person that will sort out patients as they enter the building, most notably the EMT section, AND help sort out who occupies beds in the ICU and the operating room. This person will make potentially lifesaving decisions on the fly after meeting a casualty for only a few seconds. This person must be very experienced and comfortable dealing with injured patients. By convention, this person is usually the most senior-ranking trauma surgeon.

Traditional US army training doctrine had previously assigned the dental officer as the triage officer at forward units such as aid stations or "charlie-med" units. The underlying thought process was that this person was the "least valuable" in terms of one-on-one bedside patient care and thus should do the triage. This is a mistake that was quickly understood once MASCALs with real injured and complex patients began arriving in numbers. The dentist is likely the most *inexperienced* trauma provider in the entire organization. While the temptation exists to place someone out-front who won't be missed clinically in the EMT section or the OR, the necessary skills to properly sort patients into appropriate areas of the hospital are perhaps the most important skill set in the entire CSH during a MASCAL. This renders not just the dental officer but other inexperienced providers as less than ideal to essentially lead the hospital during this situation. The triage officer should be the person who has an in-depth understanding of trauma care and who understands the principles and potential pitfalls of triage and even more importantly must be someone who is calm and focused. The triage officer should also be someone who can work with and communicate easily with the other key leaders of MASCAL care such as the senior anesthesiologist or CRNA, the chief nurse/nursing supervisor, and the hospital leadership.

In a similar way, *someone* experienced in surgery must sort out the patients who leave the EMT section and go to the operating room or the ICU. While it may make sense to use two other people perform these triage tasks, it may not be the most efficient use of personnel. For example, some facilities have used an anesthesia provider to triage to the operating room and a critical care physician to triage patients to the ICU, both of these in addition to the person out-front moving people in to the hospital. Remember, the triage task requires experience, brainpower, and a physical presence in or around the area where the most serious patients will be located—the EMT section. Because of the physical and mental portions of the task, it will, by definition, take another two people away from their area of work. The ICU doctor won't be able to actually be in the ICU guiding care, and the anesthesia provider won't be passing gas and guiding a resuscitation in the operating room if they are away from their areas of work. Utilizing this method of triaging all three areas takes three people out of the clinical fight. While some facilities have had the luxury of having such an abundance of personnel, this is usually not the case. Three separate people taken out of the clinical fight can be a major detriment in most deployed environments or in less well-resourced civilian settings. The ideal triage officer would be experienced in all three of these clinical areas, at least enough to make decisions on who goes where and when. One person has this experience—the surgeon.

While it is tempting to think that a surgeon's presence in the operating room is so valuable that taking them away from actually operating is not the best use of their time, this is actually not practically true. Most CSHs have more surgeons assigned than they have actual operating tables, and even if they don't, the task of getting the patients sorted in and out of the right EMT areas facilitates the premise of recognizing, and implementing, the *biggest bang for the buck*. This may be counterintuitive, but the practical execution of mass casualty situations has borne this *surgeon-centric* technique to be not only useful but the most efficient method of facilitating efficient movement and mitigating death.

This mindset and plan is not without its limitations. What happens when there *aren't* as many surgeons as there are operating tables? Or, worded more precisely, what happens when the clinical situation arises that the surgeon triage officer *must* step away from her triaging duties to perform a lifesaving operation? The simple answer is: Then the surgeon hands over triaging duties to the second in command (usually the DCCS or equivalent) and steps away, into the operating room. This type of leadership transition requires two things:

1. Planning ahead. Identify the person who may take over for the triage officer if this situation arises well ahead of time. Broaching the topic in the heat of a live mass casualty situation is poor planning.
2. Recognizing the clinical situation to be a *need* not a *want*. Surgeons *want* to be in the operating room. It's what they do. Some surgeons, especially ones that are experienced enough to be named the triage officer of a deployed CSH, think they have the operative experience and skill that cannot be matched and certain operative situations would best be handled by them, instead of someone less experienced. In reality, even the least experienced general surgeon has more than the required ability to open a cavity and stop bleeding. While complicated vascular reconstructions or operative decision-making can exist, they are actually very rare. Keeping the triage officer as a last resort not only facilitates the actual triage job, but it also facilitates some operative leadership as he/she can give some input to a less experienced surgeon while still not taking over a case. Still, if the situation becomes a numbers game and there are simply four surgeons for four OR beds and the last bed needs to be opened for someone who'll die without it, then one must do what one must do. Transitioning the triage officer role would then be a no-brainer. But this is very unlikely.

The good part of transitioning the triage officer role is that there is now one less thing to be triaged. By definition all the available OR beds are being used, so there is no need to triage the OR. This both makes it simpler for the new triage officer and obviates the need for that person to have operative experience.

Pitfalls of Choosing a Triage Officer

What about using an experienced emergency medicine physician to triage out-front? This would make some sense on the surface. But two things work against this concept:

1. There are usually very few (or none) emergency medicine physicians assigned to a forward military facility. Using one of likely two or less to triage out-front will take that person away from their ability to provide ATLS-like care to the injured. More importantly, it limits their ability to facilitate ATLS procedures such as intubation, chest tubes, or central lines, thus limiting their ability to be a force-multiplier in the single area that is already recognized as the *biggest bang for the buck*. In the civilian environment, the emergency medicine physicians will be the key bedside personnel in the emergency care area and particularly when the surgeons have left to go to the operating room. Preserving them for bedside care and leadership inside the emergency department is usually the best use of this resource.
2. If that person is out-front, then who is triaging the operating rooms? Most likely it is a surgeon, who is now also out of the clinical fight. In situations with limited personnel resources, which is the vast majority of deployed environments, this presents a preventable problem. Quite simply it would be a doubling of the work effort for the same product. Combined with the issue raised in item 1 above, using the emergency medicine physician is not the best choice.
3. What role does rank play in choosing the triage officer? Usually, experience in dealing with the injured, especially the war-injured, and rank go hand in hand but not always. The group of surgeons deployed in the unit at any given time will consist of a variety of backgrounds and experience. Conceivably the group could consist of a very high-ranking surgeon with very little trauma experience (e.g., an 06 reservist pediatric surgeon who hasn't done any trauma in years) and several other surgeons of much lower rank that have much more recent experience. Resist the urge to assign the higher-ranking person as the triage officer. This can present a political issue in the unit, but careful consideration of this delicate issue by a group of officers can quell any concerns of this nature. But putting this person out-front when it is not the most clinically reasonable decision could be a major mistake.

What about if a surgeon demonstrates they are *not* the best person to be the triage officer? This could happen for a variety of reasons. The most likely reason is the rank issue above. It is not uncommon for the entire surgeon group to misidentify the triage officer because the assumptions made about rank and experience are misaligned or the person simply doesn't perform well at the role when the proverbial bullets start flying. One reason for this goes beyond just experience. This is a complicated, moving machine. The triage officer must also be a good communicator and leader of people. It is not uncommon to find surgeons who have both experience and rank but are simply unable to effectively lead in a stressful situation. Regardless of the reason, if the triage officer demonstrates the job is beyond their abilities to adequately or safely perform the duties assigned, then they must be replaced. This could also be a touchy political situation, but one the officers must address privately and respectfully make a change in this leadership position. If at all possible, resist the urge to make the change *during* a mass casualty event.

What if *no* surgeons are comfortable in this role? Sadly, this is a reality in some deployed situations. Operational tempo, surgeon turnover, or long periods of peacetime could result in some deployed units having surgeons with no, or drastically less than their nonsurgeon counterparts, operational or trauma experience. But if that is the case, all the officers must come to this conclusion together, and it may be the best situation for the unit to assign a nonsurgeon as the triage officer. While this is a reality, it is not very common.

Triage Categories and Their Location

The triage category system used by the US military is the NATO DIME (delayed immediate minimal expectant) system. This has proven to be a very useful and resilient tool to triage casualties. However, there are two other categories that are not traditionally mentioned but deserve some discussion: emergent and dead.

The triage of patients will occur in the triage area initially, and then a constant revisiting of the concept will occur during the casualty's entire stay at the facility. The triage area is typically located outside the EMT section of the facility, under cover if possible (Fig. 4.1). This allows the triage officer to see each patient and move them either into the EMT section or divert them to other parts of the CSH without having to use precious EMT space. The best method for triage is for the triage officer to speak to and *touch* every casualty. The triaged patients go into different areas of the hospital according to the severity of their category: emergent, immediate, delayed, minimal, expectant, and dead (Fig. 4.2). In order to best understand appropriate clinical management and facility setup, it is a good exercise to examine each particular triage category in detail.

Emergent and Immediate

This was, and still is in many systems, just referred to simply as immediate. These patients are patients with life-threatening injuries that will need immediate assistance and ATLS-like interventions within the hour. They include patients with injuries such as:

- Traumatic brain injury
- Pneumothorax
- Life-threatening hemorrhage
- Cardiac injuries
- Penetrating injuries to the torso
- Major vascular injuries
- Airway compromise

These patients need to go to the EMT section of the CSH. However, like many things in life, there exists a spectrum of both patient injury severity and the comfort and experience of the people treating them. This is a reality that must be recognized. This concept is best exemplified in two patients, both with the same injuries:

Patient A is a 28-year-old man involved in a dismounted RPG blast. He is yelling about his leg and is wondering where his buddy is. He has an obvious amputation of his left leg at the knee with a tourniquet in place. He has penetrating

Fig. 4.1 The Triage staging area outside the EMT. From Ref. [5]

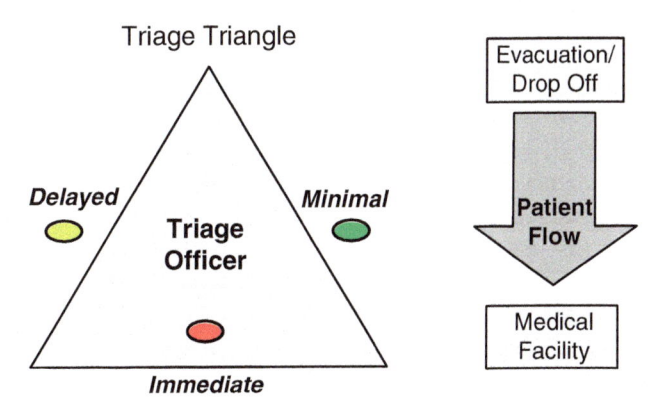

Triage and Evacuation Categories

- Standard NATO nomenclature is recommended, often called "DIME"
  - 🟡 **– Delayed** (yellow tag) – may be life-threatening, but intervention may be delayed for several hours with frequent reassessment – (fractures, tourniquet-controlled bleeding, head or maxillofacial injuries, burns)
  - 🔴 **– Immediate** (red tag) – immediate attention required to prevent death – usually "AABC" issue – airway, arterial bleed, ventilation, circulatory
  - 🟢 **– Minimal** (green tag) – ambulatory, minor injuries such as lacerations, minor burns or musculoskeletal injuries – can wait for definitive attention
  - ⚫ **– Expectant** (black tag) – survival unlikely, such as extensive burns, severe head injuries
- Triage categories differ from Medical Evacuation categories :
  - 🔴 **– Urgent** – save life or limb, evacuate within 2 hours
  - 🔴 **– Urgent surgical** – same but must go to higher Level surgical capability
  - 🟡 **– Priority** – evacuate within 4 hours, or may deteriorate into urgent
  - 🟢 **– Routine** – evacuate within 24 hours to continue medical treatment
  - 🟢 **– Convenience** – administrative movement

Fig. 4.2 Triage and Evacuation Categories. From Ref. [5]

injuries to his abdomen and left chest. He answers questions from the triage officer appropriately. He has a palpable radial pulse.

Patient B has the exact same injuries. He is missing his left leg, has a tourniquet, and has penetrating injuries to his abdomen and left chest. But he is not conscious and has no radial pulse. He does have a faint pulse in his groin.

Both of these patients present with immediate need for treatment of their injuries and need to go to the EMT section. But clearly patient B is much worse off. While the nature of his injuries is similar to patient A, he is clearly in shock and needs an intervention on his airway. Both are immediate but one is actually *emergent*. This is an important realization because it not only helps divide up space in the EMT section but helps divide personnel. Figure 4.3 shows one described setup of a traditional CSH EMT tent with all the beds arranged on one wall. Instead of all eight beds falling under the same immediate category, the first three would be *emergent* beds, setup with equipment, and personnel specifically for more lifesaving procedures on arrival. Similarly, the personnel assigned to each bed would reflect their abilities as well. It is a mistake to think all

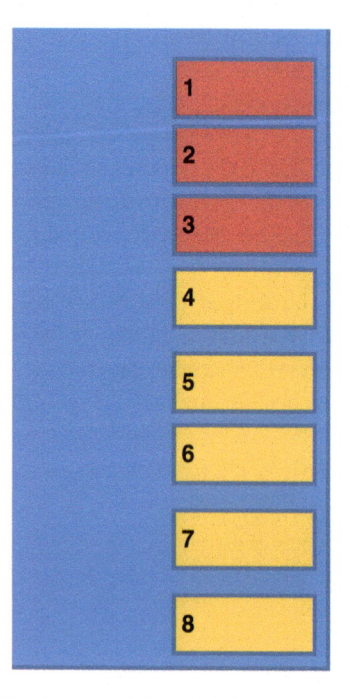

Fig. 4.3 The traditional CSH EMT tent is arranged with all the beds on one wall. An alterative approach is to having all eight beds falling under the same immediate category, the first three would be emergent beds and setup with equipment, and personnel specifically for more lifesaving procedures on arrival

providers are the same. They are not. Each medic, nurse, and doctor will have a different set of experiences and different comfort levels in executing the trauma plan and performing procedures. It is best to realize this and take advantage of it to help facilitate the mission. For example, if there are four general surgeons (one is the triage officer), two orthopedists, one urologist, two gynecologists, and one emergency medicine doctor, that would make eight doctors for eight beds, and the emergency medicine doctor could "float" and be a procedural force-multiplier. It would be foolish to think each of the eight doctors is equally experienced or comfortable managing an injured casualty. For example, many orthopedists have enough trauma experience that, with a little bit of training, could be up to speed to effectively manage even seriously injured casualties. But their ability to perform certain procedures like central lines and chest tubes, which also can be easily learned, may not be as well developed as their general surgery counterparts. For this reason the orthopedists should not be on any of the first three beds. And for the same reason, the emergency medicine physician should be "floating" and readily available to perform any procedures and then peel off and allow the rest of the management to proceed with the assigned provider (the orthopedist in this case).

Similarly, managing the airway is an experience-driven skill. Arguably the best airway managers in the world are anesthesia providers, and in this fictitious CSH, there are four anesthesia providers: one anesthesiologist and three certified registered nurse anesthetists (CRNA). One way of setting up this team is to have a CRNA at the head of each of the three emergent beds and the anesthesiologist standing by to either (1) help with the first case that rolls back to the operating room or (2) take the first case that rolls back to the operating room from any of the non-emergent beds. When a patient arrives to an emergent bed, the CRNA will either intubate them or not. Then, if they roll back to the operating room immediately, the CRNA will simply go with them and continue their anesthesia care on that bed. If the airway is established and the patient is *not* going to the operating room immediately (likely going to the ICU), then the CRNA will simply allow the patient to leave and assume their position back at their emergent bed, waiting for the next casualty. This facilitates the idea and efficiency of recognizing the difference in provider ability (which functionally translates to *bed* ability).

All this taken together dictates what the triage officer does out-front. While it makes sense to use a clinical gestalt as criteria to call one patient emergent and another immediate, more objective criteria are much easier to articulate and reliably follow. In the case of the 28CSH in Baghdad, the criteria to get into the emergent area were that the patient could not be conscious *and* could not have a radial pulse. This proved to be a good delineator of each triage category and limited both our over and under triage rates. But that is not to suggest our rates were zero. In fact, your unit should expect to make some triage mistakes. But what these objective criteria do is help limit them and stack the clinical chips in the casualty's favor, placing the most experienced people in the right place for the right patient.

Delayed

Delayed patients have injuries that will likely require some sort of surgery: washouts, fracture fixation, and laceration closures. Their injuries typically require them to be non-ambulatory but do not involve any major penetrating injuries above the knee or elbow. This will be the largest group of patients admitted to the hospital after an explosion event.

These patients are typically carried on a litter and will see the triage officer out-front. After a quick assessment, the triage officer will articulate the patient to go to the delayed area and then bypass the EMT section of the CSH. The delayed area can be in any location of the hospital. The major requirements of the delayed area are:

1. A central, preferably open location where nurses can treat the patient as well as have visibility of the overseeing physician

2. Access to the major things the patient will need in the next few hours: pain medicine (usually narcotics) and dressing supplies/splint material

In Baghdad, this was facilitated best by putting the patients in the hallway on the first floor. This was a large open area where we could put 50 or so casualties and still had access to the supplies in the OR as well as immediate assistance to the overseeing physician if needed. However, many deployed units will not be in a three-story hard building but rather a traditional tent CSH setup. In this case, the best place for a delayed area is actually in the ICW (intermediate care ward), with overflow into the common area of the pharmacy, lab, and X-ray vestibule (PLX). This was ideal because the supplies and personnel (nurses and medics) are already located in this location and the beds were already available. In makeshift areas such as Baghdad or the overflow into a PLX, casualties will be either on litters or blankets on the floor.

The initial workup and treatment of all these casualties will be done by nurses and medics, many of whom have little to no trauma experience. It is important to make sure they are appropriately trained to identify and treat common injuries. This can be done in a variety of ways to include pre-deployment training as well as participation in the practice trauma situations in the EMT section. The principles of the trauma workup in the delayed area are to undress the patient, identify injuries, keep them warm and comfortable, dress injuries as best they can, and bring up concerning findings to the delayed officer, a physician in charge of medical oversight in this area. The most ideal person for this job is a nonsurgeon assigned to the CSH, such as an internist or a nonsurgeon colocated with the CSH such as a psychiatrist, family medicine/general medical officer, or flight surgeon. Resist the temptation to put an extra emergency medicine physician, if there is one, in this job. They will be needed in the EMT section. While these physicians may also be inexperienced in trauma, they will provide invaluable help, especially in the management of the under-triaged. Almost as importantly, they provide a common sense clinical chain of command element. Issues brought to the delayed officer are evaluated, and anything that presents a surgical emergency (suspected major vascular injury, unsuspected injury to the torso, declining mental status, etc.) is then brought to the triage officer. The triage officer will then likely send one of her/his surgeons to the delayed area to evaluate the situation. It is important to behave in this sequence. One thing to avoid is any "backwards flow" back into the EMT section to facilitate workups. This could potentially be a major movement mistake as the triage officer is keeping track of EMT beds that are open or occupied. If a delayed patient is now occupying a bed the triage officer thinks is open, it could lead to confusion and delays when the triage officer puts an incoming casualty into that bed. The same principle exists for ICU patients that have surgical emergencies. Surgeons go to the ICU to evaluate them, not bring the patient back to the EMT to be evaluated.

Minimal

Patients triaged to the minimal category have minor soft tissue injuries, minor fractures from which they can still ambulate, or other injuries that require some local wound care, possibly a splint, and some oral pain control. The easiest way to triage these patients is to have them stand up out of the trucks that bring them. Anyone who can safely ambulate without much pain and has no major long bone injuries can go to the minimal area.

The minimal area is best located away from the other major functioning areas of the hospital. Any outpatient clinic-type entity located or colocated with the CSH is ideal. The staffing for this area is typically best done by a physical therapist, physical therapy tech, and/or a medic. These providers are relatively experienced in both wound care and extremity injury evaluation. Any injuries to long bones or soft tissue injuries that are beyond something that could likely heal with local outpatient wound care are brought up to the minimal area officer in charge, likely the physical therapist, and then to the triage officer.

Expectant

The traditional description of an expectant patient is best articulated in the word picture of a gunshot wound to the head in the Vietnam War: a patient with a supposedly deadly wound in an environment that cannot care for them (no modern ICU). Expectant patients are not *expected* to survive. Expectant patients, as in the word picture above, do not use precious hospital resources because those resources either don't exist or are believed to be so otherwise occupied; they can't even consider addressing that patient's needs until there is literally no other patients that could require those resources. They are essentially left to die. Sometimes, as in the case of the word picture patient, there is no other good option for the circumstance. But in today's modern military medical world, identifying an expectant patient is very, very rare especially coalition forces. Modern casualties come in two types:

1. Those that can be operated on or otherwise have a lifesaving procedure
2. Those that need to be flown somewhere to get a lifesaving operation or procedure

In the world of FSTs and split CSHs, those that fall into the latter category are almost always neurosurgical emergencies or major burns. The major difference in those patients between now and the Vietnam War is the modern ICU resuscitative care for both burns and neurosurgical emergencies. For the most part now, it is possible to control the airway, give appropriate fluid resuscitation, and get them to someone who can help within a relatively short period of time. If they have to stay at your facility for any length of time, then they get the full bore of the resuscitative effort until they can safely move out. The concept of putting them to the side and not doing anything for them is not really a reasonable plan in most circumstances.

The same thing is not true of local nationals. Depending on the medical rules of engagement, there may be a very appropriate transition from resuscitative care to comfort care. These cases are mostly neurosurgical or burn cases. For example, at different points in the war in Iraq, the lethal dose (percent burn) where 100% of the victims would not survive when left to their own community was as low as 30% with an inhalation injury and 40% without one. In those cases, the appropriate strategy was to transition care from resuscitation to comfort care, and they would die comfortably in the hospital. A similar concept existed for major head injuries in local nationals. Survival in those cases was dictated not only by the anatomic severity of the injury but also by the ability to care for them after surgery. In both cases, coalition troops and local nationals, the concept of expectant is a relative one that does not necessarily fit the traditional description as outlined in injury patterns in previous wars.

Dead

Unfortunately, death is a realistic part of war. Dealing with the dead is something inherently intrinsic to the CSH, especially in a mass casualty situation. The expectation should be that a large number of dead will either enter the facility or die shortly after arrival in a major explosive event. There must be a place for the dead in your facility. This is something that must be well thought out prior to deploying. In most cases, there is no colocated support facility to house bodies of the wounded who expire, so it is essential the officers in the MTF to develop a plan themselves. Several principles exist for the location of the bodies:

- Do not house them in a clinical treatment area for the living.
  - It is not a good idea for morale to have a dead body lying in the ICU next to live ones.
- Do not put them in a common area used for traveling from one clinical delivery area to another.
  - Hallways or vestibules are also not a good idea.
- The living soldiers and commanders will want to pay respects to the dead. Have enough space for them as well.
- Do not put them in the dining facility or the chapel. The living will need those facilities.

- The area needs to be well air-conditioned, if possible. This is a consequence of biology as much as it is a comfort.

Considering all these principles, the officers should be able to identify an appropriate space to house the dead. If there is already a formal morgue on the base, that is ideal. If not, areas such as moral, welfare, and recreation (MWR) tents and even command group conference areas are reasonable choices.

One important point of assessing a casualty's triage category is to *reassess* them constantly. In most cases there is a clear path for each casualty, but over and under-triage is a fact of mass casualty life. It is up to the triage officer to both perform this function herself/himself as well as create a culture within the organization to be approachable and able to take the clinical opinions of others.

Understanding the Roles of the Command Group or Hospital Leadership

There is no single greater function of a command group of a military treatment facility than to facilitate movement of patients out of the facility during and after a mass casualty situation. The modern military battlefield healthcare system relies on this concept. Both the deputy commander for clinical services (DCCS, chief doctor) and the director of clinical nursing (DCN, chief nurse) have key roles in planning for a mass casualty exercise, mostly in regards to nurse staffing and call-in plans and in the organization of the physician/surgeon team, to include identifying and naming the triage officer. While there are other duties that the DCN and DCCS may have during a mass casualty exercise, their main function will be purging the hospital before casualties overwhelm the facility and moving casualties out when the facility begins to fill. To facilitate this they essentially keep two lists: one for the patients in the ICW and one for the patients in the ICU. The important part of the lists isn't necessarily who is where but *how much* of each clinical area is full. Time to effective movement (how far away MEDEVAC assets are in theater), bed availability, and anticipated incoming casualties all play a role when the command group decides to begin moving people out of the facility. One rote way of executing this plan is to simply have a number, say 80%, and use that as a trigger to begin movement. When the beds in the ICU or the ICW are 80% full, begin packaging patients and calling MEDEVAC to move them.

Another function of the lists is to have redundant systems in place, not necessarily for any movement but instead to create a follow-up plan after the mass casualty incident is essentially over, and all the patients are either in the delayed area, the ICU, or the OR. At this time the triage officer, the DCCS, and the DCN together match all their lists and start walking around the facility, checking off patients as they get to them and making sure their needs are met. In situations where casualty numbers rise above 40 or 50, it is not uncommon for one person to have a list with someone on it missed by one or two of the other triad. The redundancy in this case is a safety measure that ensures every patient receives the care they need.

Because of both the safety effect and the need to have real-time ideas of the casualty burden, the best place for the DCCS and the DCN to be is right next to the triage officer in the triage area. This is not the usual position for most DCCS/DCN/surgeon physical relationships in peacetime hospital operations. Most of the time surgeons, administrative nurses, and administrative physicians are *not* in the same clinical areas. But it is an invaluable necessity in a mass casualty incident. Movement out of the facility and making sure all patients are accounted for are as important as making sure the patients are triaged and operated on appropriately.

Understanding the Rate-Limiting Step

The operating room is the rate-limiting step of a mass casualty situation. The main reason for this is twofold: there are only a few operating tables, usually four, and operations take about an hour to complete. Because of this it is very important to appropriately triage patients to the operating room. This is the responsibility of the triage officer, not the individual surgeon. Remember, the vast majority of casualties from explosion events will need some sort of surgery from washouts to major vascular operations. The best way to make this a functional part of the CSH is to have each surgeon who wants to go to the operating room *briefly* present the casualty to the triage officer, who will make a decision. Injuries to the torso with hemodynamic instability and major vascular injuries without any vascular control are the highest priority, followed by torso injuries without instability and by controlled major vascular injuries. All other injuries, including traumatic amputations and mangled extremities, can wait, providing all bleeding is controlled with tourniquets or otherwise.

The mainstay of operative management in a mass casualty situation is damage control surgery. Open the cavity, stop the bleeding, control contamination, shunt if you have to, and get OUT! Make the most conservative decisions possible, leave the abdomen and chest open with a vacuum dressing, ligate anything that can safely be ligated (all veins, essentially), and amputate any limbs with major soft tissue injuries, nerve injuries, vascular injuries, and bony injuries. The goal of the operation is to save the person's life and get them off the table, so it can be used again for the next casualty. One rule of thumb is to budget 1 h for every case. Any case going on more than 1 h should have another surgeon *scrub in*.

The rhythm of the operating room can somewhat be controlled by an active triage officer. The very nature of mass casualty incidents is that casualties come in waves. This enables the triage officer to utilizes spaces between the waves to move and check on the casualty burden as a whole. Many times they can work their way into the operating room, and both give advice/guide the case as well as simply assess the situation to get an idea of when a case will be finishing or what resources they may need. Remember, the triage officer also has an overview of resources are in the hospital, and this can help gauge what can/should be done in a current OR case. For example, the triage officer could identify a case where an extra assistant would be very valuable and will know who is available to help and assign that person if appropriate. This type of time/room management is essential to keeping cases moving and patients efficiently moving through the hospital.

Mass Casualty Pitfalls

Chest X-Rays Only

One principle of mass casualty management is to perform lifesaving things only. One pitfall would be to prioritize nonlifesaving procedures in favor of potentially lifesaving ones. In the case of X-rays, a chest X-ray is the only potentially lifesaving plane film to be performed in the EMT. Limiting films to only chest X-rays facilitates rapid evaluation and movement of patients out of the EMT. X-rays of the pelvis and long bones are not necessary. Obvious fractures should be splinted, and any suspected major pelvic fracture with hemodynamic instability should be either undergo pelvic packing and/or have a binder placed. Taking a pelvis film is, quite simply, not worth the time, especially when there is usually only one X-ray technician shooting films in the EMT. When the mass casualty incident is over and the triage officer feels comfortable, she/he can then allow all the plane films of extremities to be shot.

ER Thoracotomy

ER thoracotomy can be a lifesaving procedure, especially with penetrating injuries from an explosion. However, the vast majority of survivable injuries that require an ER thoracotomy are cardiac injuries. The reverse is also true; most other noncardiac injuries are not survivable. A pitfall to avoid is to continue on with an ER thoracotomy that has a very low likelihood of surviving. One guideline to follow in a mass casualty incident is to always open the pericardium in ER thoracotomies, but if the patient has no cardiac activity and has no cardiac injury, then simply stop the procedure and pronounce them dead. Cross-clamping the aorta and performing cardiac massage/giving epinephrine are so unlikely to be survivable that it is not an efficient use of surgeon or emergent/immediate bedtime.

Narcotic Administration

The practice of ordering narcotics in the hospital must undergo a paradigm shift to adequately and effectively treat casualties. The potential pitfall surrounding this issue is to *not* recognize this and continue on with business as usual. The usual practice of a doctor ordering a narcotic and a nurse giving it must change because the usual practice of doctor availability for orders like this will change. Nurses in the EMT, the ICU, and the ICW must have free access to narcotics and use their best judgment to help control pain. Most, if not all, patients will not arrive with any formal order sheets. Protocols within the hospital should be set up to adequately train nurses to properly dose and administer common IV and oral narcotics during a mass casualty situation.

Communication

The best communication is eye to eye. In a traditional CSH, all the tents are in close proximity to one another, so it is not terribly cumbersome for the triage officer to walk to the OR or the ICU and speak to the officers in charge of each area. The reverse is also true. However, if the space is too large or the CSH occupies a hard building on multiple floors, radios are a good solution. Depending on the security situation of the operating base in which the CSH is located, commercially available handheld radios are ideal for this situation. It is important to remember, no matter if the radio net is secure or not, the *clinical* participants should be limited to the triage officer, the operating room, the ICU, and perhaps the ICW if it is far away from the triage area. The pitfall to avoid here is to not recognize the specifics of your CSH and adjust the communication plan accordingly.

Lists

The triage officer should keep three separate lists. The triage officer's only concern is what is available and what is occupied. The details of what exactly occupies what are not important. Laminated paper and dry-erase markers are best, but some lists can be kept on a white board if it is centrally located in or near the triage area. Those three lists are:

1. A mock-up diagram of the EMT section, describing emergent and immediate beds. Empty boxes are filled when the bed is assigned and it is occupied. It is simply erased when the casualty leaves, so the triage officer only has to look down in his/her hand to see what is available and what isn't.
2. A list of ICU beds. 1–12, for example. As the triage officer moves a patient to the unit, she/he simply writes the trauma number in the space or otherwise marks it as occupied.
3. A list of OR beds. Similar to the ICU, the triage officer will mark the beds as occupied or not or can write in the trauma number or name if known.

The DCCS and the DCN also need to keep lists. These lists need to have trauma numbers and locations. One way to keep these lists is to have a simple spreadsheet with the trauma number on the row and four separate columns for EMT, ICU, OR, and ICW. As the patient moves from place to place, they can simply check the appropriate box. Pencil is best for this. The DCN needs a list of both ICU beds and ICW beds similar to the triage officer. This way, as the beds begin to fill, they will reach certain thresholds to activate the purge system of the hospital and begin the movement of patients out of the facility. The pitfalls to avoid here are (1) not making the triage officer's list easy to use (just keep it simple with space that is occupied or not occupied), (2) not recognizing the importance of the DCN's lists and the triggers to initiate movement out of the hospital, and (3) not keeping redundant lists between the DCCS and DCN.

Suggested Reading

1. Briggs S. Advanced disaster medical response manual for providers. 2nd ed. Woodbury: Cine-Med Publishing; 2014.
2. Department of Defense. Emergency war surgery: NATO handbook. Seattle: Pacific Publishing Studio; 2011.
3. Lynn M. Mass casualty incidents. New York: Springer; 2016.
4. Martin M, Beekley A. Front line surgery: a practical approach. New York: Springer; 2011.
5. Lammie JJ, Kotora JG, Riesberg JC. Combat triage and mass casualty management. In: Martin MJ, Beekley AC, editors. Front line surgery: a practical approach. New York: Springer; 2011.

Resuscitation

Phillip Kemp Bohan and Martin A. Schreiber

Introduction

Explosive blasts can produce highly variable patterns of injury. Rapidly changing pressures between tissues of different densities lead to primary injury, while damage from projectiles and surrounding structures in the proximity of the blast results in secondary and tertiary injury, respectively (see Fig. 5.1). Primary injury has been shown to affect the tympanic membranes, lungs, and hollow viscera more frequently than other organ systems; however, injuries produced through secondary and tertiary injury are dependent on a number of different variables and can be extremely unpredictable [1]. Blast injury, most commonly from improvised explosive devices (IEDs), has been the primary mechanism of injury in the wars in Iraq and Afghanistan, though recent attacks on civilian populations have also forced civilian trauma centers to resuscitate and manage blast-injured patients (see Fig. 5.2).

Resuscitation of blast-injured patients draws upon the broader principles of resuscitation in trauma but also requires an individualized approach to each patient to ensure that each type of injury is appropriately addressed. Patients noted to have shattered tympanic membranes on initial survey may also harbor profound occult lung injury from blast-associated barotrauma. Following the tympanic membrane, the lung is the most commonly injured organ in blast-associated trauma. Excessive fluid administration during resuscitation in these patients would exacerbate any underlying lung trauma and potentially result in severe respiratory distress. However, patients with extensive secondary and tertiary injuries who present with signs of hemorrhagic shock will require immediate and focused resuscitative efforts.

The broad goals of resuscitation are to restore adequate intravascular volume, augment the body's natural clotting ability, slow or prevent the development of coagulopathy, and maintain end-organ perfusion [2]. This chapter will discuss methods of resuscitation, current practice guidelines, and suggestions for the amendment of these guidelines based on specifics of the blast-injured patient and blast scenarios. Particular attention will be given to early high-ratio blood component therapy, the reemergence of whole blood resuscitation, and specific considerations for resuscitation in blast-injured patients. A significant amount of relatively new data concerning resuscitation in trauma comes from the wars in Iraq and Afghanistan. As blast injury was most common in those populations, this data applies directly to the topic of this chapter.

P. Kemp Bohan (✉)
San Antonio Military Medical Center,
Ft. Sam Houston, TX, USA

M. A. Schreiber
Division of Trauma, Critical Care, and Acute Care Surgery, Oregon Health & Science University,
Portland, OR, USA

Fig. 5.1 A combat casualty with traumatic amputation of both lower extremities secondary to blast injury. Tourniquets were placed proximally for hemorrhage control in the field

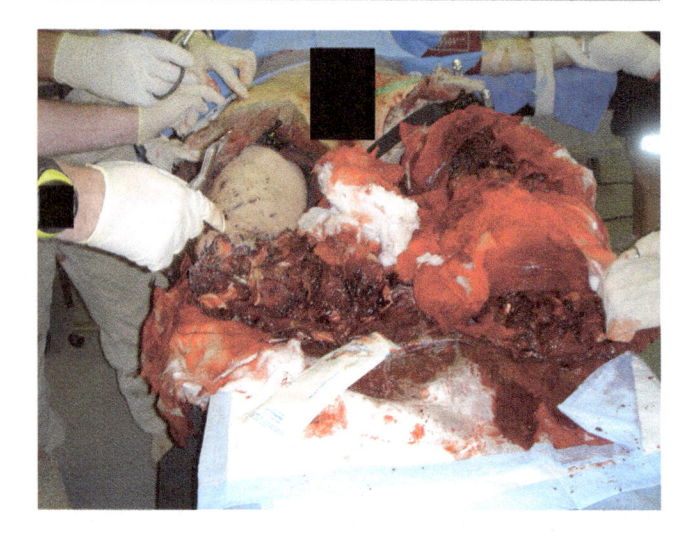

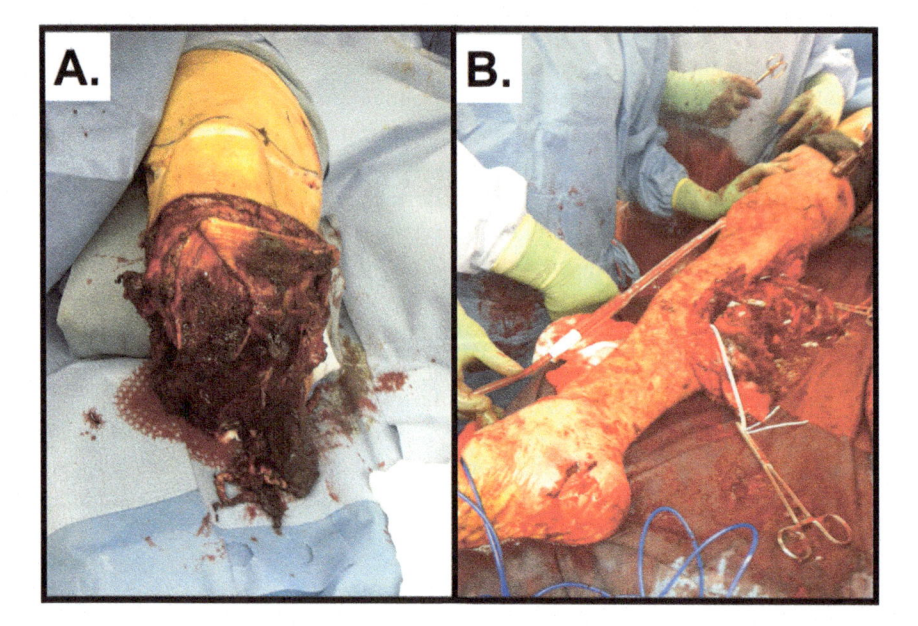

Fig. 5.2 Injuries seen after the 2013 Boston Marathon bombing including major extremity amputations (panel A) and mangled extremity injuries with significant bony and soft tissue damage (panel B) (Photos courtesy of Dr. George Velmahos)

Methods of Resuscitation

Resuscitation Fluids: Crystalloid and Colloid

Resuscitation fluids can broadly be categorized as either crystalloids or colloids. Crystalloid solutions contain varying concentrations of ions and are categorized as hypo-, iso-, or hypertonic, depending on the relative concentrations of the solution and blood. Examples of crystalloid solutions include normal saline (NS) and lactated Ringer's (LR) solution. Colloids contain large osmotic molecules designed to remain in the intravascular space. These molecules increase the osmotic pressure of the intravascular space, drawing in and theoretically holding fluid in that space

Table 5.1 Commonly available resuscitation fluids

Generic formulation	Trade name
Crystalloids	
0.9% saline	Normal saline (NS)
Compounded sodium lactate	Lactated Ringer's (LR)
Balanced crystalloid solution	PlasmaLyte
Colloids	
4% human albumin	Albumex 4
6% hetastarch in lactated electrolyte solution	Hextend
6% hetastarch in 0.9% saline	Hespan
6% hydroxyethyl starch in 0.9% saline	Voluven
4% succinylated gelatin in 0.7% saline	Gelofusine
Low molecular weight dextran in 5% dextrose	Dextran-40

Commonly encountered resuscitation fluids, divided into crystalloids and colloids. Normal saline is considered the reference crystalloid fluid, while 4% albumin is the reference colloid

to buttress intravascular volume. Examples of colloid solutions include hydroxyethyl starches, gelatins, and dextrans (see Table 5.1) [3].

Large-volume resuscitation with crystalloid for hemorrhaging patients rose to prominence in the Vietnam War and continued throughout the remainder of the twentieth century, despite reports of decreased mortality utilizing delayed resuscitation or plasma/blood product resuscitation [4]. The rise in crystalloid resuscitation corresponded with the development of technology capable of separating whole blood into components. Blood products could now be stored for longer periods of time, but emergency resuscitation with blood products became much more difficult as each product required significant preparation prior to transfusion. Crystalloid offered a quicker, cheaper means of rapidly supporting depleted intravascular volume and restoring perfusion pressure in hemorrhaging patients [5]. In addition, the logistical requirements for shipping, storing, and carrying crystalloids are much lower compared to blood products, which made them particularly attractive for application in resource-constrained settings such as the battlefield.

When comparing crystalloid to colloid as a primary resuscitative fluid, there is no appreciable difference in survival rate [6, 7]. The utilization of one fluid or the other is driven by cost and practicality. Compared to colloid, crystalloid is less expensive per unit but requires a larger transfusion volume to produce a significant change in intravascular volume status. In the civilian setting, where EMS providers are able to carry liters of NS or LR at all times, crystalloid is typically the resuscitative fluid of choice because it is cheaper. However, in the military, in austere and far-forward settings, colloids are preferred due to weight and volume considerations.

Despite the initial support for crystalloid and colloid as intravascular volume expanders, both types of resuscitative fluids are associated with a number of significant complications. First, and perhaps most importantly, rapidly restoring perfusion pressure prior to the definitive surgical control of bleeding increases the likelihood of "popping the clot" and rebleeding from the initial wound. First described in 1918 by Dr. W. B. Cannon [8], a US Army surgeon in World War I, rebleeding secondary to resuscitation only gained traction in the trauma community in the early 1990s. In 1991, Bickell et al. compared resuscitation with 80 ml/kg LR to no resuscitation in a swine hemorrhage model and found that both hemorrhage volume and mortality rate were significantly higher in the group receiving LR when compared to the untreated group [9]. Building on this data, Bickell et al. then conducted a prospective trial in 1994 that compared immediate resuscitation to delayed resuscitation following surgical control of hemorrhage in penetrating torso trauma patients who presented with a systolic BP ≤90 mmHg. The group found that survival was higher in patients receiving delayed resuscitation compared to immediate resuscitation (70% vs 62%, $p = 0.04$) [4]. This landmark study definitively demonstrated the dangers of rebleeding following resuscitation.

A second problem with crystalloid resuscitation is that while the initial bolus of volume creates enough pressure to dislodge a nascent clot, only a small fraction of the infusion actually remains within the vasculature in the ensuing minutes and hours. Up to 90% of isotonic crystalloid is ultimately "third-spaced" to extravascular interstitial spaces, resulting in tissue swelling and further organ injury [10]. This phenomenon may be exacerbated by diffuse tissue injury produced by blast injury. The important association between massive fluid resuscitation and lung injury was described first during the Vietnam War, where soldiers with no evidence of lung injury developed acute respiratory distress syndrome following aggressive crystalloid resuscitation [11]. Additional studies have noted crystalloid resuscitation to be a risk factor for abdominal compartment syndrome in trauma patients with no abdominal injury (secondary abdominal compartment syndrome) [12, 13]. Specifically in blast-injured patients, third-spacing of fluid can easily exacerbate underlying lung injury from primary blast trauma and result in rapid respiratory compromise.

Finally, large-volume crystalloid administration causes hemodilution and can exacerbate acute traumatic coagulopathy (ATC). Recent literature has demonstrated that hemodilution and ATC should be approached as two distinct entities. Hemodilution occurs with the administration of massive crystalloid volumes without compensatory supplementation of platelets, red blood cells, and clotting factors. Separately, ATC is a protein-C-mediated hypocoagulable state that can develop in severely injured patients [14–16]. While the two processes are distinct, they can be difficult to examine independently as hemodilution likely exacerbates ATC [14]. The study by Bickell et al. revealed that hemoglobin and platelet levels were significantly lower and prothrombin time (PT) and partial thromboplastin time (PTT) were significantly longer in the immediate-resuscitation group when compared to the delayed-resuscitation group at admission; [4] each of these laboratory findings points to the presence of a coagulopathy. The study was not designed to elucidate the relative contributions of hemodilution and ATC to the development of coagulopathy, though it is likely that a combination of both processes resulted in the development of a hypocoagulable state. A final important point is the rapidity with which the coagulopathy developed: coagulopathy was present in these patients as they arrived, prior to any intervention [4].

Hypotensive Resuscitation

While Bickell et al. proposed the theory of rebleeding as a result of resuscitation in their landmark study [4], no controlled experiments had been performed to formally investigate this hypothesis until Sondeen et al. [17] explored the question using a swine hemorrhage model in 2003. The group found that in pigs subjected to massive hemorrhage and then resuscitated with LR, rebleeding occurred once the systolic BP reached 94 ± 3 mmHg. The authors studied the effects of multiple injury sizes (1.5, 2.0, and 2.8 mm punch aortotomies) with the hypothesis that injury size would play a role in rebleeding. Interestingly, while larger injuries resulted in larger volumes of initial blood loss, the authors found no relationship between injury size and rebleeding systolic blood pressure. This finding further strengthened the conclusion that the propensity of a vessel to rebleed is driven predominantly by the blood pressure [17].

Hypotensive resuscitation, also known as permissive hypotension, is the judicious administration of fluids to an actively bleeding patient in order to achieve the goals of resuscitation while avoiding complications associated with rebleeding. Importantly, permissive hypotension should not be interpreted as providing absolutely no fluid resuscitation to the patient prior to gaining surgical control of bleeding. Capone et al. showed that rats resuscitated to a mean arterial pressure of 40 mmHg prior to surgical control of bleeding had similar 2.5-h mortality but improved 3-day survival when compared to rats not resuscitated with any fluid prior to surgery [18]. More recently, Hampton et al. compared outcomes among 1200 level 1 trauma patients who either received no prehospital fluids (n = 191) or any prehospital fluids (n = 1009) [19]. The authors found that prehospital fluid administration was associated with decreased in-hospital mortality (hazard ratio [HR] 0.84; 95% CI 0.72–0.98) [19].

These studies should not be viewed as antagonistic to the findings of Bickell et al. [4] Just as excessive fluid administration can lead to immediate rebleeding problems in severely injured trauma patients, no fluid administration at the time of initial injury results in a deficiency in end-organ perfusion that only manifests in the days following injury. Hypotensive resuscitation seeks to balance these two competing sets of complications by initially restoring a low but adequate perfusion pressure through fluid administration in the field and maintaining this until surgical control of bleeding can be achieved, at which time more aggressive measures to restore volume and mitigate the effects of tissue hypoperfusion can be attempted.

Damage Control Resuscitation

Damage control resuscitation (DCR) is the combination of permissive hypotension with early initiation of high-ratio blood component therapy, minimization of crystalloid usage, and rapid and definitive hemorrhage control [20]. A driving force behind the development of DCR was an improved understanding of coagulopathy in trauma patients and the recognition that hypotensive resuscitation alone did not address this coagulopathy. Early coagulopathy develops in 20–30% of severely injured trauma patients and is a harbinger of future morbidity and mortality [21, 22]. In a retrospective review of 7638 trauma patients, MacLeod et al. showed that mortality was 3.6 times more likely in patients with an abnormal PT (95% CI 3.15–4.08) and 7.81 times more likely in patients with an abnormal PTT (95% CI 6.65–9.17) on admission [21]. Similarly, Brohi et al. reviewed 1867 trauma patients and found that patients who were coagulopathic on presentation had a higher mortality (46.0% vs 10.6%, $p < 0.001$) [22]. Importantly, the authors also noted that the development of coagulopathy was unrelated to the volume of crystalloid or colloid given to a patient [22]. These patients developed coagulopathy despite limited fluid resuscitation, suggesting that hypotensive resuscitation alone was insufficient at combating ATC.

Of the four tenants of DCR, the most controversial over the past decade has been that of high-ratio resuscitation. The benefits of high-ratio resuscitation were noted first during the recent wars in Afghanistan and Iraq. Borgman et al. reviewed 246 US Army casualties, the majority of whom had suffered blast mechanism injuries, and found that rates of overall morbidity and mortality secondary to hemorrhage were significantly higher in patients resuscitated with lower ratios (1:8) of plasma and RBCs when compared to patients resuscitated with higher ratios (1:1.4) of plasma and RBCs [23]. While later retrospective studies supported this initial finding [24, 25], a weakness of these studies was the potential for survival bias: patients who lived longer received higher ratios of products, while patients who died early did so before plasma and platelets could be administered (see Fig. 5.3).

Holcomb et al. conducted the Pragmatic Randomized Optimal Platelet and Plasma Ratios (PROPPR) trial in 2015. The study was a randomized controlled trial comparing blood product ratios of 1:1:1 and 1:1:2 (plasma, platelets, and PRBCs) during initial resuscitation [26]. This prospective and randomized study design minimized the likelihood that survival bias would

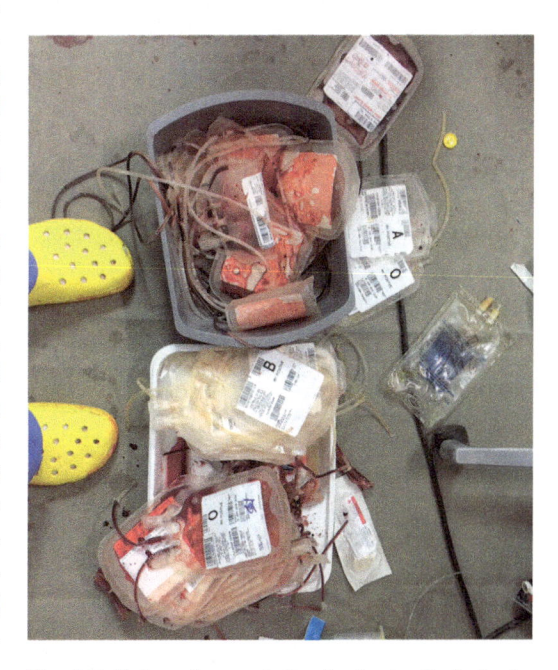

Fig. 5.3 Balanced resuscitation in theater. Early in the conflict, 1:1:1 resuscitation was found to be superior to low-ratio resuscitation. However, given the limitations of the retrospective studies and concern for survivor bias in the early literature, it was not until Holcomb et al. published the results of the PROPPR study that 1:1:1 became accepted in civilian practice

significantly impact the study results. The authors found that while there was no overall mortality benefit associated with high-ratio resuscitation, patients who received a 1:1:1 ratio of plasma, platelets, and PRBCs achieved hemostasis more frequently and had fewer early deaths due to exsanguination than patients receiving 1:1:2 ratio resuscitation [26]. Further, the authors noted that the median time to death from hemorrhage was 2.3 h [26]. Following PROPPR, 1:1:1 has become standard empiric therapy for early resuscitative efforts in most US trauma centers, although there remains a significant debate about the optimal ratio of blood products for damage control resuscitation. What has become generally agreed upon is that an early balanced resuscitation focusing on both restoring circulating red blood cell mass and providing clotting factors and platelets is clearly superior to the previous strategy of administering larger volumes of crystalloids and then packed red blood cells and delaying initiation of plasma or platelet transfusion until much later in the resuscitation.

While high-ratio resuscitation is the driving component of DCR, the same principles of minimizing supplementary fluid administration and permissive hypotension prior to definitive control of bleeding are still critical. In a retrospective analysis of 307 trauma patients with severe hemorrhage managed with high-ratio DCR, Duke et al. found that patients who received <150 mL crystalloid in the ED had lower intraoperative mortality and improved survival when compared to patients who received ≥150 mL crystalloid during the initial ED resuscitation [27]. Similarly, in a separate study, Guidry et al. evaluated fluid administration in trauma patients who received ≥4 units PRBCs and high-ratio resuscitation and found that higher volumes of crystalloid administration in the setting of DCR was associated with overall decreased survival [28]. Finally, Schreiber et al. randomized 192 trauma patients with an SBP <70 mmHg or with no palpable radial pulse in the field to receive either controlled resuscitation (250 mL initially and then 250 mL boluses for loss of radial pulse or SBP <70 mmHg) or standard resuscitation (2 L initially and then fluid as needed to maintain an SBP of 110 mmHg or greater) [29]. The authors noted that among blunt trauma patients, 24-h mortality was 3% in the controlled resuscitation group and 18% in the standard resuscitation group (OR 0.17, 95%CI 0.03–0.92) [29]. Taken together, these data suggest that while each component of DCR conveys a certain survival benefit alone, the ability to unite these various components into a single resuscitation paradigm predictably provides the greatest benefit to the patient.

The greatest limitation of component therapy lies in the process of separating and storing the components. In theory, resuscitation using a 1:1:1 ratio of components should roughly approximate resuscitation with whole blood. However, the separation of a unit of whole blood into components and the storage solutions used to preserve component longevity both result in a significant dilution of RBCs, platelets, and clotting factors. Up to 40% of coagulation factors from the whole blood unit are lost in the process; similarly, significant decreases in both platelet function and platelet number also occur [30]. When components are given back in a 1:1:1 ratio, the patient receives a much less potent version of reconstituted whole blood that produces a dilutional effect and provides only a fraction of whole blood functionality.

An additional consideration when transfusing blood products is the age of the products themselves. In non-leukoreduced, non-washed blood, breakdown products and cytotoxic elements accumulate over time and create a solution capable of producing a pro-inflammatory state in the recipient's endothelium [31]. Lipids and plasma isolated from non-leukoreduced stored blood have been shown to induce significant tissue injury in in vivo models [32]. Zallen et al. examined the relationship of age of blood to multiorgan failure by retrospectively comparing trauma patients who received between 6 and 20 units of RBCs in the first 12 h after injury. The authors found that patients who developed multiorgan failure received significantly older RBC units and that the age of RBC units was an independent predictor for multiorgan failure [33]. Thus, component therapy is limited not only by a dilution of product but by the degeneration of the product and the accumulation of pro-inflammatory markers that can exacerbate the inflammatory response already present in trauma patients.

Whole Blood Resuscitation

From World War I through the Vietnam War, transfusion with whole blood was the preferred means of resuscitation for massively hemorrhaging soldiers. Component therapy replaced whole blood transfusion following the Vietnam War not because component therapy was demonstrated to have improved outcomes but because of technologic advances that allowed for the separation and long-term storage of components [34]. Whole blood comes in two varieties: warm, fresh, whole blood (WFWB) and stored whole blood (SWB). WFWB is transfused within 24 h of the time of collection, while stored whole blood is mixed with a citrate-containing solution to prevent clot formation and then refrigerated for up to 21 days [34]. In combat environments, WFWB is the more likely source of whole blood and is drawn from a "walking blood bank" of soldiers previously screened for blood-borne disease and blood-typed to identify ABO antigens.

The recent wars in Iraq and Afghanistan have led to a resurgence in the use of whole blood as a viable method of resuscitation. Given the difficulties in maintaining a blood supply network in combat theaters, especially during the more kinetic phases of the wars, both forward surgical teams and combat support hospitals (CSHs) had limited access to platelets and plasma [35]. Further, the arrival of even one or two casualties requiring massive transfusion (>10 units PRBCs in 24 h) in quick succession could rapidly deplete the component reserve [36]. When blood components were unavailable or when demand was predicted to far outstrip the blood bank's supply of component therapy, whole blood became a reliable and necessary adjunctive therapy. One US CSH in Iraq described a massive transfusion protocol in which blood drive efforts began immediately upon the identification of a casualty requiring massive transfusion [36]. Casualties received a single massive transfusion pack (4 units PRBCs, 4 units FFP, 10 units cryoprecipitate) during the initial resuscitative effort but were transitioned to whole blood transfusion within an hour of arrival [36].

There are few randomized controlled trials that compare the outcomes of whole blood versus blood component resuscitation. In 1991, Manno et al. assessed whether WFWB was associated with improved hemostasis after cardiopulmonary bypass in children [37]. The authors randomly assigned children to receive WFWB (Group I), whole blood administered 24–48 h after donation (Group II), or RBC, FFP, and platelets (Group III, component therapy) and measured 24-h blood loss to assess the degree of hemostasis. Blood was stored either at room temperature (Group I, WFWB) or 4–6 °C (Group II, delayed transfusion). There was no significant difference between groups in the volume of blood transfused. However, mean 24-h blood loss was much lower in the groups receiving whole blood (50.9 mL/kg in Group I, 44.8 mL/kg in Group II) than component therapy (74.2 mL/kg in Group III; $p = 0.03$). The generalizability of this study to the trauma population is questionable, though this early data does suggest a benefit for patients receiving young whole blood transfusion [37].

In 2013, Cotton et al. conducted the first randomized controlled trial in the trauma setting that compared whole blood and component resuscitation [38]. Trauma patients with obvious active bleeding who required emergent uncrossmatched blood on ED arrival were randomized to receive leukoreduced whole blood stored at 1–6 °C for up to 5 days or component therapy (RBCs, plasma, and platelets). As the process of leukoreduction of whole blood results in the removal of platelets, whole blood transfusions were supplemented with apheresis platelets (modified whole blood, or mWB). The primary outcome was total blood product use in the first 24 h. The authors found no differences in the 24-h RBC, plasma, or platelet use between the two study groups, nor were there differences in the median blood volume transfused in the first 24 h. However, a significantly larger percentage of patients with traumatic brain injuries (TBIs) were enrolled in the mWB group; after excluding all patients with TBI and repeating the analysis, the authors found that the 24-h RBC, plasma, platelet, and total product use were all significantly lower in the group receiving mWB. There was no difference in 24-h or 30-day mortality between the two groups in either the overall or subgroup analysis. The authors concluded that in patients without severe TBI, mWB reduced overall transfusion volume when compared to component therapy [38].

A number of retrospective (and thus inherently limited) studies have demonstrated improved survival when comparing patients receiving WFWB to those receiving components. Nessen et al. examined survival in combat casualties who received RBCs, FFP, and WFWB to those who only received RBC and FFP and found that the addition of WFWB appeared to result in improved in-hospital survival [39]. Spinella et al. compared casualties receiving RBCs, plasma, and WFWB to those who received RBCs, plasma, and platelets and found that both 24-h and 30-day survival rates were higher in the WFWB cohort [40]. Blast injury was the most common mechanism of injury in these studies. While these data suggest WFWB is associated with a survival benefit, more rigorous clinical trials are needed to definitively demonstrate this.

The two obvious concerns when using whole blood for resuscitation are the development of an acute transfusion reaction and the transmission of blood-borne pathogens, notably hepatitis B, hepatitis C, and HIV. Transfusion reactions can occur either through host antibodies attacking donor cells or donor antibodies attacking host cells. Historically, group O blood has been considered universally compatible blood because group O RBCs should express no A or B antibodies. However, group O donor plasma can still contain anti-A or anti-B IgG that can produce a hemolytic reaction [41]. The concentrations of anti-A or anti-B can be quantified and loosely grouped into "high-titer" and "low-titer" plasma; low-titer anti-A/anti-B whole blood is considered safer as it carries a lower risk of transfusion reactions [41, 42]. A study reviewing adverse events in the UK blood services found that the rate of total adverse reactions for transfusion of any blood product is 10 events per 100,000 components, with 0.4 transfusion-related deaths occurring per 100,000 components [43]. Specifically, the risk of a hemolytic reaction due to ABO incompatibility is around 1:80,000, while the risk of a plasma incompatibility reaction is around 1:120,000 [42]. In emergency situations, the benefits of transfusion of group O donor blood to nongroup O recipients generally outweigh the low risks of transfusion reactions outlined above, particularly if low-titer anti-A/anti-B donors can be preferentially utilized [41]. Further, the study by Nessen et al. examining WB use in combat casualties revealed no increased risk of utilizing group O whole blood as a universal donor [39].

To prevent infectious disease spread during whole blood transfusion, all soldiers are prescreened prior to deployment and every 3 months during deployment. Rapid screening for hepatitis A, hepatitis B, and HIV is performed on donated blood, but no FDA-approved rapid screening tests exist, and the current tests are around 85% sensitive. Transfused units are routinely screened retrospectively in the United States, and transmission rates remain extremely low [44]. Spinella et al. noted that among 2831 samples retroactively tested, 0.11% were positive for hepatitis C and 0.07% were positive for human T-lymphotropic virus; no samples were positive for either HIV or hepatitis B [45]. The authors also found that there was no difference in the rates of disease transmission when comparing units that did or did not receive prescreening using rapid antigen testing prior to transfusion [45]. In military settings, where soldiers are frequently screened for blood-borne diseases, the ability to maintain a disease-free walking blood bank is relatively reliable, and the benefits of transfusion surpass the minimal risk of disease transmission. Civilians are not subject to the same screening requirements as soldiers. Creation of a walking blood bank among a civilian population would require careful selection of potential donors, the implementation of significant screening policies, and improved (and FDA-approved) rapid testing to evaluate whole blood samples prior to transfusion.

Current Guidelines

Point-of-Care Management

The majority of deaths secondary to hemorrhage among trauma patients occur within 24 h of injury, with the median time to death of around 2.7–3 h [26, 46]. This is particularly true in the austere or combat environment, where the majority of deaths occur in the prehospital environment or within 60 min of arrival at a forward treatment facility [47, 48]. As such, resuscitation should begin promptly and, in most cases, prior to the patient's arrival in a definitive care center. The Tactical Combat Casualty Care (TCCC) guidelines [2] detail the current military resuscitation methods and goals for point-of-care resuscitation. Published in 2014, these guidelines reflect a number of the advances previously discussed, including hypotensive resuscitation, the early use of blood products, and whole blood resuscitation in far-forward environments.

At point of injury, patients should be assessed for signs of hemorrhagic shock to determine if resuscitation is warranted. The two primary indicators of shock used in the field are the presence of altered mental status in a non-head-injured patient or the absence or diminution in the quality of the radial pulse. Casualties that do not have either of these findings on exam are most likely not in shock, and no resuscitation is provided. The recommended fluids for resuscitation according to TCCC guidelines, in descending order of priority, are whole blood; then a 1:1:1 ratio of plasma, platelets, and RBCs; then plasma alone; and finally RBCs alone. Hextend is the initial non-blood fluid recommended for resuscitation; LR and NS have the lowest priority. The resuscitation is continued until mental status and the radial pulse are restored and the casualty is moved as soon as is tactically feasible to a medical treatment facility for urgent surgical repair as needed. During transport, patients should continue to be resuscitated to 80–90 mmHg (and >90 mmHg in head-injured patients).

Civilian point-of-care resuscitation deviates slightly from the TCCC guidelines outlined above, though the same principles apply. Crystalloid, rather than colloid, will likely be the resuscitative fluid of choice when blood products are not available. Patients requiring resuscitation should be appropriately identified; EMS units contain blood pressure cuffs, and so a more accurate assessment of systolic blood pressure is possible. Some air evacuation units now carry blood products; [49, 50] if these products are available, the use of these products during transport is indicated. Whole blood, however, is not widely available in civilian populations at this time.

Definitive Resuscitation

Approaches to managing early resuscitation vary extensively among trauma centers in the United States [51]. The PROPPR trial convincingly demonstrated the benefits of high-ratio resuscitation in hemorrhaging trauma patients [26]. Yet high-ratio therapy alone is unable to address unique conditions in each patient that may be contributing to the development or persistence of coagulopathy. Therefore, definitive resuscitation should involve three components: first, initiation of empiric 1:1:1 therapy to temper the progression of coagulopathy; second, a rapid and accurate assessment of hemostatic mechanisms to characterize the patient's individual coagulopathy; and third, a transition to patient-specific resuscitation to definitively address the underlying coagulopathy.

Often, the most challenging element of definitive resuscitation is the rapid assessment of a patient's hemostatic capacity. Conventional coagulation tests, such as PT, PTT, international normalized ratio (INR), platelet count, and fibrinogen level, are substantially limited in two ways. First, the tests are time-consuming and often require 30–45 min to complete. The physiology of the patient can change substantially between the time when labs are drawn and the time when lab data is available. As a result, resuscitation based on these conventional tests lags behind any evolving coagulopathy. Second, the tests only examine a single element of coagulation in vitro rather than assessing the entire coagulation cascade in vivo.

Table 5.2 Thromboelastography parameters

Parameter	Measurement
Reaction rate (R value, R)	Quantity and quality of clotting factors
Kinetic time (K time, K)	Quantity and quality of clotting factors
α angle	Platelet and fibrinogen levels
Maximum amplitude (MA)	Overall clot strength (platelets + fibrinogen)
Lysis at 30 min (LY30)	Rate of fibrinolysis

Relevant thromboelastography (TEG) parameters to consider when managing resuscitation. Pathologic states such as acute traumatic coagulopathy (ATC) can produce derangements in multiple TEG parameters as ATC affects multiple components of primary and secondary hemostasis

A promising alternative to conventional coagulation testing is viscoelastic testing. Thromboelastography (TEG) and rotational thromboelastometry (ROTEM) dynamically assess hemostasis by applying a rotational force to a sample of whole blood and recording changes in clot strength over time [52]. The tests measure a number of different variables such as time to clot initiation, rate of clot formation, overall clot strength, and rate of fibrinolysis (see Table 5.2). A significant advantage to TEG/ROTEM is that both tests can be performed rapidly and at the bedside. Rapid TEG (r-TEG), a specific assay of TEG that uses both kaolin and tissue factor as reagents, can provide actionable information on a patient's clotting capacity within minutes.

TEG and ROTEM were initially developed for use in cardiac surgery but have recently gained traction as a feasible means of assessing hemostasis in trauma settings. Holcomb et al. compared r-TEG to conventional testing and found that r-TEG correlated well with conventional coagulation testing and was additionally more predictive of massive transfusion than either PT/INR or aPTT [53]. Other groups have independently shown that TEG/ROTEM values on admission are predictive of future blood product requirement [54–56] and the development of ATC [56].

Multiple centers have now demonstrated that TEG/ROTEM can be used to guide definitive resuscitative efforts. Gonzalez et al. [57] conducted a randomized clinical trial comparing massive transfusion directed by TEG to massive transfusion directed by traditional coagulation tests. In both groups, abnormal lab values resulted in specific transfusion interventions. The authors found that survival was higher in the TEG group than the conventional coagulation testing group ($p = 0.032$) and patients in the conventional coagulation testing group required more plasma and platelets in the first 2 h of resuscitation ($p = 0.022$ and $p = 0.041$, respectively) [57]. The authors concluded that TEG-guided massive transfusion was a more efficient and effective means of resuscitation than massive transfusion guided by conventional coagulation assays. Tapia et al. [58] retrospectively compared TEG-guided therapy to empiric 1:1:1 therapy in a similar demographic of patients requiring massive transfusion and found that 1:1:1 therapy actually worsened mortality in patients with penetrating trauma who required more than 10 units of RBCs [58]. Combined, these data suggest that TEG-guided therapy is superior to therapy guided by conventional coagulation testing and can be tailored to the individual patient in a manner that empiric therapy cannot replicate (see Fig. 5.4).

Definitive resuscitation unites empiric therapy and TEG-guided therapy. The two treatment modalities address two different elements: empiric therapy replaces what the patient is losing (whole blood) and temporizes the development of coagulopathy, while TEG-guided therapy corrects the specific coagulopathy. Empiric therapy with high-ratio 1:1:1 resuscitation should begin as close to the time of injury as possible. Once the source of hemorrhage is definitively controlled and the patient is no longer losing whole blood, TEG-guided therapy is warranted to address the residual coagulopathy [59]. Actively hemorrhaging patients typically reach the OR or the IR suite in a timely fashion; either of those areas can then serve as the "transition point" to more directed resuscitative care. The combination of these resuscitative paradigms allows for the flexibility needed to appropriately treat hemorrhagic shock.

Considerations in Blast-Injured Patients

Resuscitation in blast-injured patients must balance the goals of resuscitation with the specific pathologies of primary, secondary, and tertiary injury, the effect of the blast on systemic circulation, and the time elapsed from injury to treatment.

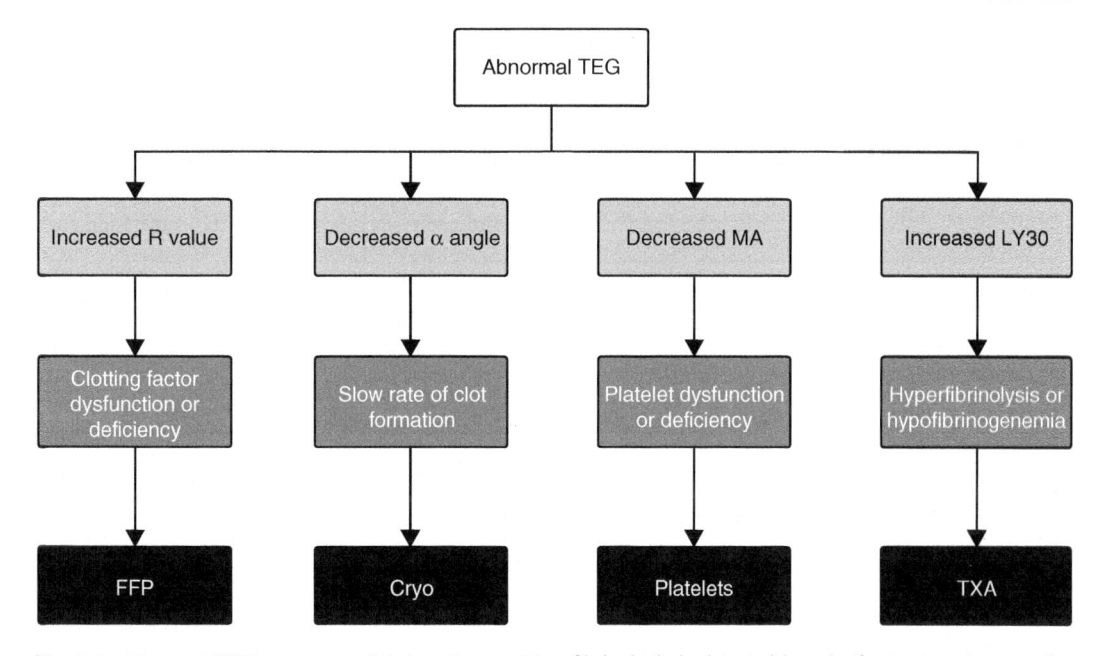

Fig. 5.4 Abnormal TEG parameters (blue) and potential therapeutic options (red). Of these, the most controversial is the management of a decreased LY30. TXA is part of resuscitation regimens at a number of institutions but must be given within 3 h of injury. ACA can be given if hyperfibrinolysis is detected later in the treatment course, but there is extremely limited data as to whether or not it provides survival benefit. FFP fresh frozen plasma, cryo cryoprecipitate, TXA tranexamic acid

Of particular concern in any blast-injured patient is primary injury to the lung as barotrauma represents a unique pathology not accounted for in the resuscitation literature described previously. Primary blast lung injury (PBLI) is due to a disruption of the alveolar septae with associated alveolar hemorrhage and impaired gas exchange [60]. PBLI typically manifests as pulmonary contusion with associated pneumothorax, pneumomediastinum, or tracheal injury. Patients with larger pulmonary contusions have a greater degree of respiratory compromise and often require mechanical ventilator support.

In any patient with PBLI, over-resuscitation should be carefully avoided as fluid overload in the setting of a compromised alveolar-capillary interface can quickly lead to pulmonary edema and acute respiratory distress syndrome (ARDS) [60]. Blood products should be preferentially administered over crystalloid in the setting of PBLI as the majority of a crystalloid transfusion will ultimately leave the intravascular space and exacerbate the underlying lung injury. Recent literature suggests that plasma helps to reconstitute the injured endothelium and glycocalyx following injury, while crystalloid causes further injury.

This protective effect results in further reduction in third-spacing and reduced organ injury [61, 62]. To ensure that patients are not over-resuscitated, hypotension and volume status should be carefully assessed, and resuscitation should be guided by both the presence of coagulopathy and the intravascular volume deficit. As soon as the goals of resuscitation are achieved, patients with PBLI should be fluid restricted until PBLI resolves.

Resuscitation in patients with either secondary blast injury (penetrating injury) or tertiary blast injury (blunt injury) can closely follow the empiric 1:1:1 therapy described above. While therapy should be initiated as early as possible, suspicion for PBLI should remain high, and patients should be assessed as early as feasibly possible for occult pulmonary injury and impaired ventilation. However, under-resuscitation of these patients is equally, if not more, detrimental to survival. Patients with PBLI and secondary and tertiary injuries will have low oxygen-carrying capacity secondary to hemorrhage and impaired oxygenation and ventilation secondary to lung injury. Garner et al. used a swine blast/hemorrhage model to compare the effects of hypotensive and normotensive resuscitation with NS in the setting of both blast injury and no blast injury [63]. The authors found that survival was significantly shorter in the hypotensive resuscitation group (~150 min) compared to the normotensive resuscitation group (~400 min; $p < 0.01$). The generalizability of this study is limited as the study used a non-survival model as well as NS as a resuscitation fluid. The findings should, however, underscore the importance of early resuscitation with blood products and the need for rapid definitive surgical control of bleeding followed by complete resuscitation.

Conclusion

Successful resuscitation should restore intravascular volume, buttress the hemostatic system, prevent coagulopathy, and maintain oxygen delivery and end-organ perfusion. Explosive injuries often produce substantial polytrauma and result in hemorrhagic shock, necessitating extensive resuscitative efforts. When possible, early resuscitation should focus on hypotensive resuscitation to maintain a low perfusion pressure without disrupting clot formation. Resuscitation with high-ratio component therapy (or whole blood, if components are unavailable) should begin en route to definitive care or upon arrival at a definitive care facility. After achieving hemorrhage control, TEG-guided therapy can be used (when available) to efficiently address the underlying coagulopathy likely present in these patients.

References

1. DePalma RG, Burris DG, Champion HR, Hodgson MJ. Blast injuries. N Engl J Med. 2005;352(13):1335–42.
2. Butler FK, Holcomb JB, Schreiber MA, et al. Fluid resuscitation for hemorrhagic shock in tactical combat casualty care: TCCC guidelines change 14-01--2 June 2014. J Spec Oper Med Peer Rev J SOF Med Prof. 2014;14(3):13–38.
3. Myburgh JA, Mythen MG. Resuscitation fluids. N Engl J Med. 2013;369(13):1243–51.
4. Bickell WH, Wall MJ Jr, Pepe PE, et al. Immediate versus delayed fluid resuscitation for hypotensive patients with penetrating torso injuries. N Engl J Med. 1994;331(17):1105–9.
5. Cohen MJ. Towards hemostatic resuscitation: the changing understanding of acute traumatic biology, massive bleeding, and damage-control resuscitation. Surg Clin North Am. 2012;92(4):877–91. viii.
6. Moss GS, Lowe RJ, Jilek J, Levine HD. Colloid or crystalloid in the resuscitation of hemorrhagic shock: a controlled clinical trial. Surgery. 1981;89(4):434–8.
7. Alderson P, Schierhout G, Roberts I, Bunn F. Colloids versus crystalloids for fluid resuscitation in critically ill patients. Cochrane Database Syst Rev. 2000;2:Cd000567.
8. Cannon WB, Fraser J, Cowell EM. The preventive treatment of wound shock. JAMA. 1918;70:618–21.
9. Bickell WH, Bruttig SP, Millnamow GA, O'Benar J, Wade CE. The detrimental effects of intravenous crystalloid after aortotomy in swine. Surgery. 1991;110(3):529–36.
10. Feinman M, Cotton BA, Haut ER. Optimal fluid resuscitation in trauma: type, timing, and total. Curr Opin Crit Care. 2014;20(4):366–72.
11. Eiseman B. Pulmonary effects of nonthoracic trauma. Introduction to conference. J Trauma. 1968;8(5):649–50.
12. Balogh Z, McKinley BA, Holcomb JB, et al. Both primary and secondary abdominal compartment syndrome can be predicted early and are harbingers of multiple organ failure. J Trauma. 2003;54(5):848–59. discussion 859-861.
13. Madigan MC, Kemp CD, Johnson JC, Cotton BA. Secondary abdominal compartment syndrome after severe extremity injury: are early, aggressive fluid resuscitation strategies to blame? J Trauma. 2008;64(2):280–5.
14. Kutcher ME, Howard BM, Sperry JL, et al. Evolving beyond the vicious triad: differential mediation of traumatic coagulopathy by injury, shock, and resuscitation. J Trauma Acute Care Surg. 2015;78(3):516–23.
15. Acute CMJ. Traumatic coagulopathy: clinical characterization and mechanistic investigation. Thromb Res. 2014;133(Suppl 1):S25–7.
16. Cohen MJ, Christie SA. New understandings of post injury coagulation and resuscitation. Int J Surg (Lond, Engl). 2016;33(Pt B):242–5.
17. Sondeen JL, Coppes VG, Holcomb JB. Blood pressure at which rebleeding occurs after resuscitation in swine with aortic injury. J Trauma. 2003;54(5 Suppl):S110–7.
18. Capone AC, Safar P, Stezoski W, Tisherman S, Peitzman AB. Improved outcome with fluid restriction in treatment of uncontrolled hemorrhagic shock. J Am Coll Surg. 1995;180(1):49–56.
19. Hampton DA, Fabricant LJ, Differding J, et al. Prehospital intravenous fluid is associated with increased survival in trauma patients. J Trauma Acute Care Surg. 2013;75(1 Suppl 1):S9–15.
20. Cotton BA, Reddy N, Hatch QM, et al. Damage control resuscitation is associated with a reduction in resuscitation volumes and improvement in survival in 390 damage control laparotomy patients. Ann Surg. 2011;254(4):598–605.

21. MacLeod JB, Lynn M, McKenney MG, Cohn SM, Murtha M. Early coagulopathy predicts mortality in trauma. J Trauma. 2003;55(1):39–44.
22. Brohi K, Singh J, Heron M, Coats T. Acute traumatic coagulopathy. J Trauma. 2003;54(6):1127–30.
23. Borgman MA, Spinella PC, Perkins JG, et al. The ratio of blood products transfused affects mortality in patients receiving massive transfusions at a combat support hospital. J Trauma. 2007;63(4):805–13.
24. Duchesne JC, Hunt JP, Wahl G, et al. Review of current blood transfusions strategies in a mature level I trauma center: were we wrong for the last 60 years? J Trauma. 2008;65(2):272–6. discussion 276-278.
25. Shaz BH, Dente CJ, Nicholas J, et al. Increased number of coagulation products in relationship to red blood cell products transfused improves mortality in trauma patients. Transfusion. 2010;50(2):493–500.
26. Holcomb JB, Tilley BC, Baraniuk S, et al. Transfusion of plasma, platelets, and red blood cells in a 1:1:1 vs a 1:1:2 ratio and mortality in patients with severe trauma: the PROPPR randomized clinical trial. JAMA. 2015;313(5):471–82.
27. Duke MD, Guidry C, Guice J, et al. Restrictive fluid resuscitation in combination with damage control resuscitation: time for adaptation. J Trauma Acute Care Surg. 2012;73(3):674–8.
28. Guidry C, Gleeson E, Simms ER, et al. Initial assessment on the impact of crystalloids versus colloids during damage control resuscitation. J Surg Res. 2013;185(1):294–9.
29. Schreiber MA, Meier EN, Tisherman SA, et al. A controlled resuscitation strategy is feasible and safe in hypotensive trauma patients: results of a prospective randomized pilot trial. J Trauma Acute Care Surg. 2015;78(4):687–95. discussion 695-687.
30. Armand R, Hess JR. Treating coagulopathy in trauma patients. Transfus Med Rev. 2003;17(3):223–31.
31. Silliman CC, Clay KL, Thurman GW, Johnson CA, Ambruso DR. Partial characterization of lipids that develop during the routine storage of blood and prime the neutrophil NADPH oxidase. J Lab Clin Med. 1994;124(5):684–94.
32. Silliman CC, Voelkel NF, Allard JD, et al. Plasma and lipids from stored packed red blood cells cause acute lung injury in an animal model. J Clin Invest. 1998;101(7):1458–67.
33. Zallen G, Offner PJ, Moore EE, et al. Age of transfused blood is an independent risk factor for postinjury multiple organ failure. Am J Surg. 1999;178(6):570–2.
34. Zielinski MD, Jenkins DH, Hughes JD, Badjie KS, Stubbs JR. Back to the future: the renaissance of whole-blood transfusions for massively hemorrhaging patients. Surgery. 2014;155(5):883–6.
35. Spinella PC, Dunne J, Beilman GJ, et al. Constant challenges and evolution of US military transfusion medicine and blood operations in combat. Transfusion. 2012;52(5):1146–53.
36. Repine TB, Perkins JG, Kauvar DS, Blackborne L. The use of fresh whole blood in massive transfusion. J Trauma. 2006;60(6 Suppl):S59–69.
37. Manno CS, Hedberg KW, Kim HC, et al. Comparison of the hemostatic effects of fresh whole blood, stored whole blood, and components after open heart surgery in children. Blood. 1991;77(5):930–6.
38. Cotton BA, Podbielski J, Camp E, et al. A randomized controlled pilot trial of modified whole blood versus component therapy in severely injured patients requiring large volume transfusions. Ann Surg. 2013;258(4):527–32. discussion 532-523.
39. Nessen SC, Eastridge BJ, Cronk D, et al. Fresh whole blood use by forward surgical teams in Afghanistan is associated with improved survival compared to component therapy without platelets. Transfusion. 2013;53(Suppl 1):107s–13s.
40. Spinella PC, Perkins JG, Grathwohl KW, Beekley AC, Holcomb JB. Warm fresh whole blood is independently associated with improved survival for patients with combat-related traumatic injuries. J Trauma. 2009;66(4 Suppl):S69–76.
41. Berseus O, Boman K, Nessen SC, Westerberg LA. Risks of hemolysis due to anti-A and anti-B caused by the transfusion of blood or blood components containing ABO-incompatible plasma. Transfusion. 2013;53(Suppl 1):114s–23s.
42. Strandenes G, Berseus O, Cap AP, et al. Low titer group O whole blood in emergency situations. Shock (Augusta, Ga). 2014;41(Suppl 1):70–5.
43. Stainsby D, Jones H, Asher D, et al. Serious hazards of transfusion: a decade of hemovigilance in the UK. Transfus Med Rev. 2006;20(4):273–82.
44. Spinella PC, Pidcoke HF, Strandenes G, et al. Whole blood for hemostatic resuscitation of major bleeding. Transfusion. 2016;56(Suppl 2):S190–202.
45. Spinella PC, Perkins JG, Grathwohl KW, et al. Risks associated with fresh whole blood and red blood cell transfusions in a combat support hospital. Crit Care Med. 2007;35(11):2576–81.
46. Holcomb JB, del Junco DJ, Fox EE, et al. The prospective, observational, multicenter, major trauma transfusion (PROMMTT) study: comparative effectiveness of a time-varying treatment with competing risks. JAMA Surg. 2013;148(2):127–36.
47. Eastridge BJ, Mabry RL, Seguin P, et al. Death on the battlefield (2001-2011): implications for the future of combat casualty care. J Trauma Acute Care Surg. 2012;73(6 Suppl 5):S431–7.
48. Martin M, Oh J, Currier H, et al. An analysis of in-hospital deaths at a modern combat support hospital. J Trauma. 2009;66(4 Suppl):S51–60. discussion S60-51.
49. Jenkins D, Stubbs J, Williams S, et al. Implementation and execution of civilian remote damage control resuscitation programs. Shock (Augusta, Ga). 2014;41(Suppl 1):84–9.
50. Holcomb JB, Donathan DP, Cotton BA, et al. Prehospital transfusion of plasma and red blood cells in trauma patients. Prehosp Emerg Care Off J Natl Assoc EMS Phys Natl Assoc State EMS Dir. 2015;19(1):1–9.
51. Etchill E, Sperry J, Zuckerbraun B, et al. The confusion continues: results from an American Association

for the Surgery of Trauma survey on massive transfusion practices among United States trauma centers. Transfusion. 2016;56(10):2478–86.
52. Whiting D, DiNardo JA. TEG and ROTEM: technology and clinical applications. Am J Hematol. 2014;89(2):228–32.
53. Holcomb JB, Minei KM, Scerbo ML, et al. Admission rapid thrombelastography can replace conventional coagulation tests in the emergency department: experience with 1974 consecutive trauma patients. Ann Surg. 2012;256(3):476–86.
54. Plotkin AJ, Wade CE, Jenkins DH, et al. A reduction in clot formation rate and strength assessed by thrombelastography is indicative of transfusion requirements in patients with penetrating injuries. J Trauma. 2008;64(2 Suppl):S64–8.
55. Kornblith LZ, Kutcher ME, Redick BJ, Calfee CS, Vilardi RF, Cohen MJ. Fibrinogen and platelet contributions to clot formation: implications for trauma resuscitation and thromboprophylaxis. J Trauma Acute Care Surg. 2014;76(2):255–6. discussion 262-253.
56. Hagemo JS, Christiaans SC, Stanworth SJ, et al. Detection of acute traumatic coagulopathy and massive transfusion requirements by means of rotational thromboelastometry: an international prospective validation study. Crit Care. 2015;19:97.
57. Gonzalez E, Moore EE, Moore HB, et al. Goal-directed Hemostatic resuscitation of trauma-induced coagulopathy: a pragmatic randomized clinical trial comparing a viscoelastic assay to conventional coagulation assays. Ann Surg. 2016;263(6):1051–9.
58. Tapia NM, Chang A, Norman M, et al. TEG-guided resuscitation is superior to standardized MTP resuscitation in massively transfused penetrating trauma patients. J Trauma Acute Care Surg. 2013;74(2):378–85. discussion 385-376.
59. Kemp Bohan PM, Yonge JD, Schreiber MA. Update on the massive transfusion guidelines on Hemorrhagic shock: after the wars. Curr Surg Rep. 2016;4(5):16.
60. Argyros GJ. Management of primary blast injury. Toxicology. 1997;121(1):105–15.
61. Holcomb JB, Pati S. Optimal trauma resuscitation with plasma as the primary resuscitative fluid: the surgeon's perspective. Hematology Am Soc Hematol Educ Program. 2013;2013:656–9.
62. Kozar RA, Peng Z, Zhang R, et al. Plasma restoration of endothelial glycocalyx in a rodent model of hemorrhagic shock. Anesth Analg. 2011;112(6):1289–95.
63. Garner J, Watts S, Parry C, Bird J, Cooper G, Kirkman E. Prolonged permissive hypotensive resuscitation is associated with poor outcome in primary blast injury with controlled hemorrhage. Ann Surg. 2010;251(6):1131–9.

Damage Control Surgery in the Blast-Injured Patient

Travis M. Polk, Matthew J. Martin, and Ronald R. Barbosa

Dismounted Complex Blast Injury

The signature injury pattern of recent conflicts in Iraq and Afghanistan is now the *dismounted complex blast injury* (DCBI) [1–3]. This dramatic injury complex typically includes at least one (and often multiple) traumatic extremity amputations and devastating injury to the other non-amputated extremities, as well as complex penetrating and blast-effect injuries of the pelvic and abdominal cavities, severe pelvic fractures, and injuries of the internal and external genitalia (Fig. 6.1). Frequently, those injured also suffer spinal fractures and/or traumatic brain injury [4]. Unfortunately, this highly lethal injury pattern portends a mortality rate up to 73% [5]. While the DCBI remains the hallmark of modern battlefield trauma, recent terror attacks at the Boston Marathon and across Europe have raised awareness of a risk to civilian population as well.

This chapter highlights the overall approach and critical aspects of damage control surgery as they pertain to the DCBI patient. A complete detailing of damage control surgery procedures for combat casualty care is beyond the scope of this discussion. Many further details for specific injuries are addressed in the corresponding book chapters.

Damage Control Principles

Throughout the history of warfare, reports from military surgeons have stressed the importance of abbreviated surgical procedure during the resuscitative period. As early as the eighteenth century, the French surgeon Larrey described that "the first 24 h is the only period which the system remains tranquil, and we should hasten during this time....to adopt the necessary remedy" in his advice on early amputation of the devastated extremity [6, 7]. Later, reports from World War II and Vietnam detailed the need for temporizing the surgical procedures performed rather than proceeding with definitive repair immediately [8, 9].

T. M. Polk (✉)
Department of General Surgery, Naval Medical Center Portsmouth, Portsmouth, VA, USA
e-mail: travis.m.polk2.mil@mail.mil

M. J. Martin
Madigan Army Medical Center, Tacoma, WA, USA

R. R. Barbosa
Trauma and Emergency Surgery Service, Legacy Emanuel Medical Center, Portland, OR, USA

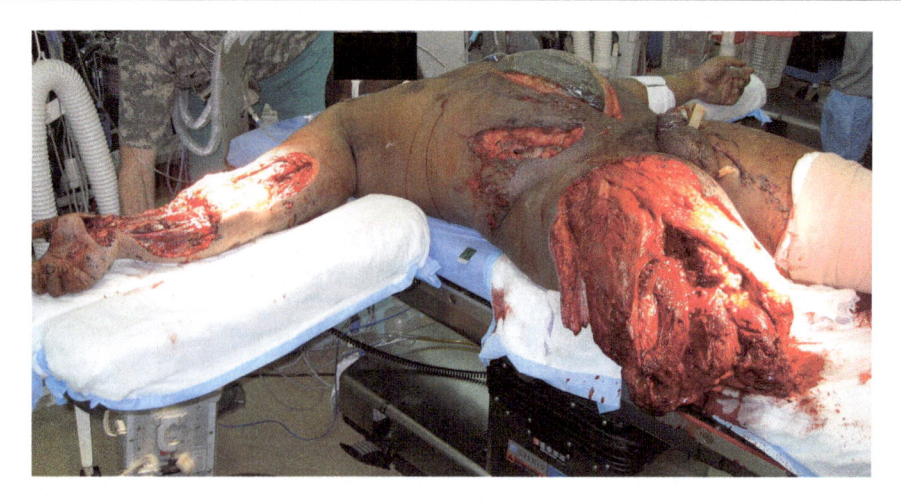

Fig. 6.1 Preoperative photo of patient with complex dismounted blast injury notable for mangled or amputated extremities, perineal/scrotal wounds, and multiple truncal fragment wounds

However, these principles were not immediately adopted in the care of the civilian trauma patients. In 1983, Stone and colleagues [10] described the concept of an abbreviated laparotomy in patients with coagulopathy and hypothermia. Later, Rotondo and colleagues [11, 12] would coin the term "damage control" surgery in their description of improved survival with abbreviated laparotomy for intra-abdominal vascular injuries. This same group went on to detail a continuum of care for the most severely injured from preoperative resuscitation and continues through to definitive management and reconstruction [13, 14]. During this same time, Kashuk and colleagues [15] began to describe the deadly physiologic consequences of the "bloody viscous cycle" of hypothermia, coagulopathy, and acidosis [16].

Today, damage control surgery implies the rapid control of hemorrhage and contamination with temporary abdominal closure, followed by further resuscitation and warming in the intensive care unit and operative re-exploration upon physiologic normalization. Initially described for abdominal trauma, the concept of damage control has been broadened to include the expeditious treatment of injuries in all body regions along with principles of hemostatic resuscitation. This broadened concept of damage control has become especially important in the military operational environment due to the devastating nature of combat polytrauma and the extended chain of evacuation where each stage may be accomplished at different physical locations (Fig. 6.2). Yet despite the complexities of this environment, several reports have suggested that damage control is equally efficacious in the military setting [17–20].

While the distribution of combat wounds by body region has remained fairly constant since World War II, the most recent conflicts have indicated that despite only 15% of the wounds being in the thoracic or abdominal region [21], over 50–70% of potentially survivable deaths on the battlefield result from non-compressible truncal hemorrhage (NCTH) [22] (Fig. 6.3). An analysis of battlefield casualties in 2008 suggested that NCTH occurs in approximately 2% of casualties with risk factors including injury patterns that include thoracic injury and solid organ injury (grade 3 or greater, named axial torso vessel, and pelvic ring disruption, hypotension, and need for emergent surgery). Of these, injury to a named torso vessel which occurred in 20% of cases conferred the highest mortality risk with an odds ratio for death of 3.4 [23].

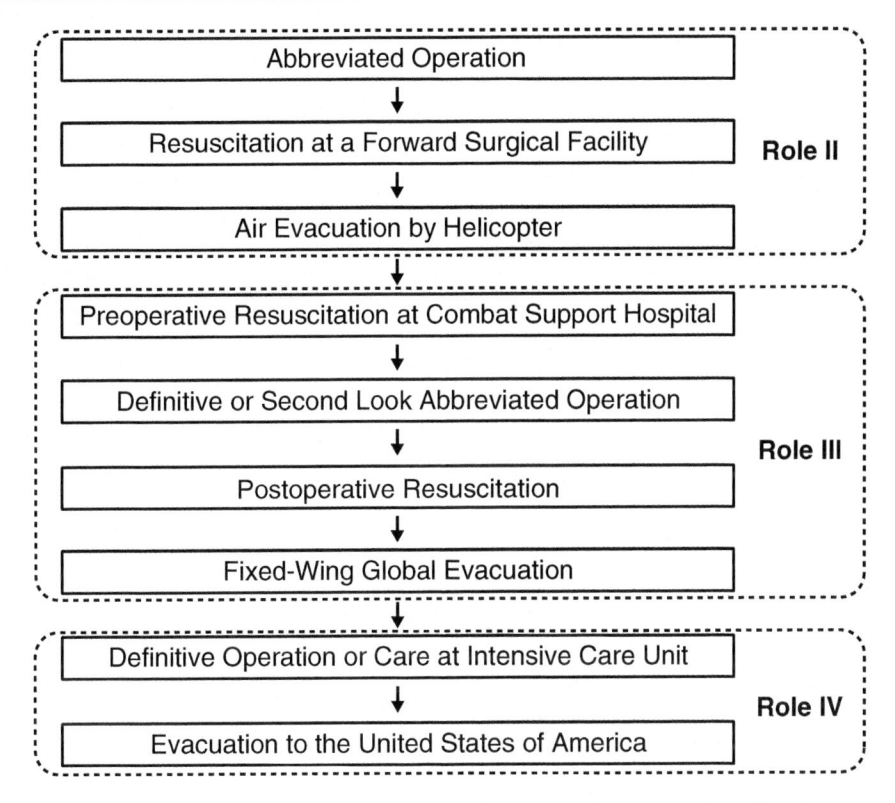

6 Damage Control Surgery in the Blast-Injured Patient

Fig. 6.2 Combat damage control stages of surgical and resuscitative care (Reproduced from Blackbourne et al. [60])

Fig. 6.3 Distribution of combat wounds by body region in OIF/OEF (Data used for figure taken from Morrison and Rasmussen [21])

Distribution of Combat Wounds by Body Region
Operation Iraqi Freedom/Operation Enduring Freedom

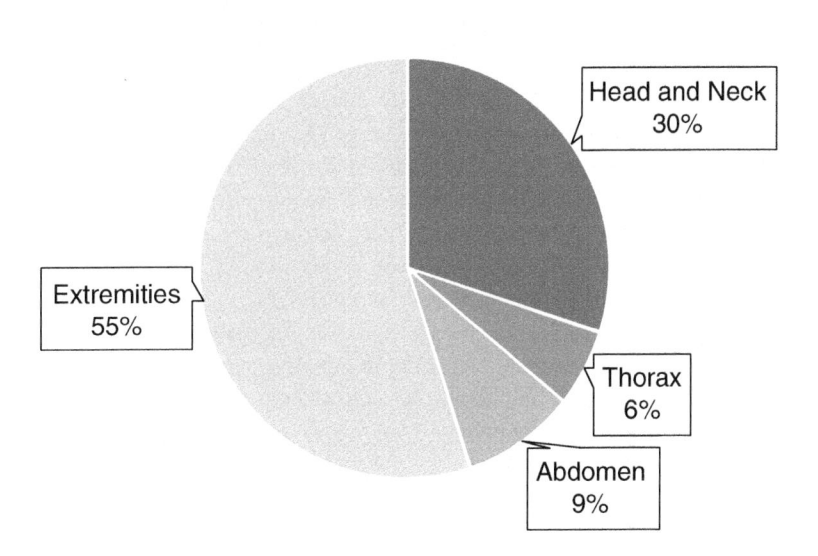

- Head and Neck 30%
- Thorax 6%
- Abdomen 9%
- Extremities 55%

Damage Control Resuscitation

As a result of lessons learned from military experiences of the last two decades, damage control resuscitation has emerged as a complimentary strategy to damage control surgery in order to address the "lethal triad" of hypothermia, acidosis, and coagulopathy [16]. This approach incorporates the early hemorrhage control, permissive hypotension, hemostatic resuscitation, and prevention of hypothermia. Hemostatic resuscitation using minimal crystalloid infusion and fixed low ratio blood products (targeting one packed red blood cell unit: one plasma, one platelet) has rapidly become the massive transfusion standard in both military and civilian settings [24, 25]. Additionally, at locations with limited availability of blood products, particularly plasma and platelets, the use of a walking blood bank to rapidly transfuse resuscitative fresh whole blood has demonstrated efficacy [26].

While fixed ratio resuscitation remains the mainstay of damage control resuscitation, there is an expanding body of experience and evidence which supports the use of thromboelastography (TEG) to assess clotting function, clot strength, and platelet contribution and to identify any evidence of significant hyperfibrinolysis. Advocates of TEG argue its use to rapidly identify or prevent acute coagulopathy of traumatic shock (ACOTS), a characteristic coagulopathy seen among severely injured patients and associated with significant mortality and morbidity. Additionally, the early administration (within 3 h of injury) of the antifibrinolytic agent tranexamic acid (TXA) is associated with improved morbidity and mortality in the setting of severe injury and major hemorrhage in both civilian and military setting [27–30]. Consequently, TXA has been added to both the joint theater trauma system and tactical combat casualty care recommendations for the treatment of life-threatening bleeding in massive transfusion situations and should be considered in all patients with large-volume bleeding or at risk of major bleeding.

One of the most important lessons learned from the battlefield experience with these severely injured patients is that they invariably have a significant amount of blood loss in the field and during transport, even if they arrive with no obvious active bleeding due to the placement of tourniquets and other hemostatic adjuncts. In addition, as these often occur in young, healthy, and physically fit soldiers, they can present with relatively reassuring vital signs despite having lost enough blood to qualify for class 3 or 4 shock (>30% total blood volume). Thus, a common mistake was to underestimate the degree of shock and to fail to begin immediate targeted resuscitation, particularly before surgical interventions were undertaken. A good general rule of thumb in these patients to estimate initial resuscitation is 4 units of blood products (four PRBC and four FFP) for each amputated or significantly mangled extremity, begun immediately after the patient arrives in the receiving area. Further resuscitation can then be tailored based on the initial response, ongoing blood loss, and surgical interventions that are required.

Approach to the DCBI Patient

The dismounted blast injury pattern includes multisystem trauma that requires an expeditious comprehensive perioperative assessment. The initial sequence of evaluation and resuscitation varies depending upon the hemodynamic status of the injured and the facility's location, capabilities, and resources available to the trauma team. However, the approach to these massively injured patients should follow traditional damage control fundamentals (Fig. 6.4). Hemodynamically unstable patients should be brought directly to the operating room for simultaneous resuscitation, exploration, and control of exsanguinating hemorrhage. Patients that remain more stable or respond to initial resuscitation may undergo initial imaging that assists in operative planning.

Due to peripheral venous access site limitations from the extent of injury and to allow for easy use of a rapid transfusion device, large-bore central venous access above the diaphragm should be rapidly obtained. The subclavian site is usually most practical since the cervical spine should be protected in these patients; however, initial standard peripheral intravenous access may be adequate to begin resuscitation until movement to the operating room (OR). If peripheral or central venous access is difficult to obtain, intraosseous (IO) access is obtained. Since the use of the com-

Fig. 6.4 Algorithm for evaluation and management of DCBI. General approach (**a**) and management with tourniquets from the field (**b**) (Adapted from Galante and Rodriguez [61])

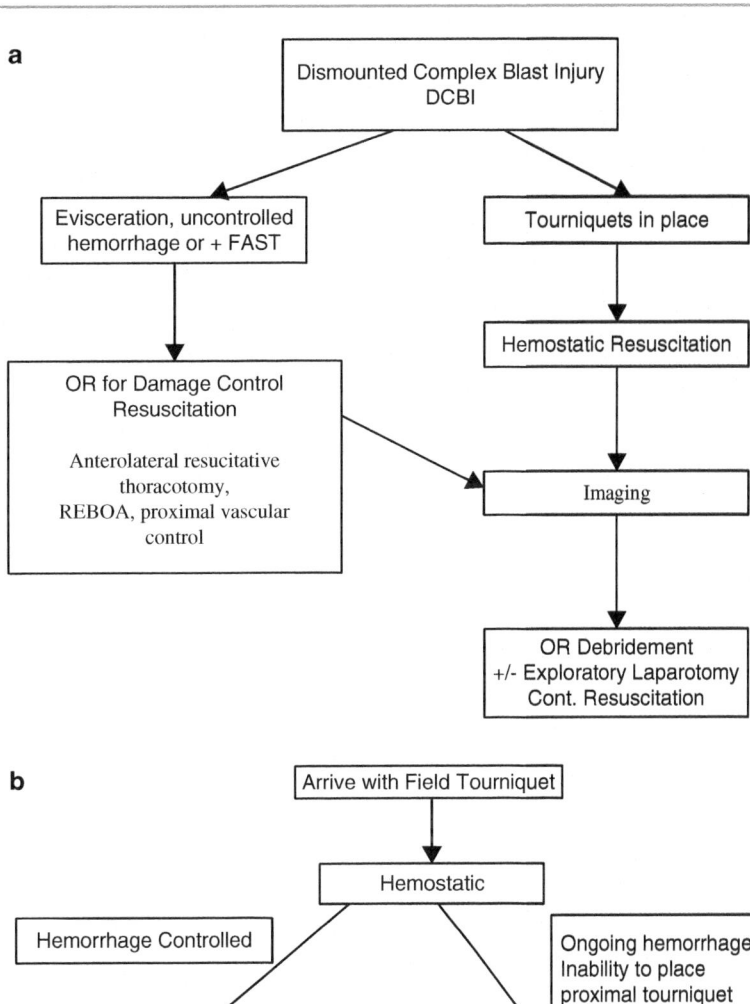

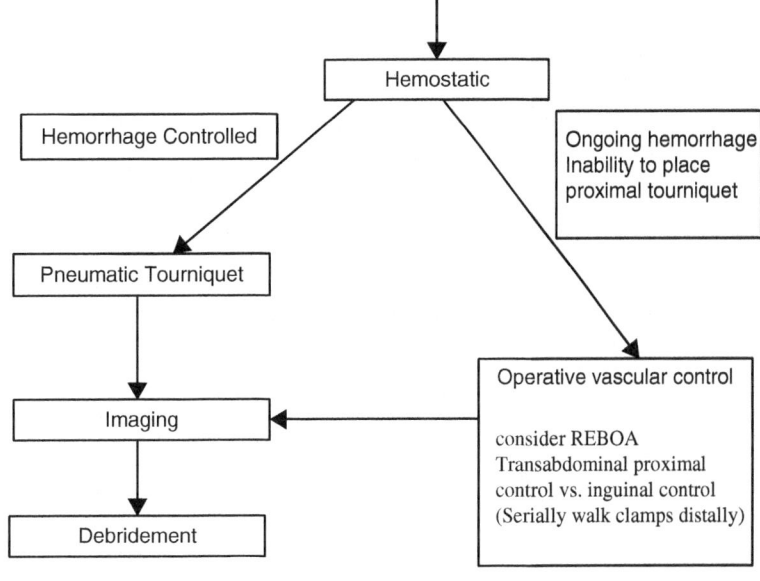

monly utilized tibial or humeral locations may be limited by injury, a sternal IO line is a reliable and effective initial conduit for administration of drugs, fluids, and blood products.

Initial damage control resuscitation starts immediately following massive transfusion protocol guidelines of a 1:1:1 ratio of packed red cell to plasma to platelets, low titer Group O whole blood or type-specific fresh whole blood via the walking blood bank. The authors prefer a starting estimation of four units of PRBCs (and appropriate matching plasma and platelets) for each amputated or mangled extremity as described above.

If adequate extremity hemorrhage control was not obtained in the field or is inadequate, this must be the first priority. Wounds initially controlled by hastily placed field tourniquets may begin to rebleed as resuscitation corrects the patient's hemodynamic lability. In most cases, field tourniquets should be exchanged for pneumatic devices upon arrival to the OR.

Airway management in the DCBI patient may be difficult because of head and neck injury, or hemodynamic instability and drug-assisted intubation must be embarked upon very cautiously. Secondary to near exsanguination, the multiple amputee has little physiologic reserve. Medication dosages must be decreased, and the team needs to be prepared for potential hemodynamic collapse and cardiopulmonary arrest. If able to adequately ventilate and oxygenate the patient temporarily, the team should consider delaying intubation until after a brief period of volume expansion with blood products.

Immediate determination of any life-threatening truncal injuries becomes the next priority. The use of ultrasound and plain radiography is useful adjuncts to evaluation, triage, and operative planning in the labile patient. Chest and pelvic films with the inclusion of abdominal and extremity films if needed may rapidly identify life-threatening injuries, fractures, or foreign bodies. Torso imaging takes priority, while extremity films can be completed as needed in the OR after hemorrhage control.

In patients who are clearly hemodynamically stable or those who have had initial hemorrhage control and operative intervention, further assessment with contrast-enhanced CT imaging that includes the head, neck, chest, abdomen, pelvis, and spine should be performed. These procedures will assist in identification of occult or missed injuries as well as guide further operative planning. Due to the mechanism of injury, patients will frequently present with multiple small fragment wounds. When the patient's wounds are too numerous to count, assessment for torso penetration and occult extremity vascular injury becomes difficult as trajectory is impossible to determine. CT or conventional on-table angiography in the operating room is a key maneuver for detection of occult vascular injury.

Unstable patients should proceed directly to the operating room for damage control surgery. Vascular access and airway management can be performed in the OR simultaneously with initiating surgical exploration. Immediate control of life-threatening hemorrhage and enteric spillage, as well as debridement of obvious contamination and devitalized tissues, should guide the initial operation.

Thoracotomy may be required for patients in extremis or those with large-volume hemothoraces. Diagnostic pericardial window should be considered in any patient with wounds concerning for possible cardiac injury, even if pericardial ultrasound is equivocal.

Decision for abdominal exploration is based upon imaging findings, obvious signs of penetrating injury, peritoneal signs, or physiologic instability without another identified source. Since advanced imaging such as CT is unavailable at many forward facilities, decisions regarding exploration are largely based on clinical exam, plain X-rays, and ultrasound. A FAST exam that is positive for free abdominal fluid should prompt abdominal exploration in this setting, regardless of the current hemodynamics.

Complex blast injuries frequently result in abdominopelvic, perineal, and genital trauma (Fig. 6.5). Rigid proctoscopy is performed to assess anorectal injury as well as cautious placement of transurethral or suprapubic bladder decompression, with retrograde urethrogram and cystogram as indicated. Pelvic fractures are often present and any instability may require temporary external fixation. Major pelvic hemorrhage can result from these fractures. Pelvic binding, external fixation, and/ or preperitoneal pelvic packing may help to reduce the pelvic volume and control hemorrhage. Injury to the external and internal genitalia is frequently encountered and a high index of suspicion maintained. Any evidence of scrotal hematoma or penetrating scrotal injury should mandate exploration. Vaginal examination should be performed in the setting of bleeding or injury in the vulva or perineum.

Once abdominal and thoracic injuries are controlled, heavily contaminated traumatic amputations and other soft tissue injuries are copiously irrigated and debrided. Definitive procedures are

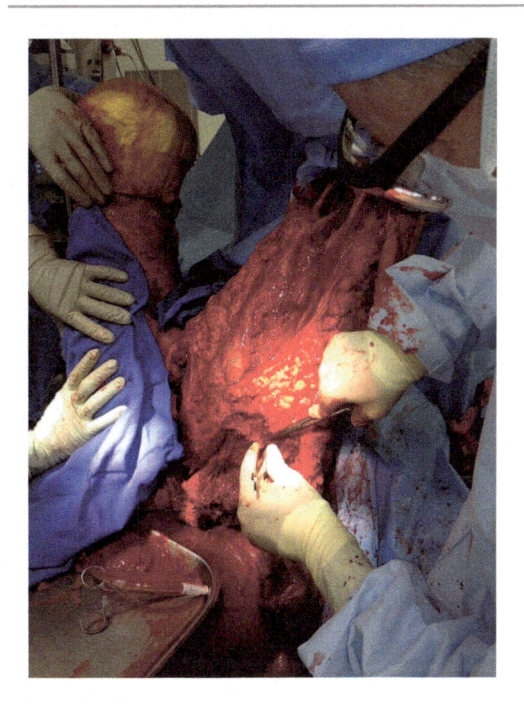

Fig. 6.5 Massive posterior degloving with injury to the anal sphincter, rectum, and scrotum. This patient was treated with a diverting colostomy. There is a contralateral transfemoral amputation

highly discouraged at the initial operation, and most wounds are rarely closed.

The resuscitative surgical phase of damage control requires efficiency and teamwork. If multiple operative teams and surgeons are available, they should work simultaneously rather than in sequence [31] (Fig. 6.6).

The environmental wound contamination of DCBI wounds is extensive and may include dirt, debris, plant matter, or even biologic material from other victims in the surrounding area (Fig. 6.7). Empiric post-injury antimicrobial coverage should be administered for the first 24–72 h with appropriate redosing for massive transfusion or prolonged operative procedures. Typically, the use of a first-generation cephalosporin such as cefazolin (or clindamycin, if allergic to penicillin) is adequate, but coverage is broadened to include metronidazole or more extensive gram-negative coverage in the presence of intra-abdominal contamination, open pelvic fracture, or perineal wounds.

These injured patients undergo serial operative examinations with careful evaluation of evolving tissue necrosis and viability prior to definitive wound management. Recurrent tissue necrosis may occur due to inadequate debridement or resuscitation, but it may also represent the development of invasive fungal infection (IFI), a highly lethal complication, and should prompt aggressive surgical and antimicrobial therapy.

Patients at increased risk for IFI include dismounted blast injury, traumatic above-knee amputation, and supermassive blood transfusion of >20 units of red blood cells given in the first 24 h following injury. Wounds are usually treated empirically with topical antifungal/antimicrobial treatment with dilute Dakin's dressings (0.025% sodium hypochlorite solution (50 mL full strength [0.5%] Dakin's in 950 mL sterile water)). If any recurrent necrosis concerning for IFI occurs, tissue cultures are obtained to assess for *Mucor* and *Aspergillus*. Systemic antifungal therapy is initiated with both liposomal amphotericin B and voriconazole. Additionally, antimicrobial therapy with broad spectrum gram-positive and gram-negative coverage is administered due to the high incidence of bacterial coinfection.

Control of Hemorrhage

Immediate control of catastrophic hemorrhage is the principal priority in the initial management of the DCBI patient. For those with compressible extremity hemorrhage, tourniquets should be applied immediately in the field since mortality increases once shock has begun [32–34]. Several junctional tourniquets are now fielded in theater, and there are now case reports of successful use [35].

While the use of a junctional tourniquet or wound packing may help temporize the profound hemorrhage, proximal control usually must be obtained via laparotomy with rapid transabdominal control of the infrarenal aorta. This is followed by the control of each common iliac artery and ultimately isolation of the bilateral internal

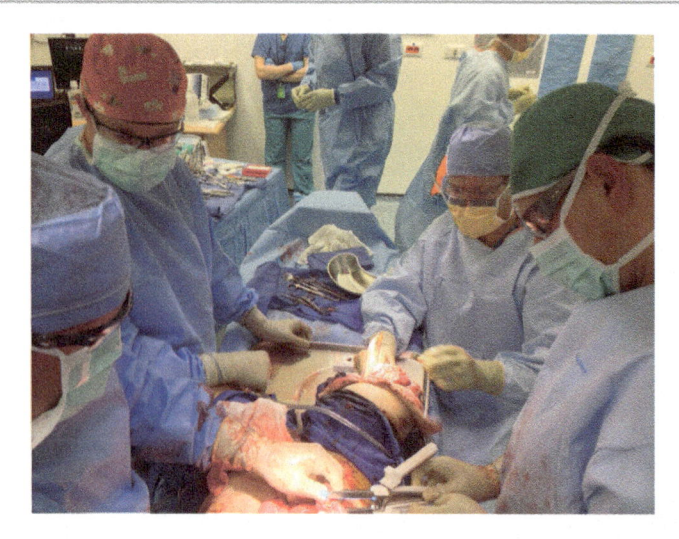

Fig. 6.6 Multiple surgeons and teams are shown operating in this triple amputee DCBI patient. Two general surgeons perform an exploratory laparotomy for proximal iliac control and abdominal damage control, while two orthopedic surgeons address debridement and hemostasis of the bilateral transfemoral amputations. A fifth surgeon (not seen) is debriding an upper extremity amputation under pneumatic tourniquet control

Fig. 6.7 DCBI wound with profound contamination with dirt, plant matter, and other debris

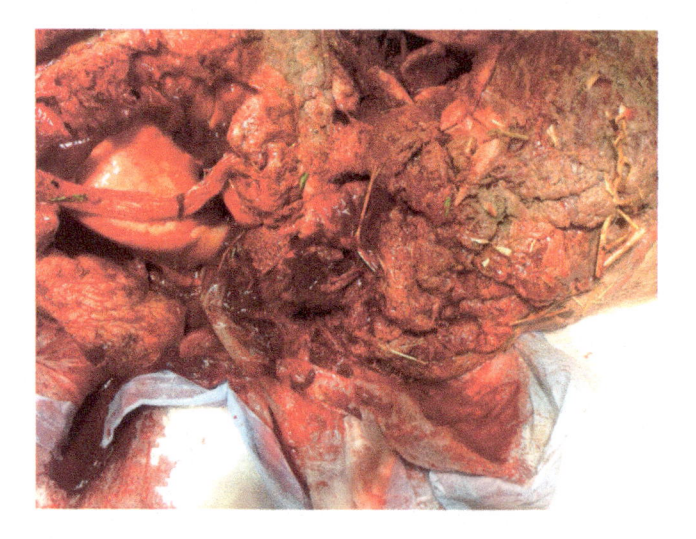

and external iliac vessels. The authors prefer the use of Rummel tourniquets or "Potts" (double-looped) vessel loops for this purpose since they can easily remain in place during an operative pause for imaging or resuscitation. The ligation of the internal iliac artery remains an option in exsanguinating pelvic hemorrhage, but should generally be avoided due to the potential for significant posterior muscle ischemia and necrosis. Alternatively, a generous groin incision with division of the inguinal ligament allows proximal control of the external iliac vessels.

Patients with non-compressible torso hemorrhage (NCTH) must have operative hemorrhage control as soon as possible. These patients should be brought immediately to the operating room for operative hemorrhage control and simultaneous blood product resuscitation. For those that arrive in extremis and hypotensive, resuscitative endovascular balloon occlusion of the aorta (REBOA) has the potential to provide temporizing proximal hemorrhage control either in the distal or proximal aorta for severe pelvic or junctional injuries or more proximally for injuries within the abdomen. As surgeons increasingly gain this skill, REBOA in the infrarenal Zone 3 may also be useful in the setting of profound pelvic hemorrhage in lieu of transabdominal hemorrhage control. Likewise, left anterolateral resuscitative thoracotomy or Zone 1 REBOA (above the diaphragm) should be performed in moribund patients, while volume resuscitation is begun [36].

Major vessel injuries should be appropriately ligated or repaired as indicated. Placement of a temporary intravascular shunt is an excellent alternative in the damage control setting that can be done rapidly, restores flow, and defers formal repair until the patient is stabilized and adequately resuscitated [37, 38]. Fasciotomies should be strongly considered in any patients with prolonged warm ischemia time or combined arterial and venous injury.

Thoracic Damage Control

Damage control within the chest follows similar principles to those utilized in the abdomen. However, in addition to hemorrhage, other life-threatening conditions must be considered. Exposure should be obtained through incisions that offer expansile exposure and access to other body cavities, such as anterior thoracotomy or sternotomy, as opposed to posterolateral thoracotomy. Niceties such as single-lung ventilation are rarely feasible in this emergent setting, although this may be feasible with main stem intubation at times. More often, simple compression and packing during exhalation are used. When significant bleeding is noted, it may be difficult at times to determine the source. Rapid temporary closure of any diaphragmatic defects will help determine which cavity is bleeding in thoracoabdominal wounds.

Thoracic penetrating injuries from penetrating wounds in the military setting require operative intervention far more often than those in the civilian setting. While most civilian wounds are often treatable with simple tube thoracostomy, many combat wounds require operative intervention. A reasonable approach is to immediately proceed to the operating room prepared to perform an anterolateral thoracotomy. A small thoracostomy incision can be made and then the chest suctioned and lavaged copiously prior to the placement of a large-bore chest tube through the incision. If substantial output persists or drains immediately, the surgeon can then proceed with thoracotomy or sternotomy [39].

Frequently, the lung is severely damaged and stapled wedge resection is the best option [40]. Air embolus should be avoided through rapid control of the injury or temporary hilar clamping. For extensive injuries, temporary hilar control can be accomplished with digital compression, hilar clamping, or the hilar twist maneuver [41]. Repair of hilar vessels in the setting of a rapidly deteriorating patient is seldom successful, and an expeditious stapled pneumonectomy may be the best option; however, the operative team must be prepared to immediately manage the associated profound cardiopulmonary dysfunction that makes this a highly lethal maneuver with a mortality of over 50% [42]. The hilum of the lung should be clamped slowly to allow the contralateral lung time to accommodate. Judicious volume resuscitation is required to mitigate the inevitable acute right heart failure [43].

Penetrating cardiac wounds may present with traumatic arrest, pericardial tamponade, or bleeding into the pleural or abdominal spaces through a hole in the pericardium. If in extremis, immediate resuscitative left anterolateral thoracotomy should be performed. Sternotomy may also be performed for more stable patients with evidence of tamponade. Temporary occlusion of bleeding may be obtained with digital pressure. Atrial wounds may be occluded with a tangential placement of a vascular clamp such as a Satinsky followed by closure with a running 3–0 suture. If unable to control bleeding digitally, defects may be temporarily occluded with a balloon catheter such as a Foley or Fogarty catheter, suture, or skin stapler [44–47]. Definitive suture repair of ventricular wounds should be performed with vertical mattress repair. This should be buttressed with Teflon or pericardial pledgets.

If greater access to the right heart or hemithorax is required, then extension of the anterolateral thoracotomy incision should be performed across the sternum and across the right chest in a "clamshell" fashion. The sternum may be divided using Gigli saw, Lebsche knife, trauma shears, or electric saw. This allows access to both pleural spaces as well as the anterior mediastinum and great vessels in the upper chest.

Temporary thoracic closure may be accomplished in a similar fashion to the abdomen, but approximation of normal anatomic position facilitates respiratory dynamics. If required, negative pressure or occlusive dressings may be applied to the chest or mediastinum, or simple en bloc closure of the skin, fascia, and muscle may be used. Care must be taken to provide appropriate drainage to the mediastinum and pleural cavities and to avoid mediastinal or cardiac compression with packs that may lead to tamponade physiology. Any sign of cardiac or pulmonary compromise during an attempted primary closure of the chest incision should prompt conversion to a damage control temporary closure method.

Abdominal Damage Control

Traditionally, damage control laparotomy is performed for those patients who present with marked physiologic derangement; however, this approach may also be required in the resource constrained environment of the battlefield or austere setting. The entire torso from chin to mid-thighs should be prepped, and a midline incision is carried from the xiphoid to the pubis. Once the peritoneal cavity is entered, the proximal aorta can be manually controlled at the diaphragmatic hiatus, while intraperitoneal blood and clots are evacuated. The abdomen can then be packed appropriately.

Attention should first be turned to evaluation for retroperitoneal hematoma with proximal and distal control of injured vessels. Access to retroperitoneal structures will require medial visceral rotation. A left medial visceral rotation will expose the entire aorta and common iliac vessels, while a rightward rotation allows access to the inferior vena cava and aorta up to the level of superior mesenteric artery. When combined with a Kocher maneuver, the entire subhepatic inferior vena cava is visualized.

Abdominal solid organ injury with DCBI may occur due to either blunt trauma from blast effect or penetration from blast fragments. Unlike the civilian setting where nonoperative management of blunt injuries has become the standard of care and nonoperative treatment of penetrating injuries has been described, the military situation favors operative exploration. In addition to increased wound severity, nonoperative management in most settings is difficult due to inconsistent imaging and interventional angiography resources and difficulties associated with the need for close observation by a surgeon throughout the chain of evacuation. Most splenic injuries will require splenectomy, while liver injuries may be controlled with packing and resectional debridement as required. As with civilian trauma, retrohepatic hematomas should not be explored unless hemostasis cannot be achieved with packing.

Combat bowel injuries are frequently destructive in nature and rarely are simple repair advisable. High-velocity projectiles produce extremely damaging wounds, but the small projectiles from a high-energy explosion will produce multiple small injuries, and care must be taken to avoid missed injuries. Despite the small nature of some of the wounds, many will have associated thermal injury that demarcates over time. Therefore, primary repair is generally not advisable and stapled resection in usually a better approach. Large mesenteric injuries may occur due to either blast-effect or penetrating injury from fragments, and this should be treated with resection of the involved segment. During the index damage control laparotomy, bowel is typically left in discontinuity.

Plans for reanastomosis and/or ostomy may be delayed until at least the second operation once the patient is more stable. If the abdomen is not able to be closed at the next operation, all tubes, drains, and ostomies should be placed as lateral as possible rather than through the rectus sheath. This lateral placement facilitates complex abdominal wall reconstruction with myofascial component separation if an open abdomen persists and results in loss of abdominal domain.

Due to the destructive nature of the wounds and frequent concomitant shock, a much lower threshold for diverting colostomy exists. The combat surgeon must not be dissuaded by the successful management of civilian colorectal trauma without diversion but instead should remember that historical data from World War I, World War II, Vietnam, and the Balkans show markedly improved mortality from over 50% to approximately 14% with the use of fecal diversion, distal rectal washout, and presacral drainage [48–50]. However, with the advent of damage control laparotomy, a selective approach to fecal diversion may be considered for less severe or isolated colon injuries. Colonic reanastomosis may be considered upon reoperation [51], although recent combat casualty experience suggests an anastomotic leak rate of 16–30% [52, 53]. Injuries to the anus, rectum, or sigmoid colon wounds should virtually always be diverted, along with severe perineal or open pelvic fracture wounds. This may be performed as a loop "end-loop" colostomy, although the distal sigmoid colon can also simply be divided and left in discontinuity during the initial procedure. Irrigation of the distal rectum and presacral drainage should be strongly considered in cases of significant contamination. In the case of severe, perianal injury, tacking of the sphincter complex and anoderm to assist in later identification and prevent proximal retraction is often useful.

Unfortunately, large abdominal wall defects occur not infrequently from IED blast. These often present with evisceration of abdominal contents and laparotomy to identify any other injuries must be performed. Definitive management of these defects can be quite challenging, but initial temporary closure with negative pressure dressings is almost always feasible.

Orthopedic and Soft Tissue Injuries

Damage control orthopedic management of DCBI casualties must focus on fracture stabilization and limb preservation and includes extensive use of external fixation techniques and aggressive debridement. Complex unstable pelvic fractures are common, and frequency correlates to the severity of amputation – resulting in a 39% incidence of pelvic fracture with bilateral transfemoral amputations (Fig. 6.8). Any blast-injured patient with an amputation should be suspected to have a pelvic fracture, and a pelvic binder should be placed in the prehospital setting or immediately upon arrival. If hemodynamically unstable, patients should be brought immediately to the operating room for preperitoneal packing with the binder in place. Additionally, the pelvis should be reapproximated with an external fixator during the first operation if possible to assist in hemorrhage control. This can be accomplished without fluoroscopy using iliac pins, and the pelvic binder can be left in place until bony stabilization is achieved. In cases of severe posterior pelvic disruption, a binder can assist with fracture stabilization until sacroiliac screws are placed during another operative session.

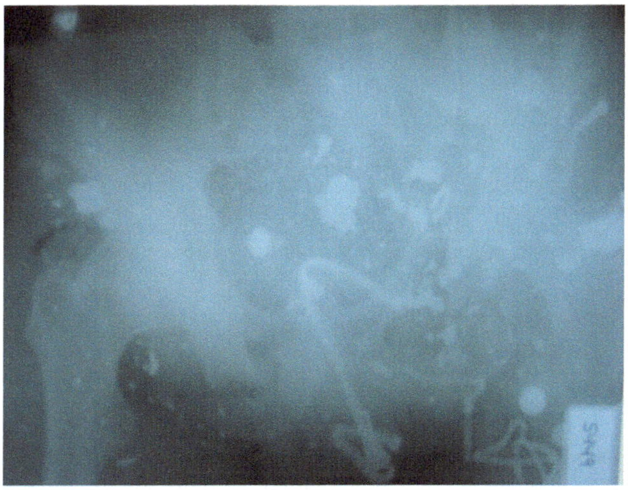

Fig. 6.8 Pelvic radiograph demonstrating severe open book pelvic fractures and multiple metallic fragments in a DCBI patient

The mortality of combined pelvic fracture and perineal wounding in this population exceeds 70%. Initial deaths occur due to hemorrhage, while later deaths are usually a result of septic complications. Hemorrhage from wounds on the buttock, perineum, or groin may be considerable due to the lack of tamponade in the pelvic preperitoneal space, and open wounds should be packed with hemostatic gauze [54, 55]. Patients in extremis should have initial proximal control vascular achieved transabdominally. If these measures fail or cross-sectional imaging shows evidence of extravasation, then angiographic embolization should be performed if available. Preperitoneal packing should be considered. Careful assessment of the rectum and genitourinary tract should be performed to assess for open pelvic fracture with a low threshold for fecal diversion.

DCBI patients often present with profound mangled extremities and traumatic amputations. Debridement of devitalized tissue is critical, and all fascial planes must be explored to irrigate blast contaminants. Foreign bodies, dirt, and debris often travel along fascial planes well away from the initial entry sites, so wounds frequently require extension for adequate exploration, irrigation, and debridement. Frequent serial debridement and low-pressure, high-volume irrigation remain the mainstay of the management of these soft tissue injuries. And closure is seldom indicated until after multiple operations. Completion amputations use a length preserving technique with salvage of all viable tissue regardless of the eccentricity of the soft tissue flap. Guillotine amputations should be avoided as well as amputation through proximal fractures. In order to maximize limb length and optimize function, fracture fixation within the residual limb should be considered if soft tissue and neurovascular structures remain intact. Wounds are dressed with moist dilute Dakin's soaked gauze and can be managed with negative pressure wound therapy once clean.

Genitourinary Injuries

The incidence of bladder, urethral, or combined genitourinary trauma approaches 25% in all patients with pelvic fractures [56, 57]; however, it soars to 72% for those with combined perineal injury and pelvic fracture [58, 59].

Fortunately, intra-abdominal ureteral injuries are uncommon. Generally, if simple repair with an absorbable suture over a double-J stent is feasible, this should be performed immediately unless the patient's burden of intra-abdominal disease or hemodynamic status mandate a damage control. Multiple damage control options exist in these situations or if the ureteral defect is not able to be easily reapproximated. The ureter can be exteriorized with a stent or small-bore feeding tube. Alternatively, ureteral ligation and nephrostomy remain a viable alternative particularly for more proximal injuries. Lastly, if severe concomitant renal injury exists, nephrectomy may be the best option in the presence of a palpable uninjured contralateral kidney.

Bladder injuries are managed in a similar fashion to civilian trauma. Gross hematuria results in high suspicion for bladder rupture, and a cystogram must be performed unless operative exploration defines an injury. Generally, intraperitoneal injuries undergo operative repair, while extraperitoneal injuries can often be managed expectantly with catheter drainage. The caveat is that with the profound perineal and pelvic injuries which occur in DCBI, many extraperitoneal bladder injuries will also require operative repair.

Urethral injuries are common and may be caused by either pelvic fracture or direct penetrating injuries. Blood at the urethral meatus, ballotable prostate, perineal penetrating wounds, and severe perineal bruising all suggest potential urethral injury. Retrograde urethrogram may be performed to evaluate urethral integrity; however, a gentle attempt at Foley catheter placement is reasonable and should be performed in the operating room by an experienced provider. If no resistance is noted and the catheter passes into the bladder, then it should be left in place. If any difficulty is encountered, a suprapubic catheter should be performed.

Management of injuries to the male external genitalia including the penis, scrotum, and testicles focuses on hemorrhage control, judicious debridement, and reapproximation of critical structures (Fig. 6.9). Penetrating penile injuries should have repair of the corpora caver-

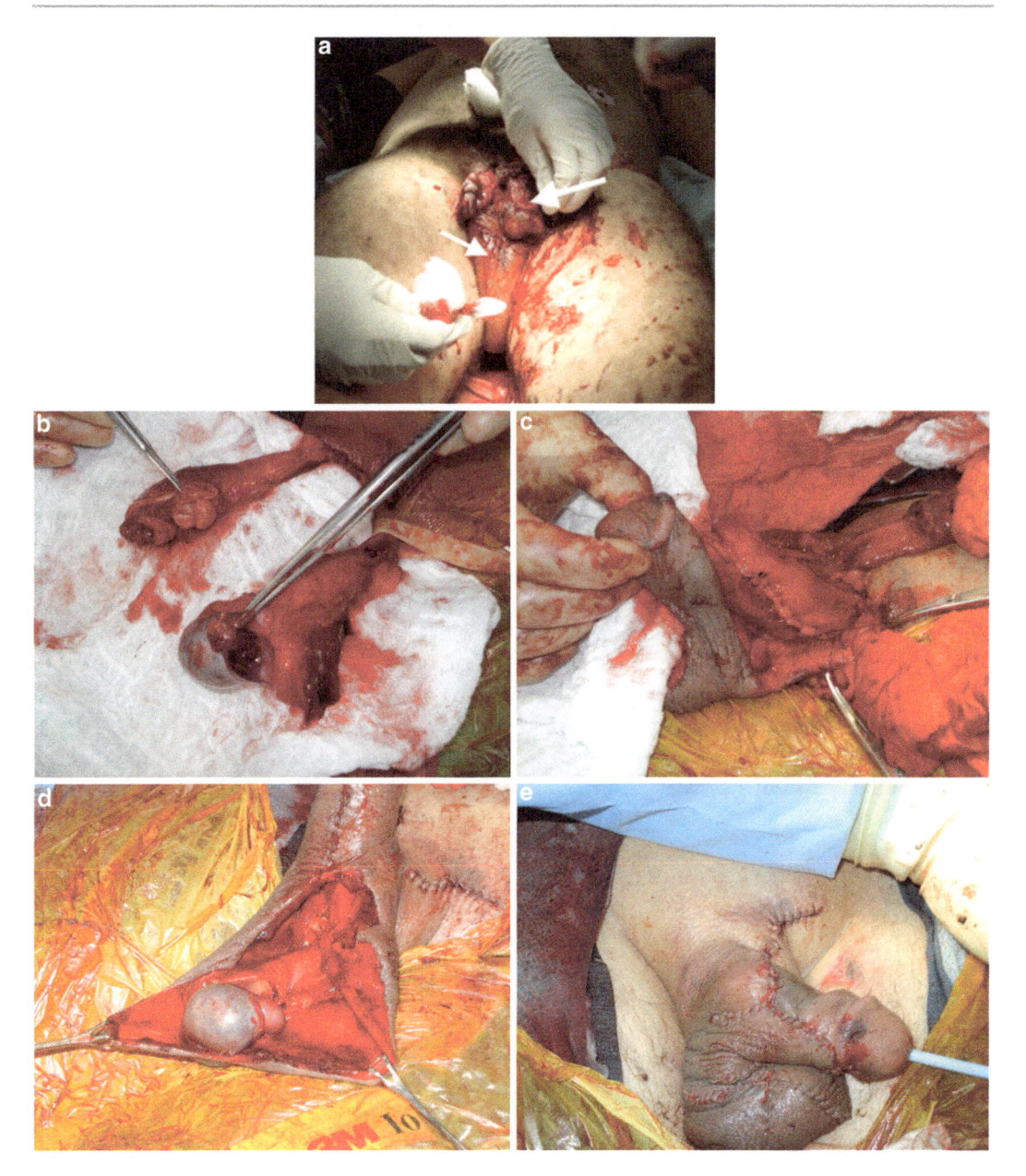

Fig. 6.9 External genital trauma from a blast injury. (**a**) There is significant injury to the penile shaft with exposure of the corpus cavernosum (large white arrow) and a large scrotal hematoma (small white arrow) that requires surgical exploration. (**b**) Complete exposure of both testicles shows the destroyed right testicle requiring orchiectomy, but the left testicle largely intact and salvaged. (**c**) The corpus cavernosum is reconstructed by reapproximation of the tunica albuginea with running absorbable suture. (**d**) Appearance after orchiectomy and penile repair and (**e**) after final closure

nosum and the partial urethral injuries with absorbable suture if feasible. Repair of the deep penile Bucks fascia over the erectile bodies is critical to future function, but care should be taken to avoid overly aggressive repair of the corpora spongiosum that may result in ischemic injury. Repair of complex penile urethral disruption should be delayed and the urinary stream diverted via cystostomy tube. The penile skin and superficial fascia can be left open in contaminated wounds and treated with moist- or vacuum-assisted dressings.

Patients presenting with penetrating scrotal wounds or notable ecchymosis should undergo bilateral scrotal exploration. Ruptured testes may be gently irrigated and nonviable seminiferous tubules debrided. The tunica albuginea should then be closed if possible. Orchiectomy should only be performed if the organ is completely devitalized. The scrotum should be reapproximated over Penrose drains if possible. If there is inadequate scrotal skin, the preferred approach is to dress the testes with a nonadherent layer and a negative pressure dressing. While the use of subcutaneous thigh pouches has been reported, the increased traction on the vas deferens and epididymal compression may cause tubular contraction and loss of harvestable potentially viable sperm [58]; therefore, the authors prefer to avoid this technique. Ultimately, skin grafting of the testes to create a neoscrotum has been a highly successful technique that is performed at a later operation.

Preparation for Transfer

One of the hallmarks of the care for the blast-injured patient in the military setting is that the patient undergoes initial stabilization and damage control surgery at the nearest capable facility, but then is rapidly evacuated to the next echelon of care or receiving facility. For the complex blast patient who almost always requires some type of urgent surgical intervention, this means that the patient may be placed into the evacuation chain immediately following surgery. Therefore, it is critical to ensure that the patient is adequately prepared for transport and that major potential problems that could arise have been anticipated and mitigated as much as possible. This should include a head to toe reevaluation to assess all known injuries, identify any potential significant missed injuries, and ensure the patient is stable enough to tolerate a prolonged transfer. The patient should not be requiring an ongoing major resuscitation or have signs of active hemorrhage, their ventilator requirements should be within the range of what a standard basic transport ventilator can provide, and adequate sedation and pain control for the transfer should be ensured. For ventilated patients, particularly those with multiple injuries and who have just undergone surgery, strong consideration should be given to administering neuromuscular blockade for the duration of the transfer flight. Finally, it is critical to ensure that there is good communication with the receiving facility and surgeon(s), preferably well in advance of patient arrival. This can be somewhat difficult in the combat setting, particularly in the early phases where there is little established reliable communication infrastructure and no universal electronic medical record. In these cases, often the low-tech and simple solutions are the best. Handwritten or printed medical notes can be packaged and sent directly with the patient, and they should outline the known diagnoses, the interventions or procedures that were performed, and the resuscitation that the patient has received. An excellent backup system is to make notations directly on the patient, typically by writing key pieces of info directly onto dressings. Figure 6.10 shows a very good example of making notations directly on the patient's abdominal dressing that conveys all of the critical information that the physicians, and particularly the surgeons, at the receiving facility need to know before they begin the next phase of care for the patient.

The "Direct to OR" Option for Blast-Injured Patients

Intuitively, severely injured patients with significant ongoing bleeding should benefit from minimizing the time to lifesaving surgical intervention. This is particularly true for non-compressible truncal hemorrhage, where there are no existing prehospital interventions that can reliably control the bleeding other than getting the patient to a surgeon as quickly as possible. However, direct evidence to support this is sparse. Recent studies suggest that delays in surgical intervention for exsanguinating torso trauma as short as 10 min increase mortality [62, 63]. The logistics required to perform an initial evaluation and then transport an unstable patient from the emergency department to the operating room can contribute to significant delays in definitive surgical control of

Fig. 6.10 Patient who underwent damage control laparotomy at a far-forward military medical treatment facility. Key information for the next echelon of care is conveyed by simple writing on dressings or bandages

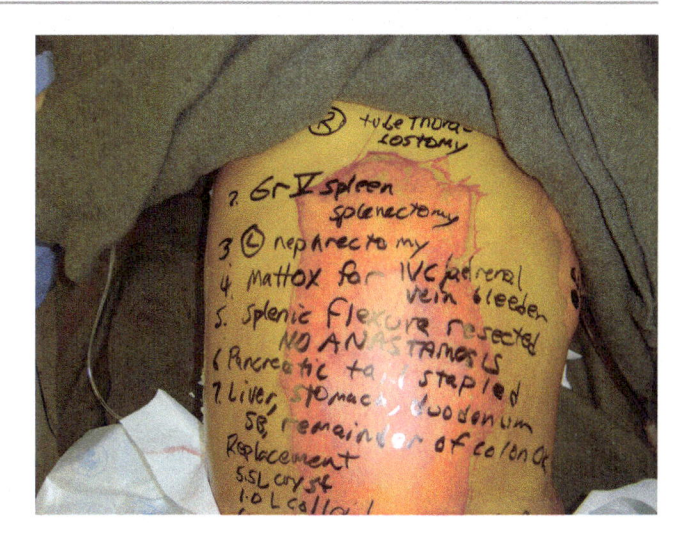

hemorrhage. Despite this, transportation of severely injured patients from the scene directly to the operating room (DOR) has been described in only a few trauma centers in the civilian environment and has not been formally characterized in the deployed setting [64, 65]. We believe that this method of triage for highly select patients who have suffered a major blast injury has clear potential benefits in terms of reducing mortality, morbidity, and other consequences of delayed hemorrhage control.

The authors (MM and RB) have extensive experience with one of the few existing "direct to OR" trauma programs in the United States and describe the foundation and fundamentals of such a program in this section. Most importantly, a DOR program can be established in any setting that has surgical assets, including the far-forward battlefield. Legacy Emanuel Medical Center is an urban Level 1 trauma center that has developed a formal policy for proceeding directly from the ambulance bay to the operating room for trauma patients meeting certain mechanistic or physiologic criteria (Table 6.1) [66, 67]. A DOR trauma activation can be requested by prehospital personnel, the ED charge nurse receiving the field report, or at the discretion of the attending trauma surgeon. The DOR mechanism is also occasionally used for non-traumatic conditions such as ruptured abdominal aortic aneurysms that require immediate surgical attention. One of the most important points for success of a DOR program is

Table 6.1 Indications for DOR activation

Penetrating injury to the neck or torso
Rigid, distended abdomen
Crush injury to the torso
Evisceration of abdominal contents
Impaled objects in the neck, torso, or pelvis
Traumatic amputations
Mangled or pulseless extremities
Profound shock (adults, SBP < 80; children, SBP < 60)
Massive blood loss on scene or en route
Cardiopulmonary arrest resulting from trauma
Discretion of EMS, ER charge RN, or trauma surgeon

that the criteria are well established and understood by all involved personnel who are responsible for making triage decisions. In the deployed setting, this decision would ideally be made by the responsible trauma surgeon or in a MASCAL scenario by the senior triage officer. The likelihood of the patient requiring triage as a DOR case can often be accurately assessed from the prehospital report and then confirmed with a very brief (1–2 min) hasty triage on arrival.

The Legacy Emanuel DOR capability was facilitated in part by cooperation between the hospital administration and trauma service in designing the physical layout of the emergency department (Fig. 6.11). Both the resuscitation bays used for normal trauma activations and the dedicated trauma ORs are located in close proximity to the patient entrance into the ER and to the

Fig. 6.11 Physical layout of the emergency department and trauma operating rooms for the Legacy Emanuel Medical Center direct to OR program, with patient movement during standard (black arrows) versus DOR (gray arrows) resuscitation

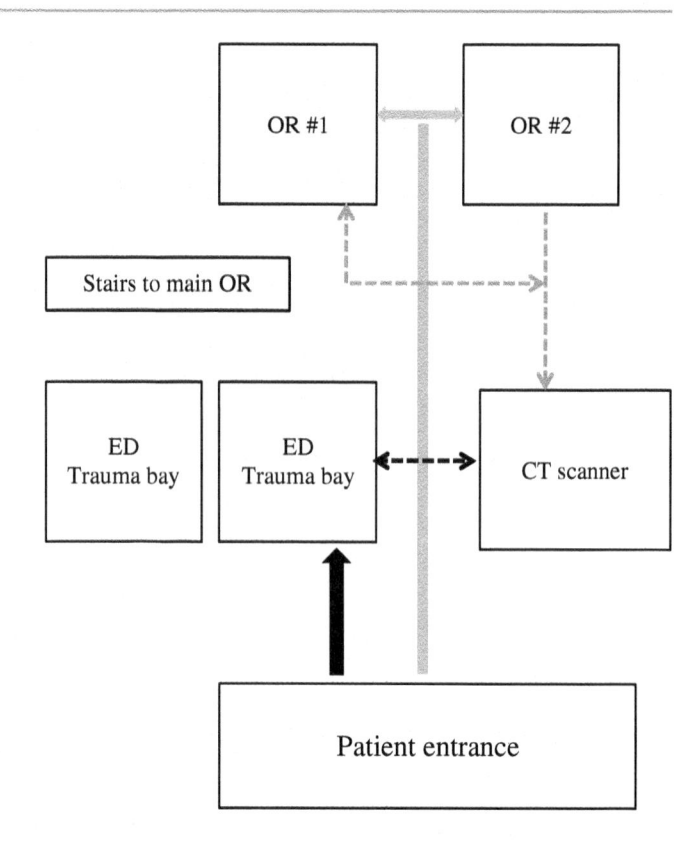

CT scanner. The trauma ORs are equipped with Level 1 transfusers and appropriate surgical instruments that are kept ready to be immediately opened. This includes basic and major laparotomy sets, a thoracotomy/sternotomy set with sternal saw, and minor and major vascular sets. The main OR is one floor below, and neurosurgical and orthopedic instruments are in close proximity.

Patients designated as DOR activations are taken from the ambulance bay or helipad into the OR and placed on the operating table where the initial evaluation takes place. By protocol these are all "highest-level" activations that include the full trauma team, including an attending anesthesiologist (Table 6.2). The ER physician does not respond to a DOR activation. If a CT is indicated during a DOR resuscitation, the patient is transported on the OR bed to the CT scanner. The CT technicians have an alphanumeric trauma pager, and less emergent scans are deferred until the disposition of the DOR patient is known. Both the attending trauma surgeon and an in-house radiology attending immediately review the CT scans.

Table 6.2 Personnel for DOR admissions

Staff trauma surgeon
Staff anesthesiologist
Senior trauma resident
Junior trauma resident (daytime only)
Trauma physician assistant [1, 2]
OR circulating nurse
OR scrub nurse or technician
Trauma resuscitation nurse
Recording nurse
Respiratory therapist
Radiology technician
OR runner

Once the initial CT scans are completed, the attending can then direct the patient back to the OR, to the intensive care unit, or to a regular emergency department trauma bay for the remainder of the evaluation.

If immediate surgical intervention is required shortly after arrival, general anesthesia is immediately induced, and sterile instruments are opened. At our institution, in the 430 cases in which immediate operation was required, the median time to the start of surgical intervention was 13 min and was <30 min in 77% of patients [66]. This compares to a minimum average of 30–45 min for emergent surgical intervention at Level 1 centers from the National Trauma Data Bank. In this analysis, we identified that DOR patients had a significantly lower actual mortality compared with predicted mortality based on their injury severity (5% vs 10%, $p = 0.01$) [66].

In our experience, about 50% of the DOR patients triaged according to the criteria listed in Table 6.1 ultimately do not need emergent surgical intervention or a significant resuscitation. Many of these are patients with a penetrating mechanism that are found to have superficial wounds and no visceral injury. After evaluation, these patients are moved from the OR to an ER room for ongoing care. Operating instruments are not opened, the OR team stands down, and patient charges are identical to a standard Level 1 trauma activation. Many DOR patients do not need immediate operative intervention but do need significant resuscitative efforts. Most of these are patients with multiple severe blunt injuries. These patients are typically kept in the OR for the initial resuscitation. This may include endotracheal intubation, placement of lines and chest tubes, evaluation by multiple specialists, massive transfusion, FAST ultrasound, obtaining X-rays and CT scans, and so forth. We have found this to be an ideal setting for a major resuscitation due to the size of the OR, superior lighting, availability of instruments and personnel, better sterile technique for procedures, and proximity to the CT scanner.

In the deployed military setting, it is also possible, and often much easier, to perform selective "direct to OR" resuscitations. The fact that the teams are typically much smaller and almost exclusively focused on trauma care makes it easier to overcome barriers or resistance to this approach. The physical setup is also typically ideal for DOR, because similar to the Legacy program, the operating room and emergency room (typically called the resuscitation or ATLS area) are in the same structure/tent or in adjoining structures. Using selective DOR resuscitation will also be even higher yield than in the civilian environment, as complex blast injury patients uniformly require some form of operative interventions and very often require emergent lifesaving interventions that are best performed in the operating room environment.

Summary

Surgical priorities for the treatment of dismounted complex blast injury follow traditional damage control principles. Immediate control of exsanguinating hemorrhage from abdominopelvic and perineal wounds takes precedence. This is followed by control of enteric spillage, debridement of devitalized tissue, and stabilization of major fractures. The surgical procedures are typically then terminated, and the patient is brought to an ICU setting for continued resuscitation, stabilization, and normalization of physiology and then either transferred to the next echelon of care or planned return to the OR at the receiving facility for further surgical procedures and definitive repairs/reconstructions. Understanding and applying the fundamental damage control surgery and damage control resuscitation principles is of utmost importance in all severely injured patients and is among the most critical components of caring for the complex blast-injured patient.

Conflicts of Interest The authors have no conflicts of interest to declare and have received no financial or material support related to this manuscript.

Disclaimer The results and opinions expressed in this article are those of the authors and do not reflect the opinions or official policy of the United States Navy, United States Army, the Department of Defense, or any other governmental agency.

References

1. Fleming M, Waterman S, Dunne J, D'Alleyrand JC, Andersen RC. Dismounted complex blast injuries: patterns of injuries and resource utilization associated with the multiple extremity amputee. J Surg Orthop Adv. 2012;21(1):32–7.

2. Mamczak CN, Elster EA. Complex dismounted IED blast injuries: the initial management of bilateral lower extremity amputations with and without pelvic and perineal involvement. J Surg Orthop Adv. 2012;21(1):8–14.
3. Andersen RC, Fleming M, Forsberg JA, Gordon WT, Nanos GP, Charlton MT, et al. Dismounted complex blast injury. J Surg Orthop Adv. 2012;21(1):2–7.
4. Office of the Army Surgeon General. Dismounted complex blast injury: report of the Army dismounted complex blast injury task force. Fort Sam Houston: Office of the Army Surgeon General; 2011. p. 1–87.
5. Cannon JW, Hofmann LJ, Glasgow SC, Potter BK, Rodriguez CJ, Cancio LC, et al. Dismounted complex blast injuries: a comprehensive review of the modern combat experience. J Am Coll Surg. 2016;223(4):652–64. e8.
6. Larrey D. Memoires de chirurgicales militaire et campagnes. Paris 1812.
7. Helling TS, McNabney KW. The role of amputation in the Management of Battlefield Casualties: a history of two millennia. J Trauma Inj Infect Crit Care. 2000;49(5):930–9.
8. Brewer LA. The contributions of the second auxiliary surgical group to military surgery during world war II with special reference to thoracic surgery. Ann Surg. 1983;197(3):318–26.
9. Jones EL. Early management of battle casualties in Vietnam. Arch Surg. 1968;97(1):1.
10. Stone HH, Strom PR, Mullins RJ. Management of the major coagulopathy with onset during laparotomy. Ann Surg. 1983;197(5):532–5.
11. Rotondo MF, Schwab CW, MD MG, Phillips GR, Fruchterman TM, Kauder DR, et al. Damage control. J Trauma Inj Infect Crit Care. 1993;35(3):375–83.
12. Rotondo MF, Zonies DH. The damage control sequence and underlying logic. Surg Clin N Am. 1997;77(4):761–77.
13. Johnson JW, Gracias VH, Schwab CW, Reilly PM, Kauder DR, Shapiro MB, et al. Evolution in damage control for exsanguinating penetrating abdominal injury. J Trauma. 2001;51(2):261–9. discussion 9-71.
14. Waibel BH, Rotondo MF. Damage control surgery. In: Peitzman AB, Schwab CW, Yealy DM, Rhodes M, Fabian TC, editors. The trauma manual: trauma and acute care surgery. 4th ed. Philadelphia: Lippincott, Williams & Wilkins; 2012. p. 74–83.
15. Kashuk JL, Moore EE, Millikan JS, Moore JB. Major abdominal vascular trauma--a unified approach. J Trauma. 1982;22(8):672–9.
16. Moore EE, Thomas G, Orr Memorial Lecture. Staged laparotomy for the hypothermia, acidosis, and coagulopathy syndrome. Am J Surg. 1996;172(5):405–10.
17. Chambers LW, Green DJ, Sample K, Gillingham BL, Rhee P, Brown C, et al. Tactical surgical intervention with temporary shunting of peripheral vascular trauma sustained during operation Iraqi freedom: one unit??S experience. J Trauma Inj Infect Crit Care. 2006;61(4):824–30.
18. Beekley AC, Watts DM. Combat trauma experience with the United States Army 102nd forward surgical team in Afghanistan††this is an original work by the authors. The opinions expressed are the authors' alone. They do not necessarily reflect the opinion of the United States government, the department of defense, the United States Army, or Madigan Army medical center. Am J Surg. 2004;187(5):652–4.
19. Patel TH, Wenner KA, Price SA, Weber MA, Leveridge A, McAtee SJ. A U.S. Army forward surgical Team's experience in operation Iraqi freedom. J Trauma Inj Infect Crit Care. 2004;57(2):201–7.
20. Place RJ, Rush RM, Arrington ED. Forward surgical team (FST) workload in a special operations environment: the 250th FST in operation ENDURING FREEDOM. Curr Surg. 2003;60(4):418–22.
21. Morrison JJ, Rasmussen TE. Noncompressible torso hemorrhage: a review with contemporary definitions and management strategies. Surg Clin North Am. 2012;92(4):843–58. vii.
22. Eastridge BJ, Mabry RL, Seguin P, Cantrell J, Tops T, Uribe P, et al. Death on the battlefield (2001-2011): implications for the future of combat casualty care. J Trauma Acute Care Surg. 2012;73(6 Suppl 5):S431–7.
23. Owens BD, Kragh JF Jr, Wenke JC, Macaitis J, Wade CE, Holcomb JB. Combat wounds in operation Iraqi freedom and operation Enduring freedom. J Trauma. 2008;64(2):295–9.
24. Borgman MA, Spinella PC, Perkins JG, Grathwohl KW, Repine T, Beekley AC, et al. The ratio of blood products transfused affects mortality in patients receiving massive transfusions at a combat support hospital. J Trauma Inj Infect Crit Care. 2007;63(4):805–13.
25. Spinella PC, Perkins JG, Grathwohl KW, Beekley AC, Niles SE, McLaughlin DF, et al. Effect of plasma and red blood cell transfusions on survival in patients with combat related traumatic injuries. J Trauma Inj Infect Crit Care. 2008;64(Supplement):S69–78.
26. Spinella PC, Perkins JG, Grathwohl KW, Repine T, Beekley AC, Sebesta J, et al. Fresh whole blood transfusions in coalition military, foreign national, and enemy combatant patients during operation Iraqi freedom at a U.S. combat support hospital. World J Surg. 2007;32(1):2–6.
27. Collaborators C-T, Shakur H, Roberts I, Bautista R, Caballero J, Coats T, et al. Effects of tranexamic acid on death, vascular occlusive events, and blood transfusion in trauma patients with significant haemorrhage (CRASH-2): a randomised, placebo-controlled trial. Lancet. 2010;376(9734):23–32.
28. Eckert MJ, Wertin TM, Tyner SD, Nelson DW, Izenberg S, Martin MJ. Tranexamic acid administration to pediatric trauma patients in a combat setting: the pediatric trauma and tranexamic acid study (PED-TRAX). J Trauma Acute Care Surg. 2014;77(6):852–8. discussion 8.

29. Morrison JJ, Dubose JJ, Rasmussen TE, Midwinter MJ. Military application of tranexamic acid in trauma emergency resuscitation (MATTERs) study. Arch Surg. 2012;147(2):113–9.
30. Morrison JJ, Ross JD, Dubose JJ, Jansen JO, Midwinter MJ, Rasmussen TE. Association of cryoprecipitate and tranexamic acid with improved survival following wartime injury: findings from the MATTERs II study. JAMA Surg. 2013;148(3):218–25.
31. Martin MJ, Beekley A. Front line surgery: a practical approach, vol. xxii. New York: Springer Publishing Inc; 2011. p. 533.
32. Beekley AC, Sebesta JA, Blackbourne LH, Herbert GS, Kauvar DS, Baer DG, et al. Prehospital tourniquet use in operation Iraqi freedom: effect on hemorrhage control and outcomes. J Trauma. 2008;64(2 Suppl):S28–37. discussion S.
33. Kragh JF, Walters TJ, Baer DG, Fox CJ, Wade CE, Salinas J, et al. Survival with emergency tourniquet use to stop bleeding in major limb trauma. Ann Surg. 2009;249(1):1–7.
34. Kragh JF, Walters TJ, Baer DG, Fox CJ, Wade CE, Salinas J, et al. Practical use of emergency tourniquets to stop bleeding in major limb trauma. J Trauma Inj Infect Crit Care. 2008;64(Supplement):S38–50.
35. Klotz JK, Leo M, Andersen BL, Nkodo AA, Garcia G, Wichern AM, et al. First case report of SAM(r) junctional tourniquet use in Afghanistan to control inguinal hemorrhage on the battlefield. J Spec Oper Med. 2014;14(2):1–5.
36. JJ DB, Scalea TM, Brenner M, Skiada D, Inaba K, Cannon J, et al. The AAST prospective aortic occlusion for resuscitation in trauma and acute care surgery (AORTA) registry: data on contemporary utilization and outcomes of aortic occlusion and resuscitative balloon occlusion of the aorta (REBOA). J Trauma Acute Care Surg. 2016;81(3):409–19.
37. Taller J, Kamdar JP, Greene JA, Morgan RA, Blankenship CL, Dabrowski P, et al. Temporary vascular shunts as initial treatment of proximal extremity vascular injuries during combat operations: the new standard of Care at Echelon II facilities? J Trauma Inj Infect Crit Care. 2008;65(3):595–603.
38. Reilly PM, Rotondo MF, Carpenter JP, Sherr SA, Schwab CW. Temporary vascular continuity during damage control. J Trauma Inj Infect Crit Care. 1995;39(4):757–60.
39. Martin M, Eastridge B. Torso trauma on the modern battlefield. In: Juan A, Trunkey DD, editors. Current therapy of trauma and surgical critical care. 2nd ed. Philadelphia: Elsevier; 2016.
40. Martin M, McDonald J, Mullenix P, Steele S, Demetriades D. Operative management and outcomes of traumatic lung resection. J Am Coll Surg. 2006;203(3):336–44.
41. Wilson A, Wall MJ, Maxson R, Mattox K. The pulmonary hilum twist as a thoracic damage control procedure. Am J Surg. 2003;186(1):49–52.
42. Bowling R, Mavroudis C, Richardson JD, Flint LM, Howe WR, Gray LA Jr. Emergency pneumonectomy for penetrating and blunt trauma. Am Surg. 1985;51(3):136–9.
43. Eastridge B, Blackbourne LH, Rasmussen TE, Cryer H, Murdock A. Damage control surgery. In: Combat casualty care: lessons learned from OEF and OIF [internet]. Fort Detrick: Office of the Surgeon General, Department of the Army, Borden Institute; 2012. p. 167–222.
44. Macho JR, Markison RE, Schecter WP. Cardiac stapling in the Management of Penetrating Injuries of the heart: rapid control of Hemorrhage and decreased risk of personal contamination. J Trauma Inj Infect Crit Care. 1993;34(5):711–6.
45. Evans BJ, Hornick P. Use of a skin stapler to repair penetrating cardiac injury. The. Ann R Coll Surg Engl. 2006;88(4):413–4.
46. Bowman MR, King RM. Comparison of staples and sutures for cardiorrhaphy in traumatic puncture wounds of the heart. J Emerg Med. 1996;14(5):615–8.
47. Wilson SM, Au FC. In extremis use of a Foley catheter in a cardiac stab wound. J Trauma Inj Infect Crit Care. 1986;26(4):400–2.
48. Ogilvie WH. Abdominal wounds in the Western Desert. Bull U S Army Med Dep. 1946;6(4):435–45.
49. Stankovic N, Petrovic M, Drinkovic N, Bjelovic M, Jevtic M, Mirkovic D. Colon and rectal war injuries. J Trauma. 1996;40(3 Suppl):s183–8.
50. MacFarlane C, Vaizey CJ, Benn CA. Battle injuries of the rectum: options for the field surgeon. J R Army Med Corps. 2002;148(1):27–31.
51. Bowley DM, Jansen JO, Nott D, Sapsford W, Streets CG, Tai NR. Difficult decisions in the surgical care of military casualties with major torso trauma. J R Army Med Corps. 2011;157(3 Suppl 1):S324–33.
52. Vertrees A, Wakefield M, Pickett C, Greer L, Wilson A, Gillern S, et al. Outcomes of primary repair and primary anastomosis in war-related colon injuries. J Trauma Inj Infect Crit Care. 2009;66(5):1286–93.
53. Duncan JE, Corwin CH, Sweeney WB, Dunne JR, Denobile JW, Perdue PW, et al. Management of colorectal injuries during operation iraqi freedom: patterns of stoma usage. J Trauma. 2008;64(4):1043–7.
54. Cothren CC, Osborn PM, Moore EE, Morgan SJ, Johnson JL, Smith WR. Preperitonal pelvic packing for hemodynamically unstable pelvic fractures: a paradigm shift. J Trauma Inj Infect Crit Care. 2007;62(4):834–42.
55. Osborn PM, Smith WR, Moore EE, Cothren CC, Morgan SJ, Williams AE, et al. Direct retroperitoneal pelvic packing versus pelvic angiography: a comparison of two management protocols for haemodynamically unstable pelvic fractures. Injury. 2009;40(1):54–60.
56. Brandes S, Borrelli J. Pelvic fracture and associated urologic injuries. World J Surg. 2001;25(12):1578–87.

57. Lowe MA, Mason JT, Luna GK, Maier RV, Copass MK, Berger RE. Risk factors for urethral injuries in men with traumatic pelvic fractures. J Urol. 1988;140(3):506–7.
58. Mossadegh S, Tai N, Midwinter M, Parker P. Improvised explosive device related pelvi-perineal trauma: anatomic injuries and surgical management. J Trauma Acute Care Surg. 2012;73(2 Suppl 1):S24–31.
59. Mossadegh S, Tai N, Midwinter M, Parker P. Improvised explosive device-related Pelviperineal trauma: UK military experience, literature review and lessons for civilian trauma teams. Bull R Coll Surg Engl. 2013;95(9):1–5.
60. Blackbourne LH, et al., editors. First to cut: trauma lessons learned in the Combat Zone. San Antonio: Borden Institute, Office of the Surgeon General, United States Army; 2012.
61. Galante J, Rodriguez C. Dismounted complex blast injury. In: Lim CRB, editor. Surgery during natural disasters, combat, terrorist attacks, and crisis situations. Switzerland: Springer International Publishing; 2016.
62. Meizoso JP, Ray JJ, Karcutskie IV CA et al. Effect of time to operation on mortality for hypotensive patients with gunshot wounds to the torso: the golden 10 minutes. J Trauma Acute Care Surg. 2016;81:685–691.
63. Barbosa RR, Rowell SE, Fox EE et al. Increasing time to operation is associated with decreased survival in patients with a positive FAST examination requiring emergent laparotomy. J Trauma Acute Care Surg. 2013;75:S48–S52.
64. Fischer RP, Jelense S, Perry JF Jr. Direct transfer to operating room improves care of trauma patients. A simple, economically feasible plan for large hospitals. JAMA. 1978;240:1731–1732.
65. Steele JT, Hoyt DB, Simons RK et al. Is operating room resuscitation a way to save time? Am J Surg. 1997;174:683–687.
66. Martin M, Izenberg S, Cole, F et al. A decade of experience with a selective policy for direct to operating room trauma resuscitations. Am J Surg. 2012;204:187–192.
67. Perchinsky MJ, Long WB, Hill JG. Blunt cardiac rupture. The Emanuel trauma center experience. Arch Surg. 1995; Martin M, Izenberg S, Cole, F et al. A decade of experience with a selective policy for direct to operating room trauma resuscitations. Am J Surg. 2012;204:187–192.
68. Perchinsky MJ, Long WB, Hill JG. Blunt cardiac rupture. The Emanuel trauma center experience. Arch Surg. 1995;130:852–857.

Hemorrhage Control

Rachel M. Russo and Joseph J. DuBose

Introduction

Over the last 15 years of war in Iraq and Afghanistan, blast injury from improvised explosive devices has proven a common mechanism of battlefield death [1]. These recent conflicts have consequently resulted in extreme injury severity compared to previous conflicts. Despite this trend, improvements in body armor and growing experience treating victims of explosive blasts have led to historically high survival rates following combat injury [2]. These advances have, however, been associated with a preponderance of patients surviving to reach forward hospital care with traumatic amputations – in some cases involving multiple extremities (Fig. 7.1). The challenges these patients represent are not unique to the battlefield, as increasing terrorist activities within the United States and Europe have increased the prevalence of patients with blast-related traumatic amputations arriving to civilian trauma bays [3, 4].

The emergency surgeon will undoubtedly encounter dramatic and troubling extremity injuries that may occur in conjunction with a multitude of apparent or occult concomitant injuries. When possible, maximizing the potential for limb preservation should be considered, even in the case of a mangled extremity or near amputation. Nonetheless, the salvage of life always takes precedence over the salvage of a limb. Until recently, patients with traumatic amputation rarely survived long enough to receive prehospital or ED care [5, 6]. However, advancements in hemorrhage control and resuscitation have allowed hundreds of patients to survive injuries previously thought to be lethal [7]. This chapter will discuss available strategies for initial hemorrhage control in the patient with multiple traumatic amputations.

Presurgical Hemorrhage Control

Tourniquet Application

The mainstay of prehospital care for the patient with traumatic amputation is the prompt application of a tourniquet. The requirement of all deployed US military personnel to carry and be trained in the application of extremity tourniquets has revolutionized survivorship for victims of traumatic amputation [8]. There remains, however, room for continued improvement. In a recent analysis of military personnel killed during Operations Iraqi and Enduring Freedom, dismounted soldiers encountering an explosive blast most frequently died from extremity and junctional hemorrhage [1, 9]. Nearly two thirds of

R. M. Russo
Department of General Surgery,
University of California Davis Medical Center,
Sacramento, CA, USA

J. J. DuBose (✉)
Department of Vascular and Endovascular Surgery,
David Grant USAF Medical Center, Travis Air Force Base, California, Fairfield, CA, USA

Fig. 7.1 Blast-injured soldier following explosion of an improvised explosive device

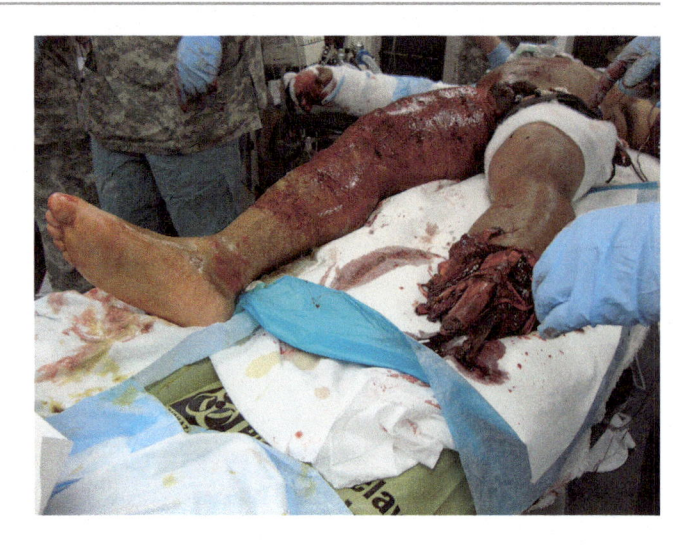

those injuries may have been anatomically amenable to prehospital interventions such as tourniquet application [10, 11]. Similar opportunities for improvement in prehospital care have been observed in civilian practice. During the Boston marathon terrorist event, for example, the use of field tourniquets was credited for the high survival rate among victims with traumatic amputations [12]. A lack of commercial extremity tourniquets, however, led prehospital providers to rely heavily on improvised tourniquets and speedy transport of patients with untreated extremity hemorrhage, resulting in patients with extremity injuries arriving to hospitals in extremis [13]. Because tourniquets have been shown to have such dramatic life-saving potential, this text dedicates a separate, important chapter to the topic.

Another related but uniquely challenging potential sequela of blast injury is junctional hemorrhage – or bleeding from extremity sources proximal to the torso that are not amenable to traditional extremity tourniquets. Unique field solutions have been proposed to help combat hemorrhage at these anatomic locations, including the Combat Ready Clamp (CRoC). The CRoC is a junctional tourniquet that has been approved by the Food and Drug Administration for inguinal hemorrhage. While the published literature on its clinical use is limited, animal studies demonstrate successful occlusion of iliac arterial injuries [14]. Its availability for civilian use is limited at this time. However, as the only currently available junctional tourniquet approved for use on the battlefield, familiarity with the device is paramount for deployed medical personnel.

Surgical Hemorrhage Control

In the initial operative care of a blast-injured casualty, operative techniques common to damage control surgery principles remain the keys to success. Exposure, packing, and resuscitation – commonly in the context of a team effort – are critical to salvage a severely injured casualty. In the setting of vascular injury associated with these wounds, however, no maneuver is more paramount to hemorrhage cessation than direct surgical vascular control [15].

When obtaining vascular control during acute extremity hemorrhage, arterial occlusion should generally be performed at the most distal site possible to achieve hemostasis in order to reduce ischemia and preserve limb length if amputation is ultimately required [15]. Ligating exposed vessels accessible through the injury may be an appealing tactic to reduce active hemorrhage. However, bleeding may continue from more proximally located injuries, and time may be wasted tying off multiple small vessels stemming from the same proximal artery. Achieving prompt hemostasis is the first priority; therefore, surgical exposure of inflow arteries outside of the area of injury may be preferable to facilitate rapid arterial occlusion when distal anatomy is distorted, bleeding is diffuse, or distal vessels are difficult to access due to the anatomy or the severity of injury.

As expedient exposure is so very critical to subsequent emergent vessel control in these settings, emphasis of common trauma exposures of these vessels must be a central focus of any chapter on hemorrhage control following blast injuries. For this reason, we will discuss effective techniques for the critical exposures that must be familiar to the surgeon treating these injuries. We also would strongly recommend that surgeons who may be called upon to care for blast-injured patients take the Advanced Trauma Operative Management (ATOM) and the Advanced Surgical Skills for Exposure in Trauma (ASSET) courses. Both courses emphasize hands-on surgical techniques for rapid control and repair of major traumatic injuries, as well as surgical anatomy and exposure techniques for all major truncal and extremity vessels.

Upper Extremity Vascular Exposure and Control

Exposure of critical upper extremity arteries represents a significant challenge, particularly when proximal control of vessel injuries is required at these locations. Anatomic challenges represented by proximal vessels navigating the thoracic cage require a thoughtful initial incision choice and the flexibility to extend incisions into the chest or neck as required to control identified injuries.

Subclavian Artery

The subclavian artery (SCA) is divided into three different anatomic segments that are each approached differently. The first, most proximal segment of the SCA extends from its origin (the aorta on the left or innominate artery on the right) to the medial border of the anterior scalene muscle. The second, middle segment extends from the medial border of the anterior scalene muscle to the retroclavicular SCA. The third, distal SCA segment extends from the clavicle to the medial border of the pectoralis minor muscle.

The proximal segment of the SCA is best approached through the chest; however, the optimal incision to provide proximal control varies based on patient stability and the side involved. Proximal control of the right SCA at the innominate artery can be obtained through a median sternotomy or right thoracotomy (described more thoroughly in "Thoracic Aorta" later in this chapter). Proximal control of the left SCA is more challenging. In hemodynamically stable patients, a trapdoor incision or a left lateral thoracotomy in conjunction with a supraclavicular incision provides adequate exposure to the takeoff of the SCA at the aortic arch. In unstable patients or those with concomitant intrathoracic injuries, hemostasis can initially be obtained by performing a left anterolateral thoracotomy and applying pressure to the apex of the left pleural cavity and, subsequently, placing a clamp at the origin of the artery from the aortic arch.

Approaching the second segment of the SCA posterior to the clavicle may be facilitated by disarticulating the clavicle from the sternum (which can be a time-consuming endeavor associated with potential complications), resecting the middle third of the clavicle, or dividing the clavicle in half (Fig. 7.2). Care should be taken to divide the clavicle in the subperiosteal plane to avoid injury to the subclavian vein, located adjacent to the inferior border of the clavicle. Since open access to this segment of the SCA is challenging and may confer additional morbidity, endovascular management of injuries in these areas is becoming more widely adopted (Fig. 7.3a, b) [16].

The distal segment of the SCA can be exposed through an infraclavicular approach and extended distally to provide access to the axillary artery in continuation (Fig. 7.4).

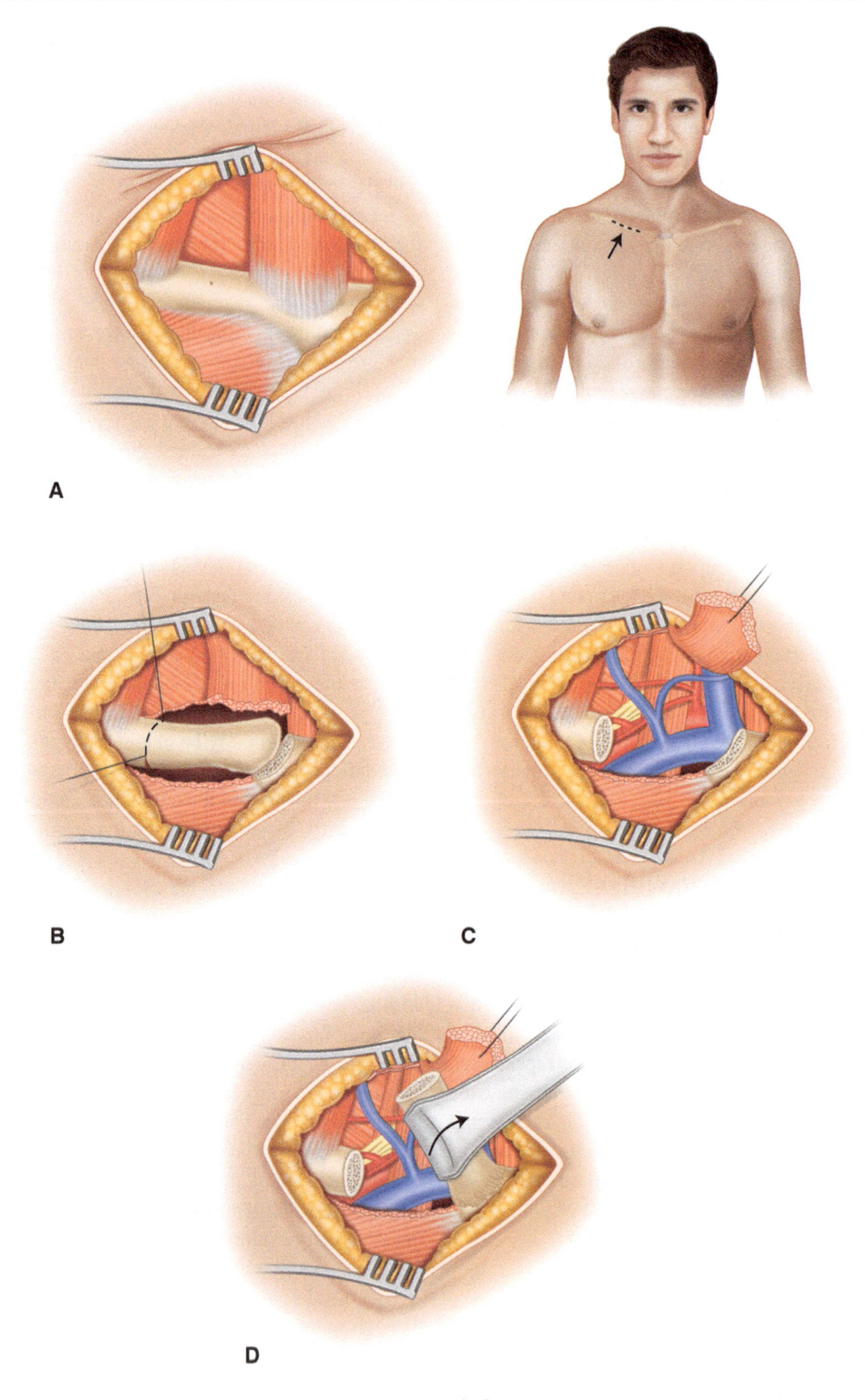

Fig. 7.2 Trans-clavicular exposure of the distal subclavian and proximal axillary arteries (**a**) Exposure of the clavicle (**b**) Division of the clavicle with a Gigli saw following circumferential dissection (**c**) Exposure of the subclavian vessels by resection of the middle third of the clavicle (**d**) Exposure of the subclavian vessels by division and retraction of the clavicle (From Dubose [43])

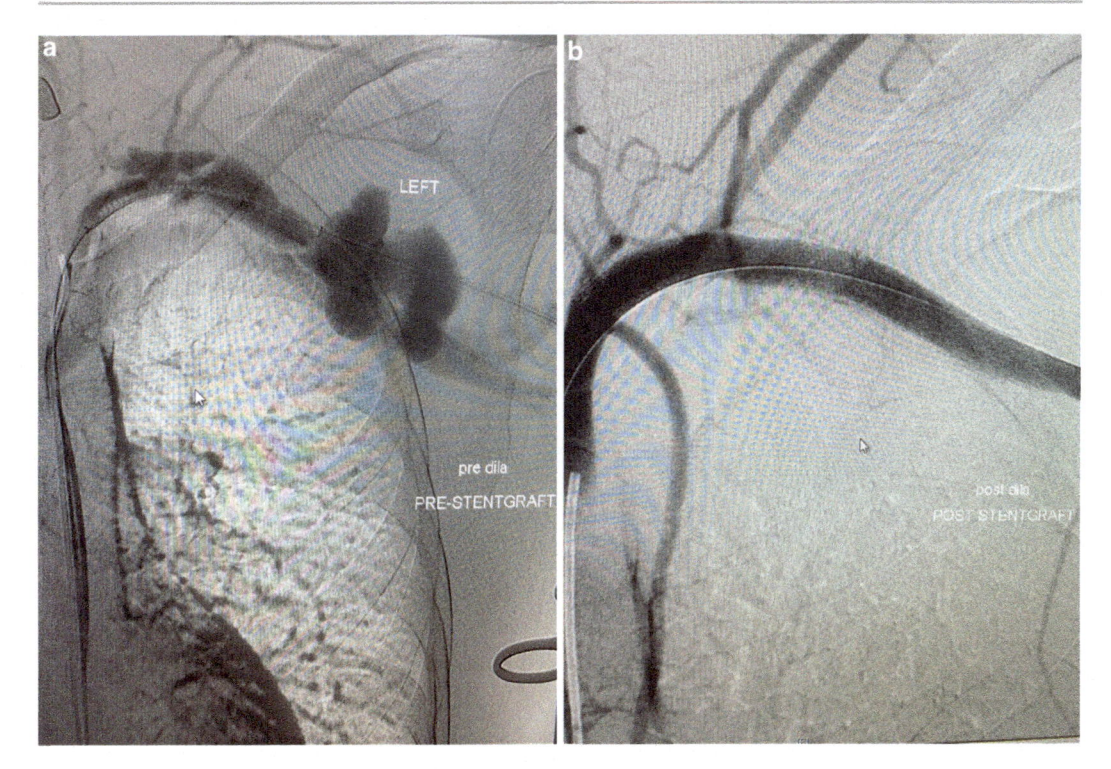

Fig. 7.3 Before and after photo of retroclavicular subclavian injury undergoing endovascular repair (**a**) Extravasation of contrast from penetrating injury to the subclavian artery evident on angiogram. (**b**) Resolution of hemorrhage following placement of a covered stent

Axillary Artery

The axillary artery originates at the lateral border of the first rib and ends at the inferior border of the teres major muscle. Like the SCA, it is divided into three parts: proximal, middle, and distal. The proximal segment is beneath and proximal to the pectoralis minor muscle with the superior thoracic artery as its single branch. The middle segment is deep to the pectoralis minor muscle and contains two branches: the thoracoacromial and lateral thoracic arteries. The distal segment is distal to the pectoralis minor muscle and contains three branches: the subscapular and anterior and posterior circumflex humeral arteries. Surgical exposure of the axillary artery in its entirety can be accomplished by way of an incision over the cephalic vein in the deltopectoral groove. If necessary, the pectoralis major and minor tendons may be divided to provide additional exposure. This incision can be extended onto the chest inferior to the clavicle to obtain proximal control at the distal SCA or be carried distally along the border of the biceps brachii to obtain distal control at the brachial artery.

Brachial Artery

The brachial artery is the distal continuation of the axillary artery that originates at the inferior border of the teres major muscle, courses along the medial border of the biceps muscle, and terminates in the antecubital fossa as it branches into the radial and ulnar arteries. Exposure is achieved through a medial longitudinal incision along the medial border of the biceps. This incision can be extended into the deltopectoral groove to provide proximal control at the axillary artery or extended distally to provide access to the radial and ulnar arteries, crossing the antecubital fossa, in an S shape to avoid later complications caused by scar contracture (Fig. 7.5). Care must be taken during mobilization of the distal segment of the

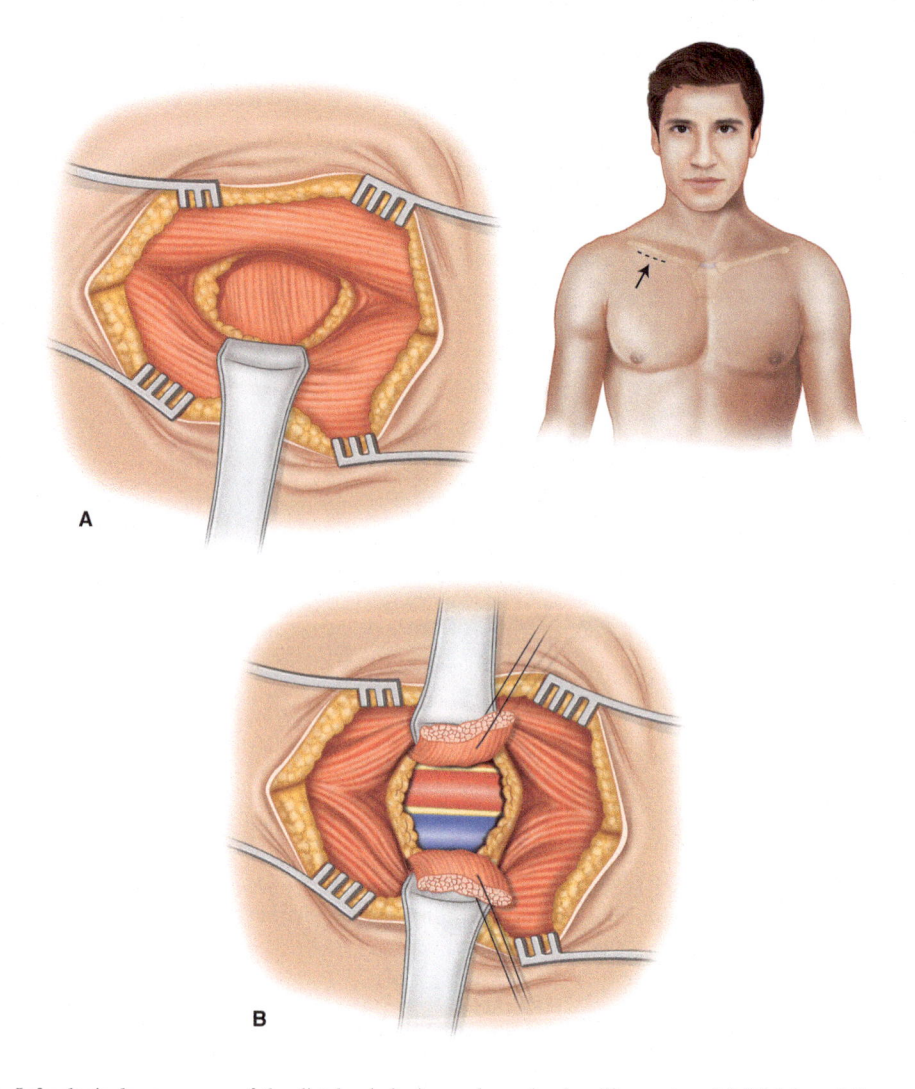

Fig. 7.4 Infraclavicular exposure of the distal subclavian and proximal axillary artery (**a**) Division of the pectoralis major (**b**) Transection of the pectoralis minor to expose the distal subclavian vessels (From Dubose [43])

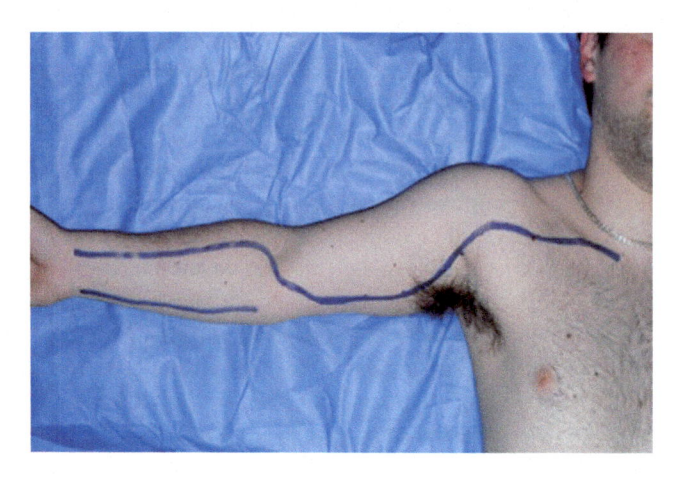

Fig. 7.5 Complete exposure of the axillary artery, brachial artery, and radial artery can be obtained through a curvilinear longitudinal incision extending from the deltopectoral groove, medial to the biceps brachii, and obliquely across the antecubital fossa toward the thenar eminence. A counter-incision can provide further exposure of the ulnar artery distal to its origin (From American College of Surgeons Committee on Trauma. ASSET: Advanced Surgical Skills for Exposure in Trauma: Exposure Techniques When Time Matters. American College of Surgeons. Chicago, IL)

brachial artery to preserve the medial nerve that courses alongside the brachial artery to provide sensory and motor function to the hand. If the patient's condition permits primary repair, it should be undertaken at the time of initial exposure. If primary repair is not possible or if the patient is hemodynamically unstable, shunting these arteries and returning for delayed repair is preferred to ligation. Ligation of the ulnar, radial, and brachial arteries can be performed with minimal residual deficit if collateral circulation remains intact.

Lower Extremity Exposures and Vascular Control

Iliac Vessels

In the setting of junctional hemorrhage, vascular exposure proximal to the inguinal ligament can be achieved through either an extraperitoneal or transperitoneal approach. The extraperitoneal "hockey-stick" or "transplant" incision can be extended proximally to provide exposure of the external iliac artery, common iliac artery, or even the aorta as necessary (Fig. 7.6). It can also be extended distally to provide exposure of the common femoral artery and its branches. If bilateral injury or concomitant intra-abdominal injuries are present, a transperitoneal approach may be preferable. During laparotomy, the iliac vessels can be exposed by medial visceral rotation and dividing the posterior peritoneum in the midline to expose the aortic bifurcation. Left medial visceral rotation is frequently preferred to right for improved aortic exposure.

Many critical structures near the iliac arteries should be identified and respected during dissection and repair. The iliopsoas muscle is readily apparent laterally with the femoral nerve lying adjacent. The ureter crosses the common iliac artery at its bifurcation and continues toward the bladder, medial to the external iliac and lateral to the internal iliac arteries. To obtain vascular control at this level, the artery should be isolated from the vein before being clamped, shunted, or ligated. The iliac veins at this location may lie adherent to the posterior surface of the arteries and are at risk of further injury during emergent exposure. The iliac veins can also be easily injured during proximal common iliac artery control.

Identified simple iliac vein injuries can often be controlled with sponge sticks and then repaired with lateral venorrhaphy. Circumferential dissection to allow the passage of vascular tapes or vessel loops should be avoided to minimize the risk of bleeding from inadvertent posterior wall injuries. Exposure of a

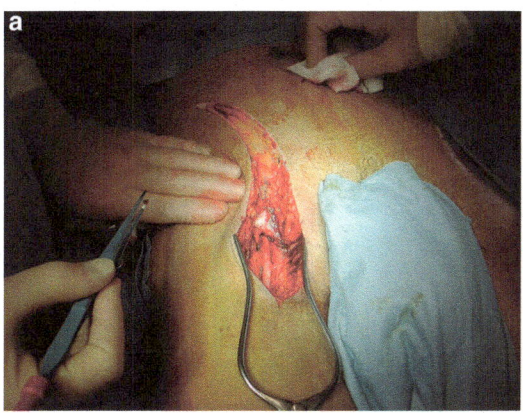

Fig. 7.6 Extraperitoneal exposure of the right iliac artery (**a**) Hockey-stick incision to expose the iliac and femoral arteries in continuation (**b**) Left is cranial. Control of the right common iliac (white), internal iliac artery (orange), and common femoral (orange) arteries. The blue vessel loop is around the ureter (Figure b from Atlas of Trauma Extraperitoneal Approach to the Iliac Vessels *Karim Brohi, trauma.org 7:12, December 2002*. Trauma.org)

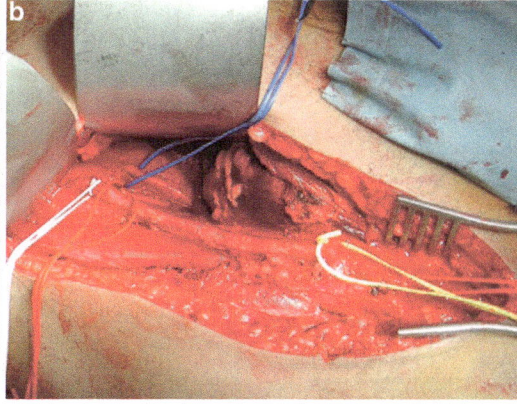

right iliac venous injury may rarely require division of the right common or external iliac artery with subsequent primary repair. The left common and external iliac arteries lie lateral to, rather crossing directly over, the iliac vein so arterial division is rarely required to obtain adequate venous exposure on the left. Iliac vein venorrhaphy is preferable, with ligation reserved for patients with multiple associated injuries, prolonged shock, or gross contamination.

Because of the significant risk of limb loss, repair of injuries to the common or external iliac arteries should be attempted if the patient's stability allows. If immediate repair is not feasible, arterial shunt placement can allow revascularization to be delayed for hours to days [7]. If iliac artery ligation is required, delayed revascularization can be achieved with an arterial bypass if performed within a few hours of ligation [17]. Extensive collateral circulation allows the internal iliac arteries to be ligated if necessary.

Common Femoral Artery

The common femoral artery (CFA) measures approximately 5 cm in length and travels halfway between the anterior superior iliac spine and the pubic symphysis, two fingerbreadths lateral to the pubic tubercle at about the midpoint of the inguinal ligament (Fig. 7.7). Exposure of this vessel begins with a longitudinal incision over the CFA, directly over the femoral pulse if one can be palpated. For trauma, a longitudinal incision is preferable to an oblique incision because it can be more easily extended to provide proximal vascular exposure as necessary.

The inguinal ligament, an important landmark in identifying the correct incision location for exposure, is two to three fingerbreadths proximal to the groin crease and overlies the medial two third of the femoral head. If the soft tissue is distorted by injury or body habitus, the bony landmarks of the anterior superior iliac spine, pubic tubercle, and femoral head can be used to approximate the location of the femoral artery. Distal extension of the incision should proceed from the inguinal ligament directly over the artery along its course, aiming toward the medial aspect of the knee to provide access to the superficial femoral artery and profunda femoris.

When placing retractors to optimize exposure, avoid traction injury to femoral nerve branches laterally or the common femoral vein medially. The femoral sheath can then be opened to expose the femoral artery. The anterior surface of the common femoral artery, which has no branches, provides an optimal initial dissection plane centered over the artery. Encountering venous structures indicates medial deviation of the dissection plane, while exposure of nerves or the iliopsoas muscle indicates deviation laterally.

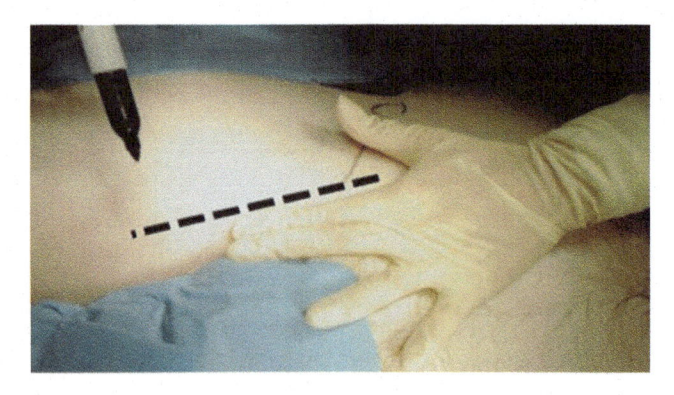

Fig. 7.7 The common femoral artery can be located in two fingerbreadths medial to the pubic tubercle. A longitudinal incision overlying the common femoral artery from the inguinal ligament extending medially toward the knee can provide exposure of the superficial femoral artery in continuation (From American College of Surgeons Committee on Trauma. ASSET: Advanced Surgical Skills for Exposure in Trauma: Exposure Techniques When Time Matters. American College of Surgeons. Chicago, IL)

7 Hemorrhage Control

This described approach should facilitate exposure to control lower extremity hemorrhage by ligating, circumferentially clamping, or shunting the CFA, profunda femoris, or SFA as necessary. As the dissection proceeds distally, an abrupt change in caliber of the CFA will be notable at the branch point of the profunda femoris and the superficial femoral arteries approximately 4 cm distal to the inguinal ligament. Better exposure of the SFA can be obtained by taking down the sartorius muscle or continuing the incision longitudinally along the anterior border of the sartorius muscle to retract it laterally as the SFA passes underneath it to reach Hunter's canal. Traction on a silastic vessel loop around the CFA can aid in improved exposure of the profunda femoris, coursing posterior-laterally, which can be ligated with relative impunity in the setting of significant hemorrhage.

If vessel control requires more proximal surgical exposure, the inguinal ligament can be divided to allow better exposure of the proximal common femoral artery. Care should be taken in this area as a major tributary to the femoral vein, giving rise to the inferior epigastric vein and the deep circumflex iliac veins, crossing over the CFA just proximal to the inguinal ligament near the takeoff of the deep circumflex iliac artery, denoting the distal extent of the external iliac artery. This vein must be identified, ligated, and divided to expose the artery at this level. The deep circumflex vessels can be ligated to provide better mobilization of the proximal CFA.

Popliteal Artery

The best emergent approach to the popliteal artery is with the patient in the supine position with the leg flexed at the knee, externally rotated, and elevated with towels or folded drapes. The longitudinal incision for exposure of this vessel is made parallel to the sartorius muscle, which is retracted posteromedially to facilitate exposure (Fig. 7.8). Division of the gracilis, semimembranosus, semitendinosus, and the medial head of the gastrocnemius will afford full exposure of the entire popliteal artery behind the knee if required.

Fig. 7.8 Surgical exposure of the popliteal artery. Division of the gracilis, semimembranosus, semitendinosus, and the medial head of the gastrocnemius will afford full exposure of the entire popliteal artery behind the knee (From Muscat et al. [44])

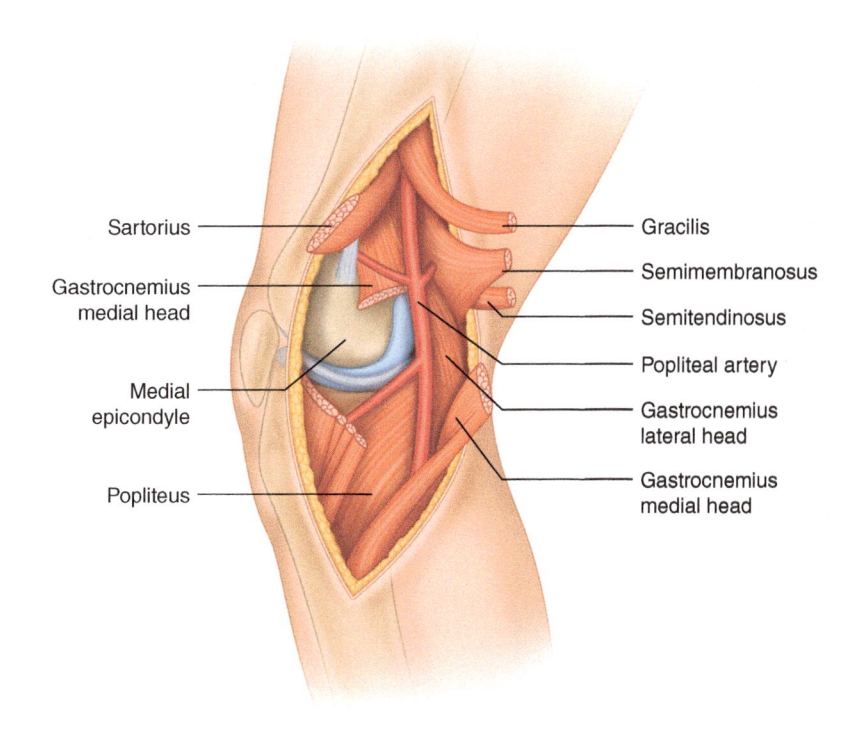

The ideal replacement conduit for the popliteal artery has yet to be identified, but autologous saphenous vein is most commonly advised. For injuries to the middle portion of the popliteal artery directly behind the knee, exposure and direct repair can be challenging. An excellent alternative is to perform a saphenous vein bypass of the injured area, with exclusion of the injured segment via ligation of the distal above-knee popliteal artery and the proximal below-knee artery.

Aorta

The aorta is divided into two main segments: thoracic and abdominal. The thoracic aorta is comprised of three sections: the ascending aorta, the aortic arch, and the thoracic descending aorta. The descending aorta begins as the aorta passes through the diaphragm and ends at the bifurcation of the common iliac vessels. Terminally, a small midline median sacral artery branches off the distal abdominal aorta at its bifurcation. For the purposes of describing levels of aortic occlusion, the aorta has three zones (Fig. 7.9) [18]. Zone 1 includes the descending thoracic aorta from the left subclavian artery to the level of the celiac artery. Zone II extends from the celiac artery to the lowest renal artery. Zone III extends from the lowest renal artery to the aortic bifurcation.

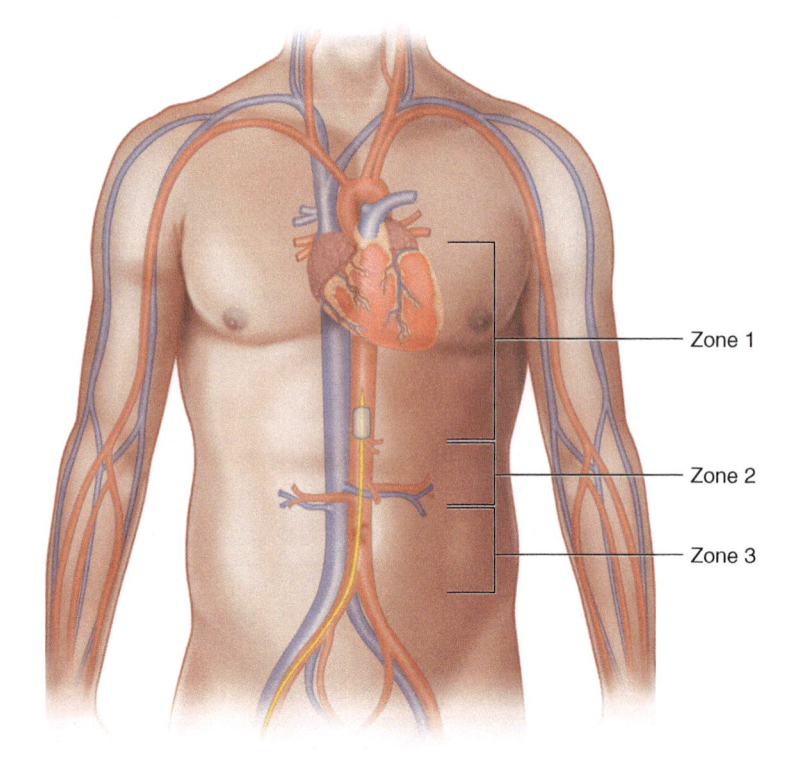

Numerous approaches to exposing the aorta have been described. The best approach varies depending on the clinical scenario, patient's condition, and level of aortic exposure required. It is important to note that, in modern practice, aortic occlusion can be accomplished through open or endovascular techniques. Open aortic occlusion can be achieved with external compression using an aortic occluder to compress the aorta against the spine or by circumferential isolation with clamp placement. Clamping the aorta without first circumferential dissection is not recommended because of the high likelihood of par-

Fig. 7.9 Zones of aortic occlusion. Zone I includes the descending thoracic aorta from the left subclavian artery to the level of the celiac artery. Zone II extends from the celiac artery to the lowest renal artery. Zone III extends from the lowest renal artery to the aortic bifurcation

tial clamping with continued hemorrhage. Endovascular repair or occlusion can be achieved with covered stents or occlusion balloons that will be described later in this chapter. The level of aortic occlusion employed should be based on the anatomic location of the injury, the patient's stability, and the ease of access.

Thoracic Aorta

Injury to the thoracic aorta can be difficult to detect and troublesome to manage in the resource-limited setting. Few patients with a penetrating thoracic aortic injury will survive long enough to receive medical care [19]. Those who do survive may present with cardiac tamponade from ascending aortic injury. Thoracic aortic pseudoaneurysms and traumatic dissections may be present in the blast-injured patient; however, they are more common after blunt injury [20]. Thoracic aortic pseudoaneurysms occur most commonly at the aortic isthmus, just distal to the origin of the left subclavian artery. Aortography has traditionally proven the gold standard for diagnosis of these injuries, but in practice CT imaging with contrast has largely emerged as the mainstay for detecting and characterizing mediastinal hematomas, intimal flaps, and pseudoaneurysms [21]. Chest x-ray may demonstrate a widened mediastinum and/or apical capping. If not recognized and repaired, traumatic aneurysms can rupture unpredictably, even years later [19].

Open exposure of these thoracic aortic injuries can be obtained through a left fourth or fifth intercostal space posterolateral thoracotomy, clamping the aorta between the left carotid artery and left subclavian artery for proximal control. Aortic occlusion in this location is associated with significant morbidity and mortality, even with short occlusion times. Aortic bypass may be necessary if occlusion is required for more than 20 min. Rates of paraplegia following this procedure vary, but have been reported to be as high as 20% when performed for elective repair of thoracic aortic aneurysms and would almost certainly be higher when performed emergently for trauma [22].

While some aortic injuries should be repaired emergently or urgently, repair of many thoracic aortic injuries can safely be delayed until control of external and cavitary hemorrhage, including evacuation of intracranial mass lesions, has been completed. Control of intra-abdominal hemorrhage should be attained with packing rather than aortic occlusion when potential aortic injury is suspected. In the acute setting, recognizing the potential for thoracic aortic injury is of the utmost importance prior to occluding the aorta to stop hemorrhage from more distal injuries. The aortic pressure created proximal to the point of occlusion can rupture a tenuous thoracic aortic injury. Generally speaking, thoracic aortic injury is considered a contraindication to endovascular aortic occlusion due to the potential for aortic rupture during wire passage and balloon positioning [23].

Left Anterolateral Thoracotomy and Clamshell Thoracotomy (Bilateral Anterolateral Thoracotomy)

For the unstable patient, access to intrathoracic structures is most quickly achieved through a left anterolateral thoracotomy performed through the fourth or fifth intercostal space (Fig. 7.10c). If palpation of the rib spaces is limited, the nipple and inframammary crease are often used as external landmarks. However, in obese patients or patients with large or pendulous breasts, these external landmarks may be unreliable. A low incision should be avoided, as it may result in inadvertent laceration of the diaphragm, abdominal cavity entry, or iatrogenic splenic injury. During end expiration, the diaphragm can be high in the chest, increasing the potential risk of intra-abdominal entry.

The anterolateral thoracotomy incision transects the serratus anterior muscle. This incision can provide rapid access to the pericardium, pulmonary hilum, and descending aorta. Intrathoracic injuries can be temporized, the aorta can be cross clamped to halt intra-abdominal hemorrhage, and cardiac compressions can be performed. Exposure of the superior and posterior mediastinum is difficult through this incision. It can be

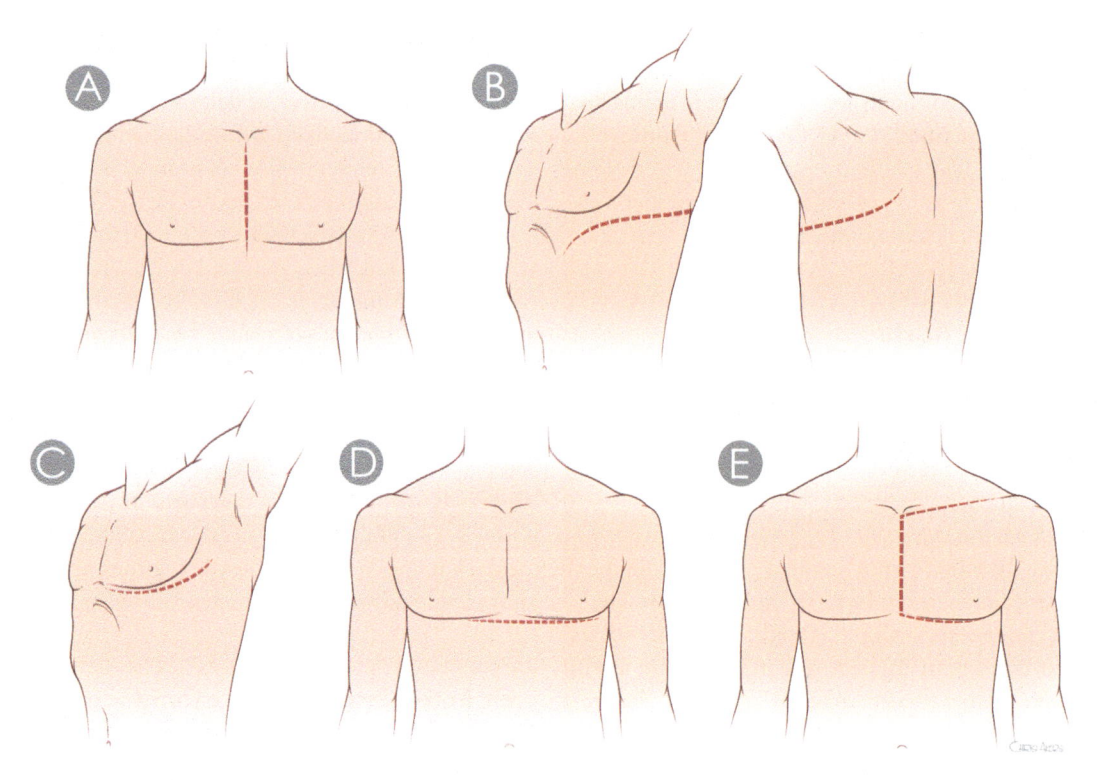

Fig. 7.10 Thoracic incision exposures: (**a**) Median sternotomy. (**b**) Posterolateral thoracotomy (**c**) Anterolateral thoracotomy (**d**) Extension of anterolateral thoracotomy across the midline for "clamshell thoracotomy." (**e**) "Trapdoor" thoracotomy (From Dubose [43])

extended with a Gigli saw or Lebsche knife across the sternum to create the "clamshell thoracotomy" for access to the right pleural cavity (Figs. 7.10d and 7.11). When utilizing this incision, care should be taken to ligate the internal mammary arteries bilaterally to avoid troublesome bleeding. A bilateral thoracotomy provides excellent access and exposure to the heart, lungs, ascending aorta, arch, and major aortic branches, particularly the innominate artery, and to the superior vena cava and innominate vein.

Posterolateral Thoracotomy

Although there is no specific standard location for the posterolateral thoracotomy incision, it is termed posterolateral because of its relationship to the latissimus dorsi muscle which it transects (Fig. 7.10b). This incision is extremely versatile and gives excellent exposure to the entire

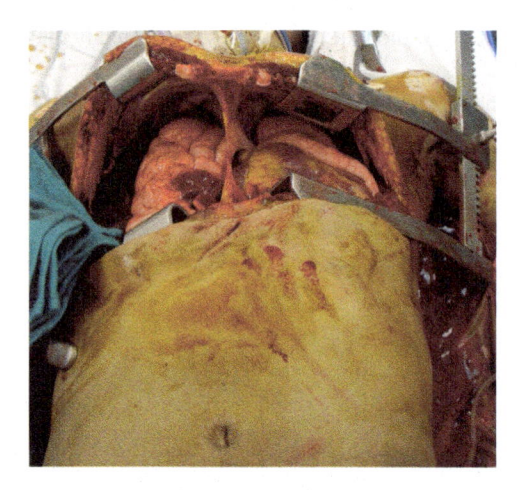

Fig. 7.11 "Clamshell" thoracotomy provides wide exposure for the unstable trauma patient

ipsilateral hemithorax if the correct interspace (depending on the desired level of exposure) is incised. For these reasons, it is the incision of choice for open elective thoracic surgery. A left posterolateral thoracotomy allows access to the descending thoracic aorta, left subclavian artery, distal esophagus, and pulmonary structures of the left chest. A right posterolateral thoracotomy provides exposure of the trachea, azygous vein, and proximal esophagus in addition to the pulmonary structures of the right chest. This incision should be used preferentially in the stable patient with an already identified injury. It is a less desirable incision for the patient in extremis because the patient must be in full lateral decubitus position and requires single lung ventilation for the best exposure. However, surgeons should not hesitate to reposition the patient from supine to lateral decubitus as necessary to gain better exposure of difficult-to-access injuries. However, one of the most important principles for trauma operations that are truly exploratory (and the exact source of hemorrhage is unclear) is to keep the patient supine to maximize exposure options and extensions into different cavities.

The skin incision is designed to allow upward retraction of the scapula when the overhanging arm is positioned out of the field. The incision begins at the anterior border of the latissimus dorsi muscle in front of the anterior axillary line and passes several centimeters below the tip of the scapula. It then extends posteriorly and cephalad midway between the posterior midline of the vertebral bodies and the medial border of the scapula. When dividing the latissimus dorsi, several muscular blood vessels may be encountered and ligated as needed. The deeper serratus anterior is divided near its muscular attachments. The trapezius or rhomboid muscle may be divided for additional exposure. After lifting the scapula with a retractor, the ribs can be palpated to select the best interspace for entry into the chest. The serratus to the second rib posteriorly is an almost always palpable landmark to aid in the proper numeric identification of interspaces. Entering the pleural space over top of the lower rib at the desired interspace will minimize the risk of iatrogenic injury to the intercostal neuromuscular bundle. Rib resection can be performed to aid in exposure.

Median Sternotomy

The median sternotomy (Fig. 7.10a) provides relatively rapid exposure of the heart and great vessels, both lungs, and the tracheobronchial tree. For this reason, it is the incision of choice for the hemodynamically stable patient with thoracic injuries. The median sternotomy is a vertical midline incision from the sternal notch to the tip of the xiphoid process. It can be extended proximally into the supraclavicular fossa and obliquely anterior to the sternocleidomastoid muscle ("trapdoor incision") to expose the innominate or carotid arteries or left subclavian artery (Fig. 7.10e). Since the patient is positioned supine, the incision can also be extended distally to the pubic symphysis to concurrently address intra-abdominal injuries. The pectoral fascia should be divided at the midline and the periosteum scored. The sternum can be divided with a power saw or Lebsche knife. Bleeding from the cut sternal edge should be controlled with bone wax or other hemostatic agents to improve visualization of the intrathoracic structures. Placing the retractor lower in the incision will aid with exposure. Slow opening of the retractor with slow spreading of the sternal edges is important to avoid injury to the innominate vein. If innominate vein injury occurs, it can be controlled by applying digital pressure from beneath the vein, compressing it against the sternum and chest wall. Other common injuries that can occur during retraction include iatrogenic rib fractures and brachial plexus injuries. Damage control surgery to control hemorrhage including aortic cross clamping can be performed through the midline sternotomy. The sternum can be temporarily closed with a negative pressure dressing or Ioban over drains while awaiting definitive repair.

Thoracoabdominal Incision

A left thoracoabdominal incision provides wide exposure of the aorta in the stable patient with a known injury. With the patient in the right lateral decubitus position and hips rotated back at least 45°, the skin incision is made from the anterior axillary line diagonally forward at the appropriate intercostal space (most commonly the seventh) toward the midline of the abdomen to end halfway between the xiphoid process and the umbilicus. The incision can be extended proximally toward the scapula or distally toward the pubic symphysis along the abdominal midline. The left hemidiaphragm is opened either radially toward the esophagus or circumferentially with a 2–3 cm rim remaining on the chest wall for subsequent closure. When incising the diaphragm, it is important to avoid phrenic nerve injury as hemiparalysis of the diaphragm portends significantly worse outcomes.

Abdominal Aorta

Abdominal aortic exposure can facilitate repair of vascular injuries to the aorta and its branches or aortic cross clamping to limit intra-abdominal, pelvic, or lower extremity hemorrhage. It is extremely important to completely mobilize the aorta prior to application of a cross clamp. Iatrogenic injury to the common iliac vein or distal inferior vena cava during dissection can be a lethal complication of aortic exposure. An aortic occluder can be used to compress the aorta against the spine to obtain rapid hemostasis until further exposure and mobilization are obtained. Blind suturing into a bleeding field is potentially disastrous. If venous injury is identified, compression with a sponge stick can provide temporary exposure. The overlying artery (aorta or iliac) can be transected to provide access to completely mobilize the vein and repair it under direct vision.

The ureters travel adjacent to the aorta and cross over the common iliac arteries, leaving them vulnerable to injury during abdominal aortic exposure by either the transperitoneal or retroperitoneal approach. Every time retractors are repositioned or a new dissection plane is entered, the ureters should be identified.

The transperitoneal approach to the abdominal aorta is the most common abdominal aortic exposure performed for trauma. The midline laparotomy incision allows for concurrent repair of other intra-abdominal injuries. Like the trauma laparotomy, the incision extends from the xiphoid to the pubis but can be extended cephalad for supraceliac exposure or combined with a midline sternotomy for wide exposure of injuries to multiple body compartments.

Supraceliac Aorta

In cases of hemodynamic instability, supraceliac aortic cross clamping can be achieved transabdominally during laparotomy. Direct access to the supraceliac aorta can be achieved by incising the diaphragm to access the chest or by dividing the triangular ligament of the liver and retracting the left lobe laterally to expose the aorta at the hiatus (Fig. 7.12). Passing a nasogastric tube can facilitate identification of the esophagus at the gastroesophageal junction. Dividing the gastrohepatic ligament, taking care to avoid injury to a replaced left hepatic artery that could be coursing beneath it, will allow the esophagus to be mobilized to the patient's left to expose the aorta. An aortic occluder can be used to compress the aorta against the spine. Alternatively, if the patient's condition allows, a clamp or umbilical tape can be used to gain vascular control after circumferentially exposing the supraceliac aorta. Alternatively, the supraceliac aorta can be exposed via a complete left medial visceral rotation, although this typically requires more time and dissection to achieve adequate exposure.

Visceral Segment

The visceral segment of the aorta is exposed through right or left medial visceral rotation. The celiac axis is best approached by a right medial visceral rotation to expose the proximal abdominal aorta. The celiac axis is surrounded by dense ganglionic and lymphatic tissue. Active bleeding in this area can be controlled with proximal aortic control in the chest through transdiaphragmatic approach or thoracotomy. The celiac axis can be ligated if the superior mesenteric artery is patent. Similarly, the common hepatic artery can be ligated if the portal vein and gastroduodenal arteries are intact. The splenic vein or artery can be ligated if necessary but should be followed by splenectomy.

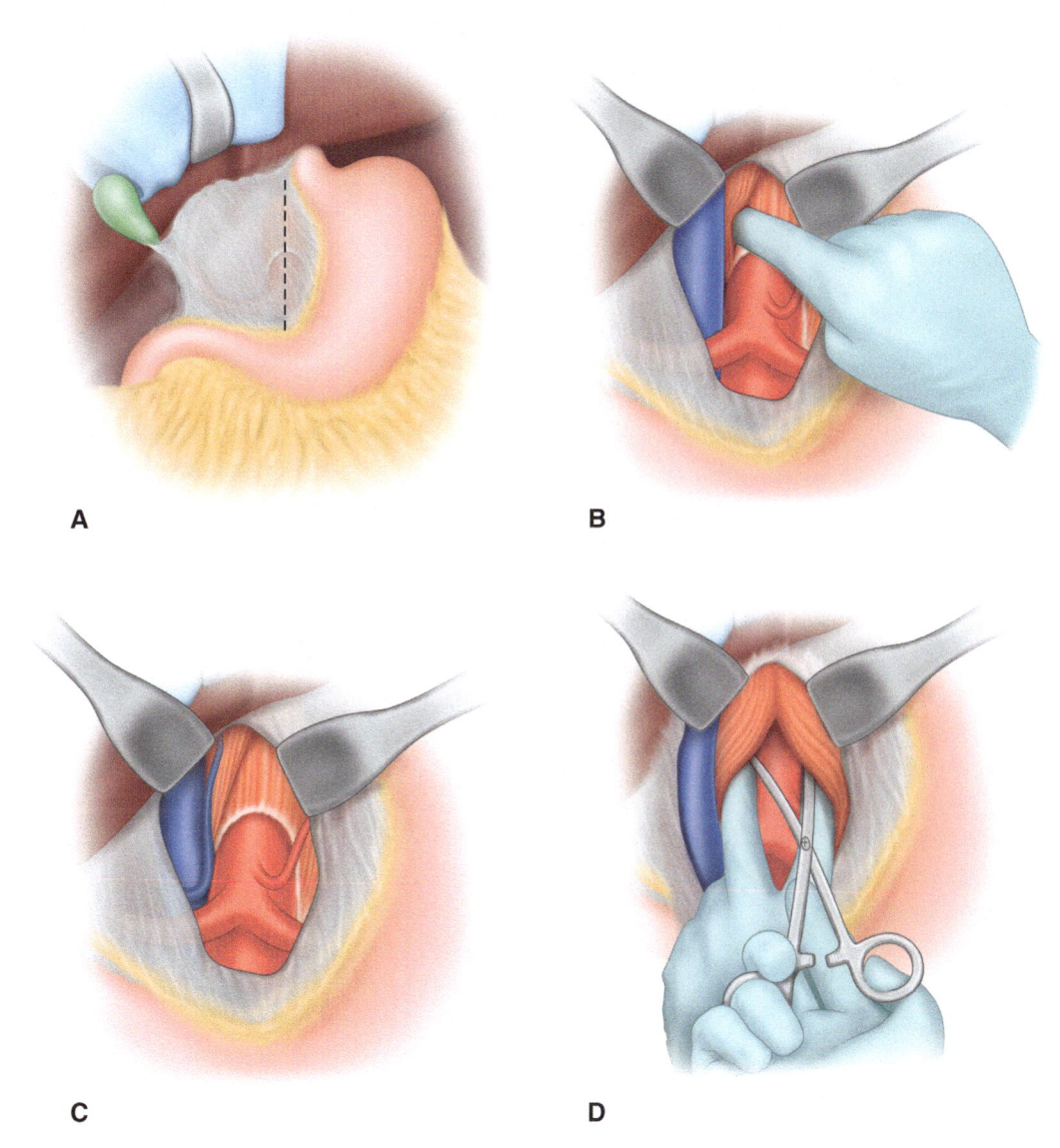

Fig. 7.12 Supraceliac aortic exposure (**a**) Dotted line indicates the location for division of the gastrohepatic ligament (**b**) The diaphragmatic crus lies posterior to the gastrohepatic ligament (**c**) Bluntly divide the fibers of the crus (**d**) Following circumferential dissection, the aorta can be clamped (From Blazick and Conrad [45])

Infrarenal Aorta

The infrarenal aorta can be isolated and clamped to control pelvic or lower extremity hemorrhage. To access the infrarenal aorta, reflect the greater omentum and transverse colon cephalad and cover them with a moist laparotomy pad. Retract the small bowel to the right to expose the ligament of Treitz. Divide the ligament of Treitz along the jejunum. Ligate the inferior mesenteric vein for improved exposure. Beware that the left renal vein will be found crossing the anterior surface of the aorta and is encountered within several centimeters after dividing the ligament of Treitz and exposing the anterior surface of the aorta.

Retroperitoneal Approach

Retroperitoneal exposure of the abdominal aorta distal to the SMA can be attained through a standard retroperitoneal incision over the 11th rib, from the posterior axillary line to the anterior border of the rectus sheath (Fig. 7.13). Exposure of the visceral segment can be achieved only if the incision is positioned over a higher rib space. The pleural cavity can be avoided if the posterior

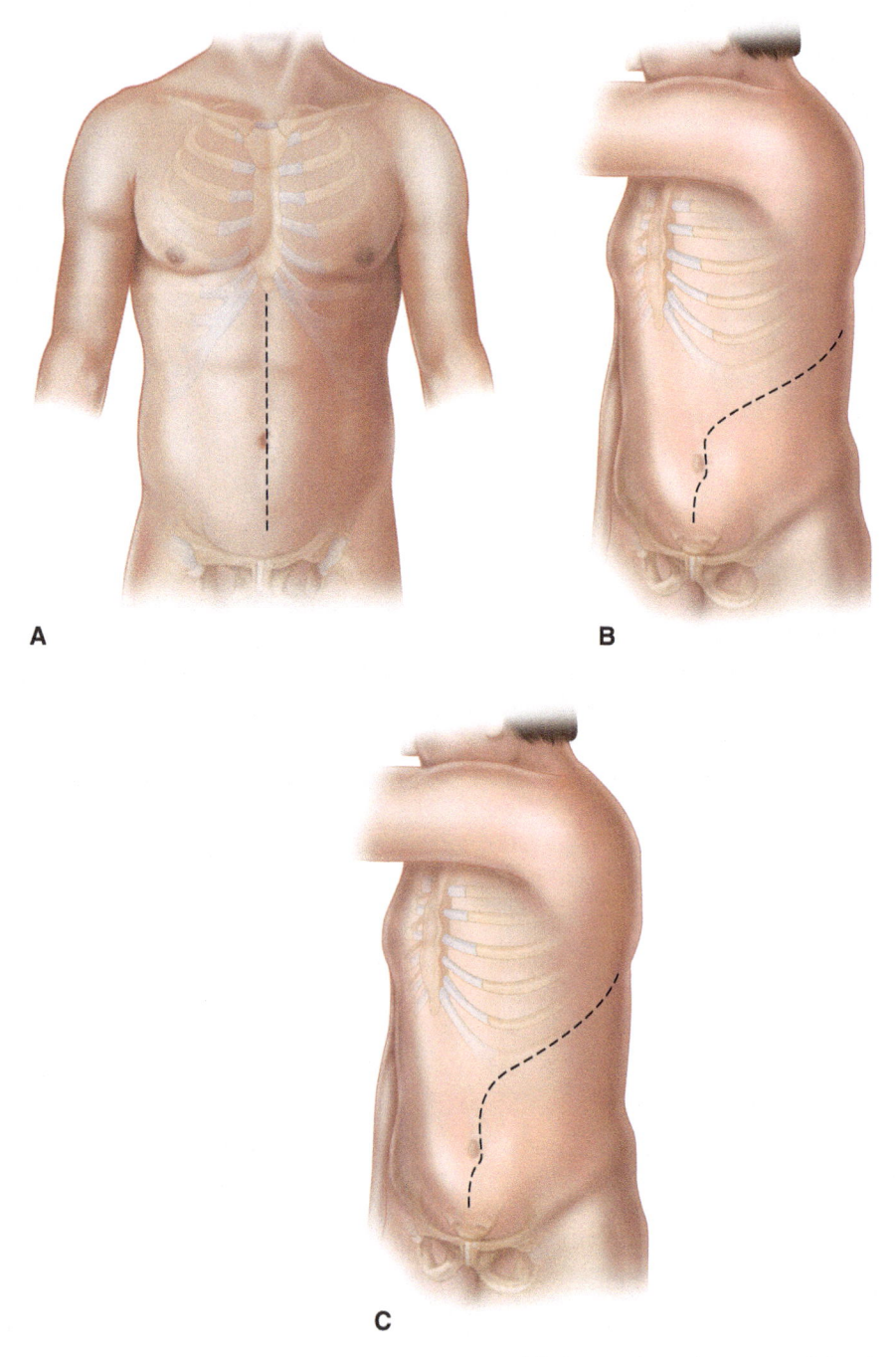

Fig. 7.13 Transperitoneal vs retroperitoneal incisions for exposure of the distal aorta. The abdominal aorta can be approached through a midline laparotomy incision (**a**) or via a retroperitoneal incision created over the 11th rib space (**b**). Retroperitoneal exposure of the visceral segment may require the incision to begin over a higher rib space (**c**) (From Blazick and Conrad [45])

extension of the incision is limited. The retroperitoneal space is entered by dividing the transversalis fascia but not violating Gerota's fascia. Resection of the distal segment of the 11th rib can facilitate identification of this plane as the transversalis fascia and transversus abdominal musculature insert at the inferior border of this rib. The aorta is most commonly approached in the retrorenal plane; however, if there is a retroaortic renal vein, the aorta can be approached anterorenally. Regardless of approach, the ureter should be identified and retracted toward the midline. The renal artery can be traced medially to identify the aorta. The renal lumbar vein should be ligated to avoid excessive bleeding when mobilizing the kidney. The infrarenal aorta can then be circumferentially exposed for clamping. The left iliac vein can course posteriorly to the aortic bifurcation and should be avoided during dissection. The left common iliac artery can be clamped with this approach, while the right common iliac artery can be controlled with a concurrently placed occlusion balloon. Circumferential control of the iliacs is not advisable through this approach, as the iliac veins are frequently adherent to the posterior aspect of the arteries and may be easily injured, compounding blood loss.

Resuscitative Endovascular Balloon Occlusion of the Aorta (REBOA)

Background

Endovascular aortic occlusion is a concept from the 1950s that has only recently gained acceptance for use in trauma patients [24]. First used during the Korean War as an adjunct to resuscitate injured patients, evolution in endovascular technology has allowed Resuscitative Endovascular Balloon Occlusion of the Aorta (REBOA) to be employed more widely and with fewer complications than in decades past [25].

Technique

Despite advancements in techniques and technology, the basic steps of performing REBOA have remained relatively unchanged. The five essential steps outlined by Stannard et al. include arterial access, balloon selection and positioning, balloon inflation, balloon deflation, and sheath removal [18]. Variations in the approach to balloon inflation and deflation have been described to reduce distal ischemia and extend the possible duration of aortic occlusion [26]. These techniques are addressed separately later in this chapter.

Arterial access, most commonly in the common femoral artery, is necessary to perform REBOA. Both open cutdown and percutaneous techniques have been described [18, 27]. After sheath placement, a balloon catheter capable of fully occluding the aorta is advanced retrograde into the aorta and inflated until distal pulses are no longer palpable. Manual proprioceptive feedback perceived as increasing resistance to inflation, a loss of distal pulses, and improvement in proximal hemodynamics signify complete aortic occlusion. Various imaging techniques including fluoroscopy, ultrasound, and x-ray have been described to confirm proper positioning (Fig. 7.14) [27–29]. The anatomic level of occlusion has important implications for the duration of occlusion that can be physiologically tolerated. It is generally recommended to begin with Zone 1 occlusion until sources of hemorrhage have been identified [30]. If bleeding is isolated to the pelvis and lower extremities, repositioning to Zone 3 occlusion can then be accomplished. Importantly, the duration of Zone 1 occlusion should be limited to as short as possible (less than an hour) to limit irreversible ischemia in distal organs and hemodynamic collapse upon reperfusion [31]. Zone 3 occlusion can be tolerated for longer with reports of survival following several hours of occlusion [29, 32–34]. Additional techniques to extend the duration of occlusion are addressed later in this chapter.

Complications from arterial injury and access remain a challenge following REBOA [33, 35]. Although continued advances in catheter technology now make it possible for catheter placement through sheaths that do not necessitate arterial repair, case reports suggest that even 7 French sheaths may result in distal thrombosis [36]. When larger sheaths are used, such as the 12 French sheath required for placement of a Coda catheter, the practitioner must be cognizant of the potential for sheath-induced limb ischemia that

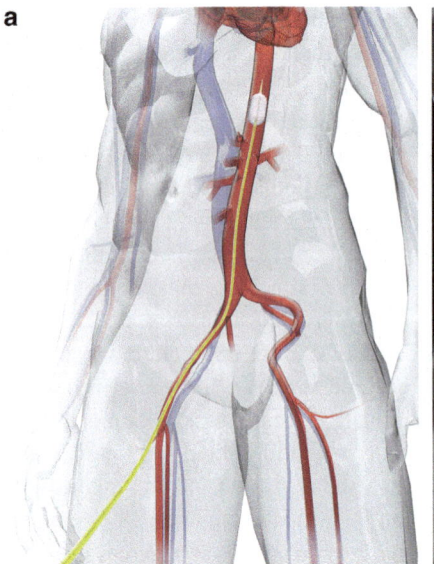

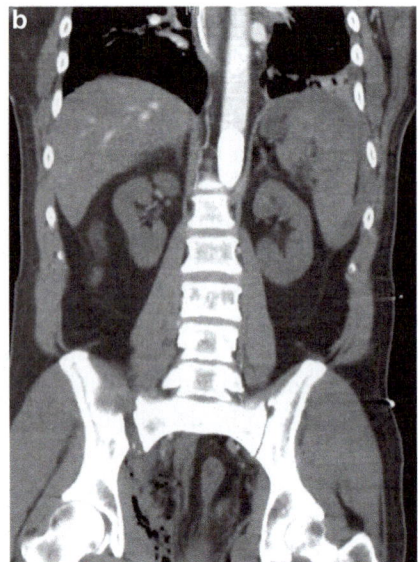

Fig. 7.14 Occlusion of the supraceliac aorta with an endovascular aortic occlusion balloon. Anatomic representation of REBOA in Zone 1 of the aorta (**a**) Anatomic representation of Zone 1 positioning (**b**) CT aortography showing contrast-containing REBOA balloon in Zone 1 of the aorta. Complete occlusion can be confirmed by absence of distal aortic contrast (Figure b from Brenner et al. [29])

has required amputation in some cases. Furthermore, all sheaths have the potential to result in pseudoaneurysms, thrombosis, distal embolization, and free extravasation at the site of insertion. Concerns for limb ischemia, challenges encountered during sheath insertion, and prolonged durations of access should all guide the practitioner to consider continued careful exploration with ultrasound or angiography if necessary to fully evaluate the femoral arteries prior to decannulation.

Mechanics and Duration of Aortic Occlusion

Regardless of endovascular or open approach, aortic occlusion creates immediate and significant alterations in physiology and blood flow throughout the body. Distal hemostasis and increases in blood pressure and blood flow to proximal organs including the heart, lungs, and brain contribute to the potential life-saving ability of this maneuver. However, not all of the effects are beneficial. Left ventricular afterload increases tremendously, myocardial oxygen consumption rises, and distal organ ischemia begins at occlusion and progressively worsens the longer occlusion continues [26]. Prolonged aortic occlusion may also result in pulmonary dysfunction including adult respiratory distress syndrome and cerebral edema. Ideally, proximal aortic occlusion should be limited to 30 min or less to avoid permanent injury [31]. Infrarenal aortic occlusion can be tolerated for hours if necessary; however, the building ischemia in distal tissue beds may induce hemodynamic instability upon the restoration of systemic circulation [32].

Techniques for Extending the Duration of Aortic Occlusion

Intermittent Occlusion

Temporarily releasing the aortic clamp or deflating the REBOA balloon may allow momentary perfusion of distal tissue beds. This technique has been described as a potential means for extending the duration of aortic occlusion with REBOA in Japan [32, 37]. However, experts hypothesize that the hemodynamic shifts resulting from rapid washout of ischemic metabolites during short periods of perfusion undermine the body's autoregulatory mechanisms and may be detrimental to patient survival [26]. Vasodilated ischemic tissue beds create a low-resistance, high-capacitance system that results in a profound loss of aortic afterload and cardiac output when occlusion is lifted, only to be immediately reversed again when occlusion is reapplied. Animal studies have demonstrated that this approach does not reduce ischemic injury or improve survival compared to complete occlusion of the same duration [37].

Partial Occlusion

As an alternative approach to providing distal perfusion, partial aortic occlusion has been studied in animal models and is starting to be described in human trauma patients [36, 38–41]. After control of major hemorrhage has been achieved (i.e., tourniquets applied, abdomen packed, chest opened), slow reintroduction of systemic circulation is begun as hemodynamically tolerated [41]. Low-volume distal blood flow is maintained until definitive hemorrhage control has been completed and the patient is hemodynamically stable enough to tolerate full reintroduction of distal blood flow. This approach is primarily described as an endovascular technique for use with REBOA; however, some surgeons have anecdotally reported performing a similar technique with manual occlusion of the aorta. Partial occlusion requires a dedicated provider to monitor the patient's vital signs and titrate aortic occlusion accordingly. The transition from complete endovascular aortic occlusion to partial REBOA requires additional attention to maintain proper balloon positioning as the loss of frictional forces between the aortic wall and the deflating balloon, combined with increased proximal blood pressure, can lead to catheter migration or prolapse [38]. Partial REBOA has been demonstrated in animal models to reduce the effects of distal ischemia and proximal overpressure injury compared to complete REBOA, but its application in human patients is only just beginning [40, 42].

Conclusion

Mechanical hemorrhage control remains a critical skill for the effective treatment of blast-injured patients with bleeding. Surgeons faced with these injuries must understand the potential and limitations of vascular control options in the acute setting – both open and endovascular.

References

1. Eastridge BJ, Mabry RL, Seguin P, Cantrell J, Tops T, Uribe P, et al. Death on the battlefield (2001–2011): implications for the future of combat casualty care. J Trauma Acute Care Surg. 2012;73(6 Suppl 5):S431–7.
2. Blackbourne LH, Czarnik J, Mabry R, Eastridge B, Baer D, Butler F, et al. Decreasing killed in action and died of wounds rates in combat wounded. J Trauma. 2010;69(Suppl 1):S1–4.
3. DePalma RG, Burris DG, Champion HR, Hodgson MJ. Blast injuries. N Engl J Med. 2005;352(13):1335–42.
4. Wolf SJ, Bebarta VS, Bonnett CJ, Pons PT, Cantrill SV. Blast injuries. Lancet. 2009;374(9687):405–15.
5. Hull JB, Bowyer GW, Cooper GJ, Crane J. Pattern of injury in those dying from traumatic amputation caused by bomb blast. Br J Surg. 1994;81(8):1132–5.
6. Hull JB. Traumatic amputation by explosive blast: pattern of injury in survivors. Br J Surg. 1992;79(12):1303–6.
7. Nessen SC, Lounsbury DE, Hetz SP, editors. War surgery in Afghanistan and Iraq: a series of cases, 2003–2007 (textbooks of military medicine). 1st ed. Washington, DC: Walter Reed Army Medical Center Borden Institute; 2008.
8. Blackbourne LH, Baer DG, Eastridge BJ, Kheirabadi B, Bagley S, Kragh JF Jr, et al. Military medical revolution: prehospital combat casualty care. J Trauma Acute Care Surg. 2012;73(6 Suppl 5):S372–7.
9. Kragh JF Jr. Use of tourniquets and their effects on limb function in the modern combat environment. Foot Ankle Clin. 2010;15(1):23–40.
10. Singleton JA, Gibb IE, Hunt NC, Bull AM, Clasper JC. Identifying future 'unexpected' survivors: a retrospective cohort study of fatal injury patterns in victims of improvised explosive devices. BMJ Open. 2013;3(8):e003130.
11. Alarhayem A, Myers J, Dent D, Eastridge B. No Time to bleed: the impact of time from injury to the operating room on survival in patients with hemorrhage from blunt abdominal trauma. AAST; Sept 2015; Las Vegas, NV.
12. Kue RC, Temin ES, Weiner SG, Gates J, Coleman MH, Fisher J, et al. Tourniquet use in a civilian emergency medical services setting: a descriptive analysis

of the Boston EMS experience. Prehosp Emerg Care. 2015;19(3):399–404.
13. King DR, Larentzakis A, Ramly EP, Boston Trauma C. Tourniquet use at the Boston Marathon bombing: lost in translation. J Trauma Acute Care Surg. 2015;78(3):594–9.
14. Kheirabadi BS, Terrazas IB, Miranda N, Estep JS, Corona BT, Kragh JF Jr, et al. Long-term effects of combat ready clamp application to control junctional hemorrhage in swine. J Trauma Acute Care Surg. 2014;77(3 Suppl 2):S101–8.
15. Cubano M, editor. Emergency war surgery. 4th ed. Fort Sam Houston: Office of the Surgeon General. Borden Institute. Department of the Army; 2013.
16. Carrick MM, Morrison CA, Pham HQ, Norman MA, Marvin B, Lee J, et al. Modern management of traumatic subclavian artery injuries: a single institution's experience in the evolution of endovascular repair. Am J Surg. 2010;199(1):28–34.
17. Kragh JF Jr, Kirby JM, Ficke JR. Chapter 9: Extremity injury. In: Savitsky E, Eastridge B, editors. Combat casualty care: lessons learned from OEF and OIF. Washington, DC: Department of the Army, Office of the Surgeon General, Borden Institute; 2012. p. 777.
18. Stannard A, Eliason JL, Rasmussen TE. Resuscitative endovascular balloon occlusion of the aorta (REBOA) as an adjunct for hemorrhagic shock. J Trauma. 2011;71(6):1869–72.
19. Smith RS, Chang FC. Traumatic rupture of the aorta: still a lethal injury. Am J Surg. 1986;152(6):660–3.
20. LF P, TW M, WC M, EJ J. Nonpenetrating traumatic injury of the aorta. Circulation. 1958;17(6):1086–101.
21. Kaewlai R, Avery LL, Asrani AV, Novelline RA. Multidetector CT of blunt thoracic trauma 1. Radiographics. 2008;28(6):1555–70.
22. Crawford ES, Svensson LG, Hess KR, Shenaq SS, Coselli JS, Safi HJ, et al. A prospective randomized study of cerebrospinal fluid drainage to prevent paraplegia after high-risk surgery on the thoracoabdominal aorta. J Vasc Surg. 1991;13(1):36–46.
23. Biffl WL, Fox CJ, Moore EE. The role of REBOA in the control of exsanguinating torso hemorrhage. J Trauma Acute Care Surg. 2015;78(5):1054–8.
24. Hughes CW. Use of an intra-aortic balloon catheter tamponade for controlling intra-abdominal hemorrhage in man. Surgery. 1954;36(1):65–8.
25. DuBose JJ, Scalea TM, Brenner M, Skiada D, Inaba K, Cannon J, et al. The AAST prospective Aortic Occlusion for Resuscitation in Trauma and Acute Care Surgery (AORTA) registry: data on contemporary utilization and outcomes of aortic occlusion and resuscitative balloon occlusion of the aorta (REBOA). J Trauma Acute Care Surg. 2016;81(3):409–19. Publish Ahead of Print.
26. Russo R, Neff LP, Johnson MA, Williams TK. Emerging endovascular therapies for noncompressible torso hemorrhage. Shock. 2016;46(3S):12–9.
27. Scott DJ, Eliason JL, Villamaria C, Morrison JJ, Rt H, Spencer JR, et al. A novel fluoroscopy-free, resuscitative endovascular aortic balloon occlusion system in a model of hemorrhagic shock. J Trauma Acute Care Surg. 2013;75(1):122–8.
28. Guliani S, Amendola M, Strife B, Morano G, Elbich J, Albuquerque F, et al. Central aortic wire confirmation for emergent endovascular procedures: as fast as surgeon-performed ultrasound. J Trauma Acute Care Surg. 2015;79(4):549–54.
29. Brenner ML, Moore LJ, DuBose JJ, Tyson GH, McNutt MK, Albarado RP, et al. A clinical series of resuscitative endovascular balloon occlusion of the aorta for hemorrhage control and resuscitation. J Trauma Acute Care Surg. 2013;75(3):506–11.
30. Holcomb JB, Fox EE, Scalea TM, Napolitano LM, Albarado R, Gill B, et al. Current opinion on catheter-based hemorrhage control in trauma patients. J Trauma Acute Care Surg. 2014;76(3):888–93.
31. Andres J, Scott J, Giannoudis PV. Resuscitative endovascular balloon occlusion of the aorta (REBOA): what have we learned? Injury. 2016;47(12):2603–5.
32. Ogura T, Lefor AT, Nakano M, Izawa Y, Morita H. Nonoperative management of hemodynamically unstable abdominal trauma patients with angioembolization and resuscitative endovascular balloon occlusion of the aorta. J Trauma Acute Care Surg. 2015;78(1):132–5.
33. Saito N, Matsumoto H, Yagi T, Hara Y, Hayashida K, Motomura T, et al. Evaluation of the safety and feasibility of resuscitative endovascular balloon occlusion of the aorta. J Trauma Acute Care Surg. 2015;78(5):897–903. discussion 4.
34. Tsurukiri J, Akamine I, Sato T, Sakurai M, Okumura E, Moriya M, et al. Resuscitative endovascular balloon occlusion of the aorta for uncontrolled haemorrhagic shock as an adjunct to haemostatic procedures in the acute care setting. Scand J Trauma Resusc Emerg Med. 2016;24(1):13.
35. Norii T, Crandall C, Terasaka Y. Survival of severe blunt trauma patients treated with resuscitative endovascular balloon occlusion of the aorta compared with propensity score-adjusted untreated patients. J Trauma Acute Care Surg. 2015;78(4):721–8.
36. Davidson AJ, Russo RM, DuBose JJ, Roberts J, Jurkovich GJ, Galante JM. Potential benefit of early operative utilization of low profile, partial resuscitative endovascular balloon occlusion of the aorta (P-REBOA) in major traumatic hemorrhage. Trauma Surg Amp Acute Care Open. 2016;1(1):e000028.
37. Morrison JJ, Ross JD, Rt H, Watson JD, Sokol KK, Rasmussen TE. Use of resuscitative endovascular balloon occlusion of the aorta in a highly lethal model of noncompressible torso hemorrhage. Shock. 2014;41(2):130–7.
38. Ho rer TM, Cajander P, Jans A, Nilsson KF. A case of partial aortic balloon occlusion in an unstable multi-trauma patient. Trauma. 2016;18(2):150–4.
39. Okumura E, Tsurukiri J, Oomura T, Tanaka Y, Oomura R. Partial resuscitative endovascular balloon occlusion of the aorta as a hemorrhagic shock

adjunct for ectopic pregnancy. Am J Emerg Med. 2016;34(9):1917.e1–2.
40. Russo RM, Neff LP, Lamb CM, Cannon JW, Galante JM, Clement NF, et al. Partial resuscitative endovascular balloon occlusion of the aorta in swine model of hemorrhagic shock. J Am Coll Surg. 2016;223(2):359–68.
41. Johnson MA, Neff LP, Williams TK, JJ DB, Group ES. Partial Resuscitative Balloon Occlusion of the AORTA (P-REBOA): clinical technique and rationale. J Trauma Acute Care Surg. 2016;81(5):S133–7.
42. Russo RM, Williams TK, Grayson JK, Lamb CM, Cannon JW, Clement NF, et al. Extending the golden hour: partial resuscitative endovascular balloon occlusion of the aorta in a highly lethal swine liver injury model. J Trauma Acute Care Surg. 2016;80(3):372–80.
43. Dubose JJ. Chapter 7: Thoracic vascular and great vessel hemorrhage: big red and big blue. In: Ball C, editor. Treatment of ongoing hemorrhage: the art and craft of stopping severe bleeding. Cham: Springer; 2018.
44. Muscat JO, Rogers W, Cruz AB, RCJ S. Arterial injuries in Orthopaedics: the posteromedial approach for vascular control about the knee. J Orthop Trauma. 1996;10(7):476–80.
45. Blazick E, Conrad MF. Chapter 22: Advanced aneurysm management techniques: open surgical anatomy and repair. In: Mulholland MW, editor. Operative techniques in surgery. Volume 2. Part 6. Section 7. Philadelphia: Wolters Kluwer Health – Lippincott Williams & Wilkins; 2015.

Blast-Related Pelvic Fractures

George C. Balazs and Jean-Claude G. D'Alleyrand

Introduction

Traumatic pelvic ring disruptions are uncommon injuries. Analyses of large trauma registries in both the United Kingdom and United States have identified pelvic fractures in approximately 8% of patients treated at trauma centers [1, 2]. Trauma patients with pelvic fractures are significantly more likely to have higher Injury Severity Scores and in-hospital mortality rates than those without them. While pelvic fractures are usually closed injuries, 3–8% of them are open in civilian trauma [2–5], with most open injuries occurring in younger individuals involved in motor vehicle accidents. Early literature on pelvic fractures reported early mortality rates of around 50% in patients with open injuries, largely due to acute hemorrhage and deep space infection [6–9]. However, series from the 1980s and 1990s reported substantially lower mortality, generally attributing this decrease to advances in hemorrhage control, soft tissue management, and resuscitative techniques [10–13].

G. C. Balazs · J. -C. G. D'Alleyrand (✉)
Department of Orthopaedic Surgery, Walter Reed National Military Medical Center,
Bethesda, MD, USA

Norman M. Rich Department of Surgery, Uniformed Services University of Health Sciences,
Bethesda, MD, USA
e-mail: jeanclaude.g.dalleyrand.mil@mail.mil

Pelvic blast injuries generate the severest form of open pelvic fractures and are associated with very high mortality rates and long-term disability among survivors. While explosive munitions have accounted for greater than 70% of combat injuries in recent conflicts [14, 15], advances in body armor have increased the survival rate among wounded servicemembers [16, 17]. In addition, the modern era has also seen an increased frequency of explosive munitions used against civilian populations [18]. Consequently, both military and civilian surgeons should be familiar with the basic principles of management and reconstruction in these complex, critically ill patients.

Pelvic Anatomy and the Effect of Explosive Blasts

The two hemipelves are connected to each other anteriorly at the symphysis pubis and to the sacrum posteriorly via the sacroiliac joints. The pelvic ring is reinforced by stout ligaments both anteriorly and posteriorly and is divided into two sections. The true pelvis contains the pelvic cavity and is comprised of the ischium, the pubis, and the portion of the ilium caudal to the arcuate line. The false pelvis surrounds the lowest portions of the abdominal cavity and is comprised of the ilium cephalad to the arcuate line. Multiple large caliber vessels pass through the pelvis supplying the lower extremities, as do the lumbar and sacral neural plexuses. When the pelvis is fractured or penetrated, all of these structures are at risk, potentially resulting in massive hemorrhage, organ failure, and permanent neurologic compromise.

Most pelvic ring disruptions occur via direct compression or through a traction mechanism, as with forced abduction of the hip, with most civilian pelvic injuries occurring in motor vehicle accidents, industrial mishaps, or falls from a height [19]. Young and Burgess classified pelvic fractures based on the direction of forces applied to the pelvis and the resulting modes of bony and ligamentous failure (anterior-posterior compression, lateral compression, and vertical shear) [20]. However, many fracture patterns do not conform to this classification system, which is why many surgeons prefer to use the Tile classification [21–23], which triages pelvic disruptions based on overall ring instability: stable, rotationally or translationally unstable, or unstable to both rotation and translation.

Pelvic blast injuries are fundamentally different from typical civilian pelvic fractures, so traditional classification and treatment schemes have limited utility. Blast-related fractures occur via a number of mechanisms, including compressive forces and penetrating trauma. Associated wounds are typically extensive, potentially including a substantial burn component, depending on blast proximity and the nature of the munitions. Hollow viscus rupture secondary to the primary blast wave and embedded environmental debris dramatically increase the contamination burden of wounds. Wounds are rarely, if ever, limited to the pelvis and extremity amputations are common [24]. Patients are critically ill, more prone to atypical infection, and require extensive surgical care over a period of months or years. Return to normal function is highly uncommon, even with optimal care.

In short, pelvic blast injuries represent a unique injury pattern that requires a comprehensive initial assessment, immediate lifesaving interventions, ongoing reassessment to monitor for complications and missed injuries, and long-term multidisciplinary care by surgical, medical, and rehabilitative specialists.

Prehospital Care

Most patients with a pelvic blast injury will die at the point of injury. Ramasamy et al. (2012) reviewed the records of 89 UK military personnel with a blast-injured pelvis; only 29 (33%) survived long enough to return to the United Kingdom [24]. Bailey et al. reviewed the records of 104 combat casualties with pelvic fractures who died of their wounds. Seventy-six percent of the injuries were due to blast mechanisms, and 77% were considered non-survivable on the basis of the injuries sustained [25]. Hollow viscus injury and large caliber vessel injury are significantly more common in penetrating pelvis injuries, as are proximal lower extremity amputations [23, 24, 26, 27]. Despite the fact that solid organ and cardiopulmonary injuries are far more common in blunt pelvic fractures than in penetrating pelvic trauma, patients with a blast-injured pelvis will die at a significantly higher rate than those with either closed pelvic fractures or perineal soft tissue wounds without fracture [26]. In most cases, these deaths occur due to massive hemorrhage, as opposed to multi-organ injury, since modern body armor is extremely effective at protecting the head, thorax, and abdomen. It is vital that treating personnel understand the extremely high mortality rates associated with this injury, since early, rapid intervention provides the only chance of survival. No factors are more important for patient survival than urgent transport to a higher level of surgical care and rapid hemorrhage control at the time of injury [16, 24].

Intrapelvic hemorrhage occurs through one of two mechanisms. Large vessel hemorrhage may occur from penetrating shrapnel or from gross fracture fragment displacement. In such cases, it is difficult to control bleeding even in an operating room setting; in the prehospital environment it is nearly impossible to manage these types of wounds and patients expire rapidly. Fortunately, this comprises the minority of cases, even in blast injuries [28]. More commonly, the small-caliber venous network in the pelvis will bleed as the pelvic ring is disrupted. While these vessels can usually be controlled via tamponade, proximal vascular control is infrequently necessary for hemostasis.

The volume of the pelvic cavity in the setting of an intact pelvic ring has been estimated at 1.5 L, meaning that the transfusion of 4–6 units of packed red blood cells may be sufficient to maintain adequate hemodynamics if the intrapelvic bleeding tamponades itself. However, with the loss of pelvic ring integrity, the potential space of the pelvic cavity dramatically increases, in some cases in excess of the entire intravascular volume [29, 30]. In high-energy pelvic fractures, rupture of the parapelvic fascia, sacroiliac ligaments, and pelvic floor may permit hemorrhage extravasation into the subcutaneous tissues, perineum, retroperitoneum, and the proximal lower extremities [31, 32]. With open fractures, the ability to tamponade is further inhibited by the communication of the intrapelvic space with the environment.

The goal of emergent management of these injuries is to minimize and stabilize the size of the intrapelvic space. Thus, the two key lifesaving interventions are the application of a circumferential binder and the sealing of open wounds. Binding of the pelvis may be accomplished with either a prefabricated binder or a simple bed sheet, wrapped and clamped tightly at the level of the greater trochanters. Inexperienced personnel will often apply binders at the level of the iliac crest, but this should be scrupulously avoided, since not only will such placement not facilitate tamponade, but it may also increase intra-abdominal pressure and decrease the ability to adequately ventilate patients [33]. In the hospital setting, before tightening the device, it is important that assistants manually close down the pelvic volume by pulling on the overlapped ends of the binder while reducing any shortening or malrotation of the lower extremities. This method generally requires three people: two on either side of the pelvis and a third manipulating the lower extremities via the feet. In a prehospital environment, however, this is often not feasible, and the focus should be the application of the binder as quickly as possible with maximal force to close down the intrapelvic space [34].

Sealing of open wounds should be accomplished with whatever dressings are available. In order to tamponade hemorrhage in patients suspected of having an open pelvic fracture, dressings should be forcefully inserted into open wounds until no more dressings can be inserted. If available, using long rolls of gauze, tied end-to-end, is preferred and facilitates retrieval at a later time. The Committee on Tactical Combat Casualty Care (TCCC) recommends the use of hemostatic dressings such as chitosan-based products when addressing compressible hemorrhage not amenable to extremity tourniquets [35], although these dressings require sustained, vigorous pressure at time of application in order to work effectively [36].

First responders may be reluctant to perform these interventions due to concerns about soft tissue damage from compressing the fractured pelvis with a binder or of increasing the chances of late sepsis by placing non-sterile packing into open wounds. However, within the UK armed forces, where all blast-injured casualties are presumed to have a pelvic fracture and are placed in a binder at the point of injury, no significant problems due to over-reduction or fracture displacement have been reported to date [37]. It must be emphasized that these patients are by definition in extremis. Thus, all concerns about later complications are secondary to the need for immediate lifesaving interventions. No matter how quickly a binder and dressings are applied, patients with a blast-related pelvic fracture sustain substantial blood loss and will be in some degree of hypovolemic shock. Adequate resuscitation, management of other injuries, and rapid transportation to facilities with surgical care are equally necessary to maximize chances of survival.

Acute Surgical Care

All patients with an unstable, blast-related pelvic injury require surgical intervention to maximize their chances of survival. At a minimum, receiving facilities need to have both orthopedic and general surgery capabilities. Care provided in the trauma bay should be limited to a primary ATLS survey and necessary interventions that can be performed rapidly [16]. In general, the blast-injured patient's vital signs, mechanism of injury, and clinical examination should provide sufficient information to the treating surgeon to indicate them for operative care, and any additional preoperative diagnostics or interventions should be limited to those guiding or assisting intraoperative care. The airway should be secured if not already done so, adequate intravenous or intraosseous access obtained, and hemostatic resuscitation begun or continued. Anterior-posterior radiographs of the pelvis and chest will provide important preoperative information and may give surgeons an early understanding of bony injury patterns affecting their ability to stabilize the patient. A focused abdominal sonography for trauma (FAST) ultrasound may be useful to evaluate for intra-abdominal or pericardial injury but carries a high risk of false-negative results in the setting of a pelvic fracture and will often not provide useful additional information in the setting of a blast-injured pelvis [38, 39]. Laboratory studies and advanced imaging such as computerized axial tomography (CT) may be considered, but should never delay transport to the operating room for a patient who is in extremis, as urgent transport to the operating room is the primary priority.

The first goal of the surgeon in the operating room is hemostasis, and this begins before the skin is incised. Even previously stable patients can rapidly exsanguinate during otherwise routine preparation in the operating room. Transfer to the OR table can dislodge tenuous clots, temporary cessation of resuscitation fluids can allow a patient with ongoing blood loss to become hypovolemic, and removal of the pelvic binder for skin preparation will end its tamponade effect and may allow renewed bleeding into the pelvic cavity.

In many cases, an external fixator can be placed prior to wound exploration or entering the pelvic cavity. This should be done before the pelvic binder is removed, because the binder will hold the pelvic volume reduced as pins are placed and bars are tightened. A properly placed binder will leave the iliac crest exposed. Placement of pins in the iliac crest is preferred for initial stabilization, since it can be accomplished without fluoroscopy and is much faster than placement of supraacetabular pins [32]. The use of three pins in each gluteal tubercle should provide sufficient control even if one pin is not placed properly into the ilium. In very urgent cases, lifesaving surgical hemostasis can be achieved with a pelvic wrap in place. This may require judicious windows to be cut out of the material, which is easier to do when using a sheet instead of a commercial binder, and this reduces the degree of sterility that can be maintained during the procedure.

A triangular configuration of spanning bars is optimal, since lower profile constructs may inhibit access to the injured pelvis, impede laparotomy, or constrict the abdomen as it swells during the early postoperative period. Once bony stabilization is achieved, a midline laparotomy incision should be used to gain access to the pelvic space and hemostasis obtained. In most cases this can be accomplished with pelvic packing, which is much more effective if the ring has already been stabilized with an external fixator. Unlike closed pelvic fractures with hemodynamic instability, there is generally no role for angiography in the acute management of pelvic blast injuries. Angiography requires specialized facilities and equipment, does not generally allow for the concurrent surgical procedures necessary to stabilize blast-injured patients, and is generally effective for only arterial, not venous, bleeding. Pelvic packing and direct control methods are preferred for the blast-injured pelvis, where extensive surgical debridement will facilitate direct access to injured structures.

In cases where large caliber vessel injury is present or bleeding is so extensive that packing is ineffective, the surgeon should attempt to obtain proximal control. It is critically important that proximal vessel ligation be performed at the lowest possible level, since all downstream tissues are at extremely high risk of necrosis. This can create near-insurmountable reconstructive challenges at a later date, limiting the availability of

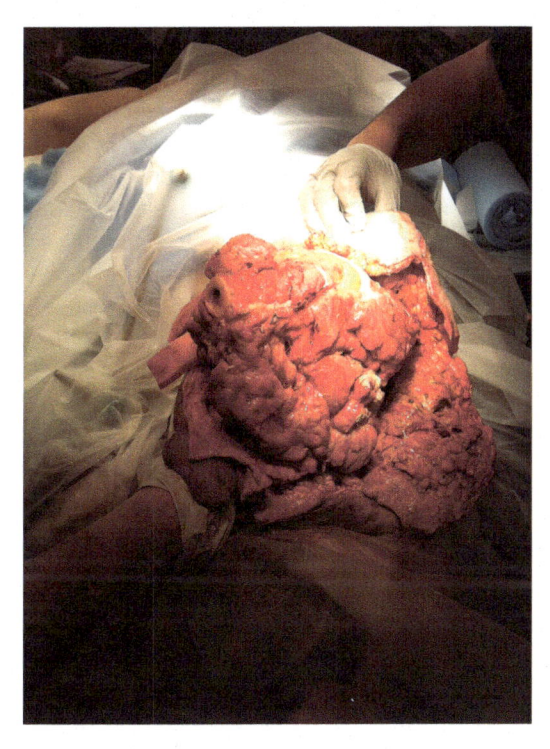

Fig. 8.1 This patient required ligation of his bilateral common iliac vessels during initial resuscitation. The resulting ischemia, combined with the evolving zone of injury and angioinvasive fungal infection, left him with no tissue available for closure. Positioned here in the right lateral decubitus position, his short residual femur and extensive soft tissue degloving are evident

local muscle and fasciocutaneous flaps and potentially requiring a more proximal limb amputation or even hemipelvectomy for soft tissue closure [40] (Fig. 8.1). That being said, we have encountered patients where ligation of the common iliac artery was necessary to control life-threatening hemorrhage. In these extreme cases, the challenges of future reconstruction are secondary to the dire need for emergent hemostasis.

Following hemorrhage control, initial debridement should be performed. The pelvis is a challenging body cavity to debride, owing to blind tissue planes adjacent to critical structures and multiple potential spaces. In a blast injury, contamination burden should be presumed to be high, and every effort should be made to ensure that all pockets of nonviable material are identified and removed. Several studies have demonstrated lower rates of pelvic sepsis and secondary muscle necrosis with thorough debridement [41–43]. Attention should also be paid to any regions of degloved skin, which must be explored and debrided. If possible, incision placement for debridement should also consider future operative approaches for bony fixation, though this is not possible in all situations. The thoroughness of this initial debridement needs to be balanced with limiting operative time to minimize hypothermia-induced coagulopathy and the amount of transfused blood products needed. In the US military, our tendency is to use sterile saline via gravity lavage, as this is often faster than pulsed lavage and comparisons of the safety and efficacy of the two techniques suggest that gravity lavage yields equivocal, if not better, results [44–46].

Historically, soft tissue management of open pelvic fractures emphasized the need to leave wounds open to allow them to drain, in order to prevent fluid accumulation and subsequent abscess development. While this principle of delaying definitive closure remains generally true, modern soft tissue management also considers future reconstruction and minimizing wound size to facilitate eventual closure or coverage. We attempt to save skin whenever possible, and although the skin edges are always debrided back to healthy borders at time of closure, in the debridements leading up to closure, we will preserve abraded or necrotic skin if that helps facilitate temporary coverage between surgical procedures, provided that there is no suspicion of fungal elements in the subcutaneous fat. We liberally use retention sutures to maintain soft tissue tension and prevent further wound retraction in the days between debridements, as long as the skin tension does not risk injury to underlying structures. We have also had good experience with negative pressure wound therapy (NPWT), which allows for fluid drainage while simultaneously promoting tissue perfusion and preventing wound retraction. However, since these devices apply negative pressure to the entire wound bed, they may increase bleeding if applied to fresh wounds with large areas of exposed capillary beds, such as after a thorough debridement in an acutely injured patient, or if applied to intact but

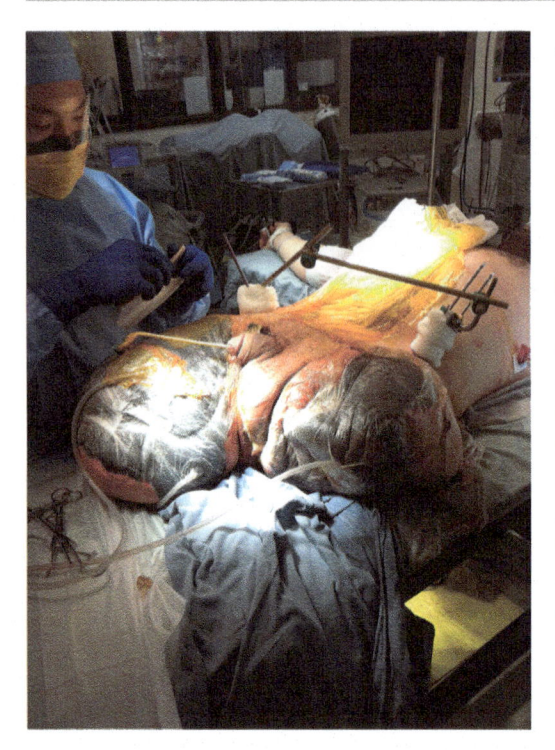

Fig. 8.2 The patient from Fig. 8.1, after hip disarticulation. Obtaining an adequate seal with NPWT of wounds, this close to the perineum can be quite challenging

exposed larger caliber vessels. Additionally, it can be very difficult to generate and maintain a NPWT seal around external fixator pins and the perineum (Fig. 8.2). For these reasons, it is sometimes preferable to use a bead pouch technique.

In cases of gross contamination or infection, we emplace vancomycin- and/or tobramycin-impregnated polymethylmethacrylate beads on nonabsorbable suture. In the less common cases of invasive fungal infection, we have also placed amphotericin-impregnated beads, though this is preceded by a consideration of the risk of nephrotoxicity. Multiple cases of invasive fungal infections following blast injury have been treated by military surgeons [47], so we routinely send fungal cultures as part of our debridement protocol to detect this uncommon but frequently fatal complication, with a low threshold to start local and/or parenteral antifungal therapy. When the decision is made to use antibiotic beads, we usually create a bead pouch with an occlusive dressing, rather than covering the beads with a NPWT dressing, to minimize the removal of the antibiotic "broth" [48]. There is also limited evidence that antibiotic beads, compared to NPWT dressings, may have lower late infection rates at dramatically reduced cost [49].

The initial surgery on the pelvis should generally be limited to hemostasis, debridement and provisional external fixation, although laparotomy or acute bladder repair/suprapubic catheter placement may also be necessary. Diverting colostomy has been intermittently advocated in the setting of open pelvic fractures due to the risks of fecal contamination of the pelvic cavity and open perineal wounds [9, 21]. This remains controversial, with mixed evidence on whether this actually reduces infection risk [50–53] and substantial concerns about the morbidity of the diversion procedure and later reanastomosis [54]. There is stronger evidence for diverting colostomy in the presence of rectal, colonic, or vaginal injury, or Faringer zone I injuries [51, 55].

Internal skeletal fixation should almost never be performed at the index surgery, given the substantially higher rates of infectious complications and premature hardware removal with early definitive open reduction and internal fixation [24]. In rare cases, percutaneous fixation of large fragments may be appropriate, such as with isolated iliac crest fractures that cannot be controlled with an external fixator.

Once initial surgery is complete, patients require ICU-level care for hemodynamic monitoring and respiratory support. In cases of aggressive local infection or concerns of developing sepsis, patients may require daily operative debridement, but we typically repeat operative debridements every 48–72 h, depending on the degree of contamination and severity of injury. In the interim, continued aggressive resuscitation, advanced imaging, and laboratory studies should be performed.

Reconstructive Care

Traditional teaching is that highly contaminated open fractures should be serially debrided until the wound bed is clean and free of infection, after which primary closure or flap coverage may be performed. Prior studies have shown gram-positive bacterial colonization of wounds close to the time of injury and predominantly gram-negative colonization in wounds that are more evolved [56–58]. However, isolates obtained from wound cultures frequently do not match the bacterial profile of subsequent infections [56, 59], and the use of pre- and post-debridement wound cultures has not been recommended [60]. As such, surgeons are left to use their clinical judgment on when to definitively close or cover these traumatic wounds. There are some studies that correlate certain proinflammatory biomarkers, such as procalcitonin, with suitability for wound closure [61–63], but assaying for these markers has not found its way into mainstream clinical practice as of this time. For the reconstructive surgeon managing a patient with a blast-injured pelvis, this lack of available, applicable evidence creates substantial difficulties in objectively determining appropriate timing and methods of fixation and closure.

Historically, open pelvic fractures have had very high rates of deep space infection, and it has been observed that this is generally the cause of most late deaths. Consequently, the traditional teaching has been that internal fixation is rarely, if ever, appropriate [20, 64, 65]. Tile argued that the presence of any skin lesion or anorectal injury created an unacceptable risk of infection and mandated the use of external fixation as definitive treatment [66]. The experience of the military orthopedic surgeons with blast injuries seems to support this perspective. The massive contamination of wounds resulting from explosive munitions results in high rates of both early and late infections, even with optimal surgical care [67, 68]. The 10% overall rate of combat-related wound infections is substantially less than that seen in combat-related pelvic blast injuries, where case series have reported rates of 83–86% [24, 40]. The major concern with this approach to treatment is that external fixation is frequently insufficient to restore anatomic alignment of the pelvis following blast injury. This is especially true in the setting of posterior ring disruptions, where an external fixator provides insufficient stability to maintain the sacroiliac joints in a reduced position.

Other authors have advocated for judicious use of internal fixation in the setting of open pelvic fractures, arguing that percutaneous fixation of the sacroiliac joint or limited plating of the anterior symphysis provides superior maintenance of reduction with minimal increase in the hardware infection. Dong et al. [69] reported on 41 open pelvic fractures, of which 45% underwent open reduction and internal fixation following serial debridement. While injury severity, soft tissue injury pattern, and initial Glasgow Coma Scale were predictive of mortality, the use of internal fixation was not [69]. A separate multicenter retrospective analysis of 39 open pelvic fractures at US and Canadian civilian trauma centers did not find internal fixation to adversely affect outcome or increase the need for secondary procedures [23]. However, great care should be taken when attempting to rely on these reports in the setting of blast injury, where contamination burden is much higher, early infection is more frequent, and rates of late infection are poorly defined.

If the decision is made to definitively treat patients with external fixation alone, surgeons must accept that the weight-bearing ring may remain unstable or malunited, creating pain with attempted sitting, standing, or ambulation. It is unclear, however, whether this is an actual clinical problem. In a series of 29 blast-injured patients with open pelvic fractures, none of the 8 patients definitively treated with external fixation required a late osteotomy or stabilizing pelvic procedure, whereas 4 of the 7 patients treated with internal fixation required premature hardware removal due to deep space infection [24]. As the authors point out, "removal of internal fixation from the pelvis after complex soft-tissue reconstruction is not a trivial procedure." Our general approach is to assess the adequacy of reduction in an external fixator, the expected functional status of the patient, and the maturity of the wound environment. External fixators are converted to supraacetabular frames when feasible, due to their superior control of the pelvic ring, and we will often place iliosacral screws once the wounds have evolved and the process of soft tissue closure has begun. However, the benefits of restoring pelvic continuity are always weighed against the risks of internal fixation.

Closure of wounds is similarly individualized. The goal of soft tissue reconstruction is the coverage of exposed bone with tissue that is adequately padded to resist shear forces. Most wounds are not amenable to primary wound closure, but often a partial closure can be achieved, minimizing the size of the area requiring flap coverage. If deeper tissue layers can be closed over exposed bone, adjunctive treatments such as dermal substitutes may facilitate final coverage with skin grafting [70–72] (Fig. 8.3). Local rotational flaps may be unavailable due to a paucity of viable tissue or due to a desire to preserve local tissue in order to optimize function. Accordingly, free-flap coverage may provide the best option for wound coverage, although options for vascular anastomoses may be limited in the blast-injured pelvis. Our plastic surgery partners have utilized anterolateral thigh, rectus femoris, and gracilis flaps with good results. Rectus abdominis flaps should be avoided when possible due to the associated reduction in core strength [73].

Outcomes of Treatment

Patients sustaining blast injuries of the pelvis face significant physical and emotional challenges. As discussed above, the majority of patients will die at the point of injury, with the remainder remaining at risk of early exsanguination and late sepsis. Associated injuries are extremely common and remain another substantial source of disability and mortality [27]. While advances in treatment may have improved survival rates, these patients remain challenging to manage throughout their care, thus reasonable expectations of functional recovery should be fostered in patients and their families from very early in their course.

Perhaps the biggest source of non-orthopedic morbidity in surviving patients is genitourinary injury. Prior to the recent conflicts in Iraq and Afghanistan, up to one-third of GU injuries were renal, usually secondary to gunshot wounds and shrapnel injuries of the kidneys or ureters, although improvements in body armor for military personnel have caused upper GU tract injuries to become less common [74]. As a result of the increasing usage of improvised explosive devices during these most recent conflicts, 5% of all combat casualties sustained GU injury, and up to 25% of patients with a pelvic blast injury had a traumatic partial or complete loss of genitalia [26, 75]. Primarily affecting men, such injuries threaten not only testosterone production but also sexual and urinary function, as well as future fertility [74, 76, 77]. As of 2013, more than 1300 American servicemembers had sustained genitourinary injuries

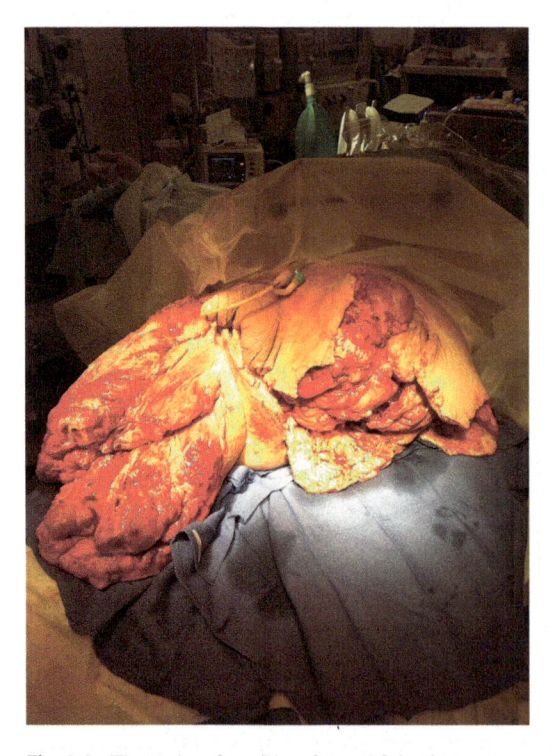

Fig. 8.3 The patient from Figs. 8.1 and 8.2, after conversion to modified hemipelvectomy. A hip disarticulation had been sufficient to address his angioinvasive fungal infection. However, his ischium was partially skeletonized, and he was not a candidate for any wound coverage aside from STSG. Performing a more proximal resection allowed primary coverage over the weight-bearing portion of his pelvis, facilitating his sitting without pain or recurrent skin breakdown

in Iraq and Afghanistan, with 147 sustaining loss of at least one testicle [78].

The initial management of these injuries focuses on standard principles of hemorrhage control, through debridement, and urinary diversion [79]. Orchiectomy is performed in cases of significant testicular trauma, as prior attempts at testicular salvage were generally unsuccessful [79]. When at all possible, sperm banking prior to testicular debridement is institutionalized in the UK armed forces but is not a standard practice in the United States [80]. At least one author has identified concerns about future fertility as more important to combat casualties than eventual sexual function [74]. Longer-term management of severe lower GU injuries focuses on genital reconstruction and hormone replacement.

Another source of long-term morbidity is impaired ambulation. While most patients surviving combat-related open pelvic fractures regain some degree of ambulatory function [27], a return to functional ambulation is difficult or impossible for many of them. In a series of 17 patients with open pelvic fractures following civilian trauma, Ferrera and Hill found that nearly half of patients required some sort of assistance to ambulate [13]. Patients with open pelvic fractures due to explosives likely do far worse. There is a strong association with lower extremity amputation(s), which are frequently high transfemoral amputations [16]. More proximal amputations increase the metabolic expenditure necessary to ambulate, and high transfemoral amputees are very difficult to fit with prosthetics. In the less common cases of hip disarticulation or traumatic hemipelvectomy, patients may have no capability for independent ambulation [40, 73].

Additional challenges for patients may include post-traumatic stress disorder, fecal incontinence, need for permanent colostomy, late infection, and heterotopic ossification causing skin breakdown or difficulty with sitting and prosthetic wear. Our experience has been that early engagement of multiple subspecialists is the key to maximizing functional outcome in the long term.

Conclusion

Pelvic blast injuries are devastating injuries that are frequently associated with severe comorbidities such as limb amputation, traumatic brain injury, and injury to abdominal and pelvic organs. The majority of patients will die at the point of injury due to massive hemorrhage, though in some cases this can be prevented by the rapid application of a pelvic binder and hemostatic dressings. Upon arrival to a trauma center, surviving patients require care from numerous surgical subspecialists. Initial management focuses on hemorrhage control and debridement, with intermediate and late efforts devoted to prevention of infection, bony stabilization, and soft-tissue coverage. Even with optimal care, survivors typically require multiple late procedures for management of GU injuries, colorectal injuries, and amputation management. While most survivors are able to return to independent living, decreasing levels of function and difficulties with independent ambulation are common.

References

1. Giannoudis PV, Grotz MR, Tzioupis C, et al. Prevalence of pelvic fractures, associated injuries, and mortality: the United Kingdom perspective. J Trauma. 2007;63(4):875–83.
2. Yoshihara H, Yoneoka D. Demographic epidemiology of unstable pelvic fracture in the United States from 2000 to 2009: trends and in-hospital mortality. J Trauma Acute Care Surg. 2014;76(2):380–5.
3. Hanson PB, Milne JC, Chapman MW. Open fractures of the pelvis. Review of 43 cases. J Bone Joint Surg (Br). 1991;73(2):325–9.
4. Dente CJ, Feliciano DV, Rozycki GS, et al. The outcome of open pelvic fractures in the modern era. Am J Surg. 2005;190(6):830–5.
5. Black EA, Lawson CM, Smith S, Daley BJ. Open pelvic fractures: the University of Tennessee Medical Center at Knoxville experience over ten years. Iowa Orthop J. 2011;31:193–8.
6. Perry JF Jr. Pelvic open fractures. Clin Orthop Relat Res. 1980;151:41–5.
7. Maull KI, Sachatello CR, Ernst CB. The deep perineal laceration-an injury frequently associated with open pelvic fractures: a need for aggressive surgical management. A report of 12 cases and review of the literature. J Trauma. 1977;17(9):685–96.

8. Rothenberger D, Velasco R, Strate R, Fischer RP, Perry JF Jr. Open pelvic fracture: a lethal injury. J Trauma. 1978;18(3):184–7.
9. Raffa J, Christensen NM. Compound fractures of the pelvis. Am J Surg. 1976;132(2):282–6.
10. Davidson BS, Simmons GT, Williamson PR, Buerk CA. Pelvic fractures associated with open perineal wounds: a survivable injury. J Trauma. 1993;35(1):36–9.
11. Richardson JD, Harty J, Amin M, Flint LM. Open pelvic fractures. J Trauma. 1982;22(7):533–8.
12. Govender S, Sham A, Singh B. Open pelvic fractures. Injury. 1990;21(6):373–6.
13. Ferrera PC, Hill DA. Good outcomes of open pelvic fractures. Injury. 1999;30(3):187–90.
14. Belmont PJ, Owens BD, Schoenfeld AJ. Musculoskeletal injuries in Iraq and Afghanistan: epidemiology and outcomes following a decade of war. J Am Acad Orthop Surg. 2016;24(6):341–8.
15. Penn-Barwell JG, Roberts SA, Midwinter MJ, Bishop JR. Improved survival in UK combat casualties from Iraq and Afghanistan: 2003–2012. J Trauma Acute Care Surg. 2015;78(5):1014–20.
16. Mamczak CN, Elster EA. Complex dismounted IED blast injuries: the initial management of bilateral lower extremity amputations with and without pelvic and perineal involvement. J Surg Orthop Adv. 2012;21(1):8–14.
17. Mazurek MT, Ficke JR. The scope of wounds encountered in casualties from the global war on terrorism: from the battlefield to the tertiary treatment facility. J Am Acad Orthop Surg. 2006;14(10 Spec No.):S18–23.
18. Covey DC, Born CT. Blast injuries: mechanics and wounding patterns. J Surg Orthop Adv. 2010;19(1):8–12.
19. Mc Cormack R, Strauss EJ, Alwattar BJ, Tejwani NC. Diagnosis and management of pelvic fractures. Bull NYU Hosp Jt Dis. 2010;68(4):281–91.
20. Burgess AR, Eastridge BJ, Young JW, et al. Pelvic ring disruptions: effective classification system and treatment protocols. J Trauma. 1990;30(7):848–56.
21. Brenneman FD, Katyal D, Boulanger BR, Tile M, Redelmeier DA. Long-term outcomes in open pelvic fractures. J Trauma. 1997;42(5):773–7.
22. Pascarella R, Del Torto M, Politano R, Commessatti M, Fantasia R, Maresca A. Critical review of pelvic fractures associated with external iliac artery lesion: a series of six cases. Injury. 2014;45(2):374–8.
23. Jones AL, Powell JN, Kellam JF, McCormack RG, Dust W, Wimmer P. Open pelvic fractures. A multicenter retrospective analysis. Orthop Clin North Am. 1997;28(3):345–50.
24. Ramasamy A, Evans S, Kendrew JM, Cooper J. The open blast pelvis: the significant burden of management. J Bone Joint Surg (Br). 2012;94(6):829–35.
25. Bailey JR, Stinner DJ, Blackbourne LH, Hsu JR, Mazurek MT. Combat-related pelvis fractures in non-survivors. J Trauma. 2011;71(1 Suppl):S58–61.
26. Mossadegh S, Tai N, Midwinter M, Parker P. Improvised explosive device related pelvi-perineal trauma: anatomic injuries and surgical management. J Trauma Acute Care Surg. 2012;73(2 Suppl 1):S24–31.
27. Purcell RL, McQuade MG, Kluk MW, Gordon WT, Lewandowski LR. Combat-related pelvic ring fractures in survivors. CurrOrthop Prac. 2017;28(2):173–8.
28. Huittinen VM, Slatis P. Postmortem angiography and dissection of the hypogastric artery in pelvic fractures. Surgery. 1973;73(3):454–62.
29. Moss MC, Bircher MD. Volume changes within the true pelvis during disruption of the pelvic ring--where does the haemorrhage go? Injury. 1996;27(Suppl 1):S-A21–3.
30. Ghanayem AJ, Wilber JH, Lieberman JM, Motta AO. The effect of laparotomy and external fixator stabilization on pelvic volume in an unstable pelvic injury. J Trauma. 1995;38(3):396–400. discussion 400-391.
31. Dyer GS, Vrahas MS. Review of the pathophysiology and acute management of haemorrhage in pelvic fracture. Injury. 2006;37(7):602–13.
32. Suzuki T, Smith WR, Moore EE. Pelvic packing or angiography: competitive or complementary? Injury. 2009;40(4):343–53.
33. Bonner TJ, Eardley WG, Newell N, et al. Accurate placement of a pelvic binder improves reduction of unstable fractures of the pelvic ring. J Bone Joint Surg (Br). 2011;93(11):1524–8.
34. Lee C, Porter K. The prehospital management of pelvic fractures. Emerg Med J. 2007;24(2):130–3.
35. Anonymous A. TCCC updates: tactical combat casualty care guidelines for medical personnel: 3 June 2015. J Spec Oper Med. 2015;15(3):129–47.
36. D' Alleyrand JC, Dutton RP, Pollak AN. Extrapolation of battlefield resuscitative care to the civilian setting. J Surg Orthop Adv. 2010;19(1):62–9.
37. Jansen JO, Thomas GO, Adams SA, et al. Early management of proximal traumatic lower extremity amputation and pelvic injury caused by improvised explosive devices (IEDs). Injury. 2012;43(7):976–9.
38. Arvieux C, Thony F, Broux C, et al. Current management of severe pelvic and perineal trauma. J Visc Surg. 2012;149(4):e227–38.
39. Ballard RB, Rozycki GS, Newman PG, et al. An algorithm to reduce the incidence of false-negative FAST examinations in patients at high risk for occult injury. Focused assessment for the sonographic examination of the trauma patient. J Am Coll Surg. 1999;189(2):145–50. discussion 150-141.
40. D'Alleyrand JC, Lewandowski LR, Forsberg JA, et al. Combat-related hemipelvectomy: 14 cases, a review of the literature and lessons learned. J Orthop Trauma. 2015;29(12):e493–8.
41. Kudsk KA, Hanna MK. Management of complex perineal injuries. World J Surg. 2003;27(8):895–900.
42. Kudsk KA, McQueen MA, Voeller GR, Fox MA, Mangiante EC Jr, Fabian TC. Management of

42. complex perineal soft-tissue injuries. J Trauma. 1990;30(9):1155–9. discussion 1159–1160.
43. Birolini D, Steinman E, Utiyama EM, Arroyo AA. Open pelviperineal trauma. J Trauma. 1990;30(4):492–5.
44. Investigators F, Bhandari M, Jeray KJ, et al. A trial of wound irrigation in the initial management of open fracture wounds. N Engl J Med. 2015;373(27):2629–41.
45. Owens BD, White DW, Wenke JC. Comparison of irrigation solutions and devices in a contaminated musculoskeletal wound survival model. J Bone Joint Surg Am. 2009;91(1):92–8.
46. Nikfarjam M, Weinberg L, Fink MA, et al. Pressurized pulse irrigation with saline reduces surgical-site infections following major hepatobiliary and pancreatic surgery: randomized controlled trial. World J Surg. 2014;38(2):447–55.
47. Lewandowski LR, Weintrob AC, Tribble DR, et al. Early complications and outcomes in combat injury-related invasive fungal wound infections: a case-control analysis. J Orthop Trauma. 2016;30(3):e93–9.
48. Stinner DJ, Hsu JR, Wenke JC. Negative pressure wound therapy reduces the effectiveness of traditional local antibiotic depot in a large complex musculoskeletal wound animal model. J Orthop Trauma. 2012;26(9):512–8.
49. Warner M, Henderson C, Kadrmas W, Mitchell DT. Comparison of vacuum-assisted closure to the antibiotic bead pouch for the treatment of blast injury of the extremity. Orthopedics. 2010;33(2):77–82.
50. Faringer PD, Mullins RJ, Feliciano PD, Duwelius PJ, Trunkey DD. Selective fecal diversion in complex open pelvic fractures from blunt trauma. Arch Surg. 1994;129(9):958–63. discussion 963-954.
51. Lunsjo K, Abu-Zidan FM. Does colostomy prevent infection in open blunt pelvic fractures? A systematic review. J Trauma. 2006;60(5):1145–8.
52. Pell M, Flynn WJ Jr, Seibel RW. Is colostomy always necessary in the treatment of open pelvic fractures? J Trauma. 1998;45(2):371–3.
53. Woods RK, O'Keefe G, Rhee P, Routt ML Jr, Maier RV. Open pelvic fracture and fecal diversion. Arch Surg. 1998;133(3):281–6.
54. Pachter HL, Hoballah JJ, Corcoran TA, Hofstetter SR. The morbidity and financial impact of colostomy closure in trauma patients. J Trauma. 1990;30(12):1510–3.
55. Grotz MR, Allami MK, Harwood P, Pape HC, Krettek C, Giannoudis PV. Open pelvic fractures: epidemiology, current concepts of management and outcome. Injury. 2005;36(1):1–13.
56. Tong MJ. Septic complications of war wounds. JAMA. 1972;219(8):1044–7.
57. Murray CK, Roop SA, Hospenthal DR, et al. Bacteriology of war wounds at the time of injury. Mil Med. 2006;171(9):826–9.
58. Weintrob AC, Roediger MP, Barber M, et al. Natural history of colonization with gram-negative multidrug-resistant organisms among hospitalized patients. Infect Control Hosp Epidemiol. 2010;31(4):330–7.
59. Brown KV, Murray CK, Clasper JC. Infectious complications of combat-related mangled extremity injuries in the British military. J Trauma. 2010;69(Suppl 1):S109–15.
60. Murray CK, Obremskey WT, Hsu JR, et al. Prevention of infections associated with combat-related extremity injuries. J Trauma. 2011;71(2 Suppl 2):S235–57.
61. Chromy BA, Eldridge A, Forsberg JA, et al. Wound outcome in combat injuries is associated with a unique set of protein biomarkers. J Transl Med. 2013;11:281.
62. Forsberg JA, Potter BK, Polfer EM, Safford SD, Elster EA. Do inflammatory markers portend heterotopic ossification and wound failure in combat wounds? Clin Orthop Relat Res. 2014;472(9):2845–54.
63. Hawksworth JS, Stojadinovic A, Gage FA, et al. Inflammatory biomarkers in combat wound healing. Ann Surg. 2009;250(6):1002–7.
64. Tang P, Meredick R, Prayson MJ, Gruen GS. External fixation of the pelvis. Tech Orthop. 2002;17(2):228–38.
65. Tile M. Pelvic ring fractures: should they be fixed? J Bone Joint Surg (Br). 1988;70(1):1–12.
66. Tile M. Fracture of the pelvis. In: Schatzker J, Tile M, editors. The rationale of operative fracture care. Berlin: Springer; 1987.
67. Tintle SM, Shawen SB, Forsberg JA, et al. Reoperation after combat-related major lower extremity amputations. J Orthop Trauma. 2014;28(4):232–7.
68. Blyth DM, Yun HC, Tribble DR, Murray CK. Lessons of war: combat-related injury infections during the Vietnam war and operation Iraqi and enduring freedom. J Trauma Acute Care Surg. 2015;79(4 Suppl 2):S227–35.
69. Dong JL, Zhou DS. Management and outcome of open pelvic fractures: a retrospective study of 41 cases. Injury. 2011;42(10):1003–7.
70. Seavey JG, Masters ZA, Balazs GC, et al. Use of a bioartificial dermal regeneration template for skin restoration in combat casualty injuries. Regen Med. 2016;11(1):81–90.
71. Valerio IL, Masters Z, Seavey JG, Balazs GC, Ipsen D, Tintle SM. Use of a dermal regeneration template wound dressing in the treatment of combat-related upper extremity soft tissue injuries. J Hand Surg. 2016;41(12):e453–60.
72. Helgeson MD, Potter BK, Evans KN, Shawen SB. Bioartificial dermal substitute: a preliminary report on its use for the management of complex combat-related soft tissue wounds. J Orthop Trauma. 2007;21(6):394–9.
73. D'Alleyrand JC, Fleming M, Gordon WT, Andersen RC, Potter BK. Combat-related hemipelvectomy. J Surg Orthop Adv. 2012;21(1):38–43.
74. Davendra MS, Webster CE, Kirkman-Brown J, Mossadegh S, Whitbread T. Blast injury to the perineum. J R Army Med Corps. 2013;159(Suppl 1):i1–3.

75. Williams M, Jezior J. Management of combat-related urological trauma in the modern era. Nat Rev Urol. 2013;10(9):504–12.
76. Harvey-Kelly KF, Kanakaris NK, Obakponovwe O, West RM, Giannoudis PV. Quality of life and sexual function after traumatic pelvic fracture. J Orthop Trauma. 2014;28(1):28–35.
77. Jones GH, Kirkman-Brown J, Sharma DM, Bowley D. Traumatic andropause after combat injury. BMJ Case Rep. 2015;2015:bcr2014207924.
78. Janak JC, Orman JA, Soderdahl DW, Hudak SJ. Epidemiology of genitourinary injuries among male U.S. service members deployed to Iraq and Afghanistan: early findings from the Trauma Outcomes and Urogenital Health (TOUGH) project. J Urol. 2016;197(2):414–9.
79. Sharma DM, Bowley DM. Immediate surgical management of combat-related injury to the external genitalia. J R Army Med Corps. 2013;159 (Suppl 1):i18–20.
80. Nnamani NS, Janak JC, Hudak SJ, et al. Genitourinary injuries and extremity amputation in operations enduring freedom and Iraqi freedom: early findings from the Trauma Outcomes and Urogenital Health (TOUGH) project. J Trauma Acute Care Surg. 2016;81(5 Suppl 2 Proceedings of the 2015 Military Health System Research Symposium):S95–S99.

Thoracic Injuries

Ryan P. Dumas and Jeremy W. Cannon

Thoracic injury is common in both military and civilian settings representing a primary or a contributing factor in up to 75% of all trauma-related deaths [1]. Most patients with thoracic injuries who reach medical care are able to be managed with non-operative measures and supportive measures and in some cases a tube thoracostomy [2, 3]. This chapter will highlight some important exceptions and additional considerations in the setting of blast injury.

Demographics of Thoracic Blast Injury

Over the past 15 years, 4–12% of trauma patient in the Iraq and Afghanistan conflicts sustained thoracic injuries with a mortality of approximately 10% [2–4]. By comparison, retrospective series of thoracic trauma in Vietnam, Korea, and Bosnia observed a mortality of 2–3%. Improvement in prehospital care, rapid evacuation, and protective equipment have led to more severely injured patients presenting to hospitals earlier. Historically these patients may have succumbed to their injuries on the battlefield but instead are now living to survive transport but ultimately may not survive their hospitalization in some cases.

In reviewing blast-specific demographics in thoracic injury, it is important to note that the exact incidence of blast thoracic injury from the modern conflicts is difficult to fully ascertain as the Joint Theater Trauma Registry (JTTR) simplified the classification of trauma to blunt or penetrating mechanisms and removed "blast"-specific injuries as a mechanism in 2007. Of the 2049 thoracic injuries reviewed by Ivey et al., over 60% were caused by explosive devices [3]. Historic data from terrorist attacks in the 1980s and 1990s report the incidence of blast lung injury to be anywhere from 3% to 15% [5]. However, the incidence appears to vary widely from series to series likely due to the clinical nature of the diagnosis as well as nonstandard definitions and inconsistent reporting.

Pulmonary contusions of all types—peripheral and central—represent a significant injury pattern from blast or explosions. They were the second most common injury in Ivey et al. (50.2%) and most common injury in the both Propper (31.8%) and Keneally (46.4%) series [2–4]. Blast lung as a specific subset of blast or explosive injuries to the chest has also been reported in several series with a reported incidence between 1.4% and 11% [3, 6, 7].

R. P. Dumas · J. W. Cannon (✉)
Division of Traumatology, Surgical Critical Care & Emergency Surgery, Perelman School of Medicine at the University of Pennsylvania,
Philadelphia, PA, USA
e-mail: jeremy.cannon@uphs.upenn.edu

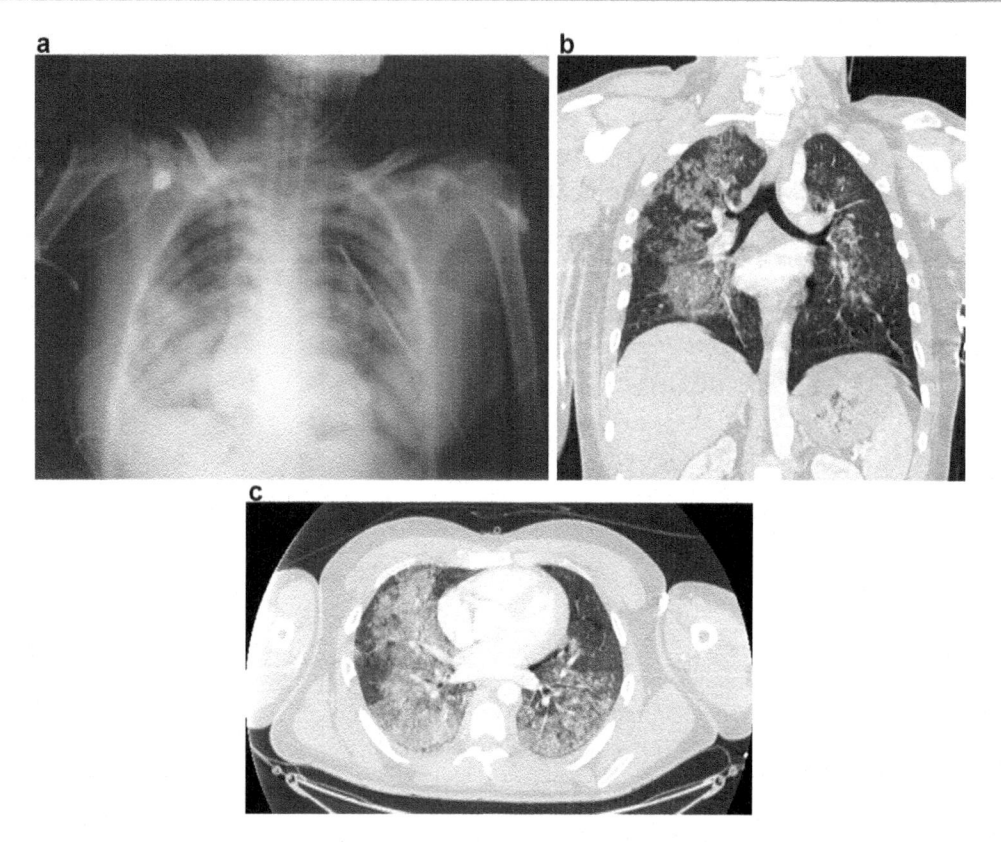

Fig. 9.1 Blast lung perihilar contusion. This contusion pattern creates the classic "batwing" appearance on CXR (**a**) with central parenchymal involvement clearly demonstrated on chest CT (**b, c**). Reproduced with permission from Hirshberg et al. [20], License # 4026721412383 (**a**) and from the American Thoracic Society. Copyright (**c**) 2017 American Thoracic Society. Johnston AM and Ballard M, Am J Respir Crit Care Med. 191(12):1462–1463, Jun 15, 2015. The American Journal of Respiratory and Critical Care Medicine is an official journal of the American Thoracic Society (**b, c**)

Initial Evaluation and Management of Thoracic Blast Injury

Thoracic Primary Blast Injury (PBI)

Primary blast injury is the most well-studied and well-described type of blast injury. It predominantly affects air-tissue interfaces such as the lungs, small and large bowel, as well as the tympanic membranes. The tympanic membrane is the most sensitive, whereas the lung requires significantly higher pressures to result in injury. Other less commonly affected systems include the central and musculoskeletal systems.

The term "blast lung" describes a severe, central pulmonary contusion that is characterized by hypoxia, hemorrhage, edema, and direct alveolar and vascular injury [8–10]. A transient spike in intrathoracic pressure caused by the blast wave displaces the chest wall toward the spinal column resulting in shearing and stressing forces resulting in a characteristic chest x-ray pattern often referred to as a "batwing" (Fig. 9.1a).

Pathophysiology

Shockwave injury was first described as early as the eighteenth century; however, a detailed understanding of the pathophysiology of blast injury on the body in general and the lung in particular did not emerge until after World War I. In 1924, Johns Hopkins physiologist D.R. Hooker first described the "Physiologic Effects of Air Concussion" [11]. He noted that "men subjected to the concussion of large shells often developed a condition of 'shock' which was unrelated to obvious traumatism since no external or internal wounds were clinically demonstrable." His observation and studies laid the foundations for subsequent experimentation and the study of blast injury. He would go onto expose animals to various explosions and correlate postmortem findings with distance from the blast epicenter.

Furthering Hooker's work, Oxford anatomist Dr. Zuckerman published his experimental study of blast injury in *The Lancet* in 1940. He described a spectrum of lung injury on postmortem analysis of animals killed by high-explosive blast. He described "severe patches of hemorrhage" as well as "hemorrhages that often follow the line of the rib." His microscopic analysis revealed torn alveolar walls and hemorrhage "originating in torn alveolar capillaries." Zuckerman ultimately concluded that "it is the pressure component of blast which bruises the lungs by its impact on the body wall," and he determined that the extent of lung injury directly correlated to the distance from the blast epicenter [12].

As detailed in Chap. 2, injury from a blast wave occurs from three distinct mechanisms: spallation, implosion, and inertia [10, 13]. In the lung, exposure to the blast wave and overpressure results in sever disruption of the airway epithelium, the vascular endothelium, and the alveoli resulting in intrapulmonary hemorrhage and potentially even air emboli [14]. Hemorrhage-induced free radical formation can also exacerbate the post-traumatic inflammatory response [15]. Ultimately, parenchymal damage results in a shunt, worsening V/Q mismatch and poor pulmonary compliance. The evolution and timing of lung insult following blast injury is detailed in Table 9.1.

Table 9.1 Timeline of blast lung injury

Inciting event	Clinical manifestation	Time from initial injury (hours)
Primary blast wave Alveolar destruction Shearing and stress forces Edema, hemorrhage Elaboration of host inflammatory mediators	Impaired gas exchange	0
Upregulation of host immune response Worsening edema Oxidative stress	Worsening gas exchange	3
Epithelial cell damage Decreased surfactant	Decrease pulmonary compliance and increased resistance	12–24
Endothelial cell damage	Worsening pulmonary mechanics	24

Adapted from Kirkman and Watts [15]

Initial Clinical Presentation

Primary blast injury to the lung is a clinical diagnosis that is supported by adjunct laboratory and radiographic data. It is important to realize however that not every patient will have symptoms, 22–50% of patients with blast lung injuries had symptoms in a review by Mackenzie et al., and only 28% of patients have hypoxia upon initial presentation [7, 16].

When symptoms do occur, clinical features of blast lung include but are not limited to dyspnea, cough, hypoxia, and cyanosis. The thoracic overpressure can also result in bradycardia, hypotension, and apnea followed by rapid shallow breathing. This constellation of findings is an immediate and direct response to the blast wave hitting the thoracic cavity and is thought to be mediated by the pulmonary C fibers and a corresponding vagal response [10, 14, 15].

Air emboli and bronchopulmonary fistula are known complications of severe blast lung injury and are thought to be responsible for many on-scene deaths following traumatic blast injury [8]. Additionally, communication between intraparenchymal airspace and pleural airspace leads to hemothorax and/or pneumothorax. To minimize these risks, initial responders should preferentially use noninvasive methods to support gas exchange [17]. If air embolism is suspected, the patient should be positioned in the left lateral decubitus position and 100% oxygen should be administered to facilitate absorption [18].

Assessment upon Arrival to Medical Care

With the caveat that some patients with blast lung injury have no symptoms, the physical examination of patients with suspected blast injury can be very informative. Patients who present with significant foamy oral secretions should immediately prompt concern for significant pulmonary edema and underlying pulmonary pathology [19]. On the other side of the spectrum, given a history consistent with an exposure to a blast, absent physical exam findings should do little to reassure the patient in the absence of adjunct data and the benefit of observation over time.

If the patient is hypoxemic or in respiratory distress, the airway should be immediately secured. In the setting of shock, absent breath sounds, or crepitus on the chest wall, thoracostomy tubes should be placed liberally using a standard open technique. Once the airway is secured and positive pressure ventilation strategies are initiated, lung compliance and resistance should be measured on the ventilator. Severe blast injury patients may have markedly reduced lung compliance even early in the course of the resuscitation; thus, we recommend the early use of low stretch lung-protective ventilator strategies in these patients.

The diagnostic modality of choice for rapid assessment of the thorax is the chest radiograph. The results of radiographs should, however, be interpreted with caution as up to 30% of patients with significant blast injuries to the chest can have a normal initial chest radiograph as the initial abnormalities can take up to 6 h to appear. Furthermore, it has been well documented that radiographs in patients with blast injury evolve and may worsen as a patient's injury "blossoms" over as much as 48 h [10].

The most common finding on plain x-ray in patient with blast injury is diffuse loss of translucency with focal opacities found in 27.1% [16]. In severe cases, the chest x-ray will demonstrate a pathognomonic "batwing" or "butterfly sign" representing bilateral, perihilar contusions [5, 10, 13, 14, 17, 19, 20]. If a "batwing" is seen on chest radiographs, this typically starts to clear in 5–7 days [13].

CT scan should be used as an adjunct in all hemodynamically stable patients with a significant injury burden and a high clinical suspicion for thoracic injury. In addition to invaluable information about the lungs, heart, and major blood vessels, CT scanning will provide a very good assessment of thoracic bony injuries like rib and thoracic spine fractures (Fig. 9.1b, c).

Prognosis and Injury Prevention

Should the causality survive the initial explosion and not succumb to hemorrhage or traumatic brain injury, the prognosis of blast lung survival ranges from 73% to 97% [10, 16, 17, 20, 21]. The majority of patients with significant blast lung injury will, however, require mechanical ventilation (76%), and most will require ventilator support within 2 h of presentation [17]. The average ICU length of stay of patients with blast lung was 12 days in one series [20].

Like acute respiratory distress syndrome (ARDS), a classification of blast lung injury (BLI) has been created. In 1999, Pizov et al. proposed a classification system based on three parameters: hypoxia, chest radiograph findings, and presence of barotrauma (i.e., pneumothorax or bronchopleural fistula) (Table 9.2). Like ARDS, they classified BLI as mild, moderate, or severe and concluded that such a classification can help predict patients that are likely to require advanced modes of ventilation [21].

Table 9.2 Blast lung injury classification

Mild	$S_PO_2 > 75\%$ without supplemental O_2 Noninvasive modes of ventilation Pneumothorax possible Bronchopleural fistula rare
Moderate	$S_PO_2 > 90\%$ on 100% FiO_2 Possible need for positive pressure ventilation PEEP of 5–10 cmH_2O Pneumothorax common
Severe	$S_PO_2 < 90\%$ on 100% FiO_2 Advanced modes of ventilation High PEEP > 10 cmH_2O Pneumothorax common Bronchopleural fistula common

Adapted from Pizov et al. [21]

The role of body armor in protecting casualties from the various types of blast injury remains a topic of active debate. Although body armor has been shown to protect casualties from penetrating projectiles, some studies suggest that body armor may worsen blast injury outcomes [22, 23]. However, others argue that this finding is a statistical artifact. By selecting out those patients who historically would have died from secondary blast (penetrating chest wounds), now patients with both survivable and non-survivable primary blast are presenting to medical treatment facilities [5].

Secondary Thoracic Blast Injury

Not only are explosives designed to generate enormous deleterious blast waves but their secondary effects are designed to be devastating as well. A significant burden of injury results from fragmentation of the explosive devices themselves. Furthermore, improvised explosive devices (IEDs) are frequently augmented with nails, ball bearings, or other projectiles designed to inflict additional secondary injuries. Much like bullets, these missiles can travel at tremendous speeds and cause significant injury. Unlike the unique physics and pathophysiology of primary blast injury, secondary blast injury from resultant projectiles much more closely resembles the injury patterns seen in the civilian population sustaining penetrating injury.

An important consideration in patients who have sustained significant secondary blast injury is large chest wall defects or open chest wounds that may mandate immediate operative intervention (Fig. 9.2). Once these injuries are identified, application of a three-sided dressing or a commercially designed chest seal is very helpful in attempts to restore pulmonary mechanics. These dressings serve as a makeshift Heimlich valve allowing air to leave the pleural space but not re-enter upon inspiration. Ivey et al. reported the incidence of open chest wounds to be 12.9% [3]. Contemporary retrospective series from both recent and past conflicts fortunately reveal that injuries to the great vessels, heart, bronchus, and esophagus are rare with an incidence ranging from 0.2% to 2.6% [2].

Although assessment of the injured patient should still proceed in adherence with ATLS guidelines, penetrating thoracic injury should immediately heighten the practitioner's concern for pneumothorax with possible tension physiology and for life-threatening cardiac injuries. If available, ultrasound examination of both the pericardium and both thoracic cavities should be performed promptly. If the absence of lung sliding is detected, there should be a low threshold for placement of a tube thoracostomy on the affected side. Furthermore, identification of pericardial fluid should prompt performance of a pericardial window, thoracotomy, or sternotomy to evaluate for cardiac lacerations. One important limitation of bedside ultrasonography is the presence of significant subcutaneous air in patients

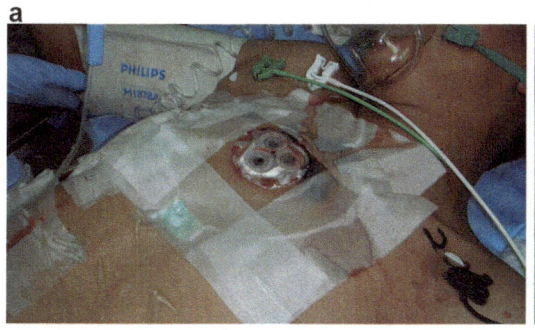

Fig. 9.2 Large chest wound resulting from secondary blast injury. This injury was temporarily closed with a commercial dressing with a built-in one-way valve which allows free egress of air from the chest (**a**). Under the dressing was a large, open chest wound which was ultimately closed with rotational pectoral flaps after surgical exploration of the mediastinum (**b**)

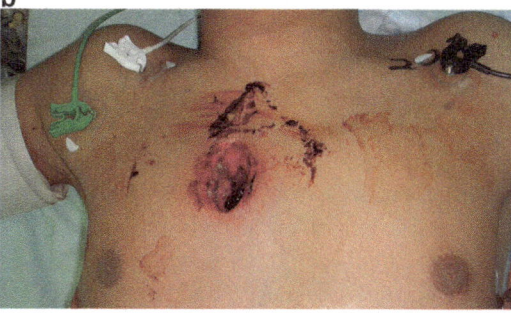

with chest wall trauma, rib fractures, and associated pneumothoraces. The presence of subcutaneous air will cause scattering of ultrasonic waves and impede image acquisition [24]. Chest radiography is also essential to the complete evaluation of patients with secondary blast injuries of the chest to evaluate for pneumothorax and hemothorax accumulation. In stable patients, CT scan is very useful in helping to identify potentially occult injuries or projectiles that may be missed on physical exam.

Large fragments and other pieces of flying debris can create significant soft tissue injuries of the chest wall and can disrupt respiratory mechanics through various mechanisms. These include destructive diaphragmatic injuries, large chest wall defects, and unstable rib fracture patterns. In general, these wounds should be addressed at the earliest possible opportunity with operative debridement of contaminated and devitalized soft tissues and, in cases of penetrating wounds near the diaphragm, exploration of the wound to evaluate for diaphragmatic integrity. Diaphragmatic injury mandates exploratory laparotomy to rule out concomitant abdominal pathology. Because these secondary wounds are typically heavily contaminated, they generally require multiple operative procedures as the zone of injury evolves in order to assure control of contamination and to minimize the risk of wound failure from premature closure.

Tertiary Thoracic Blast Injury

Explosions cause immediate disruption of surrounding buildings, structures, and vehicles, and casualties are also thrown by the effects of large blasts. These mechanisms result in tertiary blast injury. The winds generated by the blast are largely responsible for this form of blast injury. Even small explosions may generate winds up to 145 mph [9].

Thoracic trauma sustained from tertiary blast injuries is similar in injury pattern to blunt thoracic trauma. Casualties need to be evaluated for rib fractures, thoracic spine fractures, aortic injury, pulmonary lacerations as well as aerodigestive tract injuries. Management of these injuries is typically non-operative unless they are combined with additional injuries that require operative intervention. Although rib plating has not been described in a combat setting, combat casualties with severe tertiary blast injury with chest wall instability or severe deformities may benefit from such interventions at level IV or V facilities as indicated by several recent reports in the civilian literature [25, 26].

Quaternary Blast Injury

Quaternary blast injuries are sustained as a result of exposure-related insults. This injury pattern encompasses burns, inhalation injury, and exacerbations of preexisting conditions from elements like dust or asbestos. In the Keneally et al. retrospective series, burn was the third most common mechanism of injury, and patients with combined thoracic and burn injury had the highest mortality [4].

Perhaps the most relevant form of quaternary blast injury in the military setting and throughout wartime history has been inhalational injury. The development of ARDS in the setting of inhalational injury was recently studied in the military population by Belenkiy et al. in 2014. They found that inhalational injury was a significant predictor for the development of moderate to severe ARDS (OR 1.90) [27].

Inhalation injury should prompt concern in every practitioner as it has been shown to increase patient mortality by up to 20% [28]. Bronchoscopy is an invaluable tool to not only diagnose but grade inhalation injury. Inhalation injury grade has been shown in multiple studies to correlate with mortality as well as mechanical ventilation requirements. Therapy should focus on aggressive respiratory support and the use of bronchodilators, inhaled anticoagulants, and mucolytic agents as adjunct treatments [29].

ICU Management of Thoracic Blast Injury

The ICU management of thoracic blast injury is principally focused on those patients requiring conventional or advanced mechanical ventilation, fluid resuscitation, and close monitoring of their respiratory status. As previously mentioned, a significant number of patients with primary blast injury to the lungs will require mechanical ventilation. Despite the need for invasive ventilation, studies have shown that most patients are managed with conventional modes [30].

Hypoxia in the setting of blast lung should be managed like ARDS with lung-protective ventilation, low stretch tidal volumes, titration of PEEP and FiO2, and permissive hypercapnia. Ventilator settings should be titrated to the lowest possible tolerated mean airway pressure to help reduce barotrauma with continuous pulse oximetry and serial arterial blood gas analysis used to further adjust settings. Clinicians should also remember that increases in peak pressures may exacerbate or precipitate air embolism through already damaged lung. Unfortunately, the treatment of air embolism opposes that of ARDS which favors high PEEP and low FiO2. In the case of serious blast injury without evidence of pneumothorax but the need for mechanical ventilation, placement of bilateral prophylactic chest tubes should be considered. Chest tubes should be left on suction for at least the first 24 h to monitor for ongoing hemorrhage and evacuate any residual intrapleural blood. In the event of profound hypoxia, ongoing respiratory failure, and the absence of significant myocardial dysfunction, candidates should be considered for venovenous extracorporeal membrane oxygenation (vvECMO) cannulation (Fig. 9.3).

Advances in pump and gas exchange membrane technology have generally made ECMO more safe as well as compact. As such, ECMO has played an increasingly greater role in the military setting for patients with significant respiratory failure. For example, at the Landstuhl Regional Medical Center in Germany, the Acute Lung Injury Rescue Team (ALIRT) is a team of medical providers that facilitates inter-facility transfers of patients requiring ECMO [31].

Volume resuscitation of a patient with thoracic trauma can be challenging as the surgeon must balance a tenuous respiratory status with hemorrhage. Resuscitation end points should focus on achieving hemostasis while correcting lactic acidosis and maintaining urine production. As suggested by the work of Bickell et al., aggressive initial fluid management may worsen outcomes in patients who have sustained torso trauma [32], and as such permissive hypotension continues to be an area of debate in trauma circles. The applicability of permissive hypotension in blast injury, however, has been questioned as investigators have argued that blast injury physiology is different than that of regular traumatic injuries [33]. Regardless, resuscitation should be hemostatic in nature while avoiding excessive crystalloid administration as the harmful effects of crystalloid have been well described [34, 35]. Ideally, viscoelastic measures of coagulation function (e.g., TEG and ROTEM) should be used to refine the resuscitation following the initial empiric phase of blood product administration [36].

Fig. 9.3 ECMO initiation in a combat facility. Photo courtesy Dr. Sandra Wanek

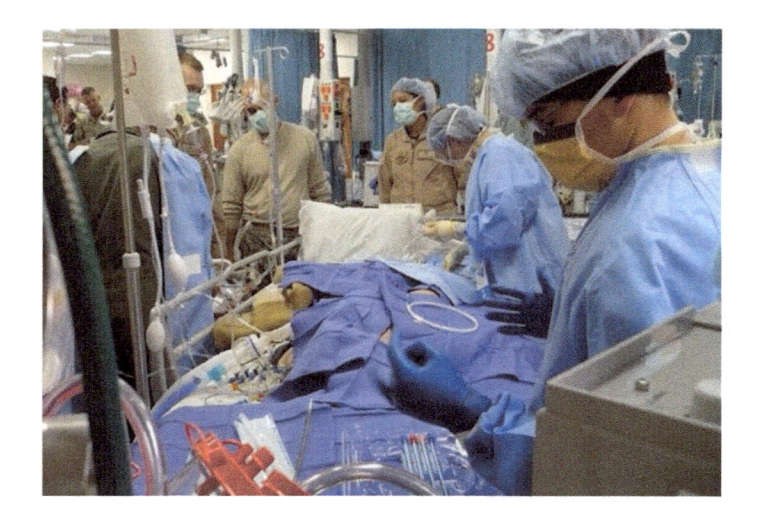

Despite injury severity and complexity, patients with combat-related blast thoracic injuries generally do well. Although there are several retrospective series addressing the epidemiology of thoracic injuries in modern combat theaters, no study specifically exams long-term outcomes and rehabilitation of these wounded soldiers. Such an investigation would be very helpful to identify treatment strategies going forward and study their subsequent outcomes on patients.

Conclusion

This chapter details the presentation and recommended management for the spectrum of blast injury to the chest. Survivors of blast events should be rapidly evacuated for surgical evaluation and management. Given the unique physics of the blast wave and its ability to cause destructive injury without external signs of trauma, surgeons and other medical providers along the continuum of care should have a high suspicion for occult primary blast injury following exposure to a blast. Furthermore, more obvious injuries from secondary blast often require operative management and should be treated as an immediate threat to life. Finally, tertiary and quaternary blast injuries are also associated with significant morbidity and frequently require advanced inpatient care. With a thorough evaluation to include adjunctive imaging and operative intervention, where indicated, followed by advanced critical care measures, survival from even the most severe forms of thoracic blast injury is possible. Future efforts should focus on evaluating potentially preventable death from thoracic blast and on long-term outcomes of these severe injuries.

References

1. Meredith JW, Hoth JJ. Thoracic trauma: when and how to intervene. Surg Clin N Am. 2007;87(1):95–118.
2. Propper BW, Gifford SM, Calhoon JH, McNeil JD. Wartime thoracic injury: perspectives in modern warfare. Ann Thorac Surg. 2010;89(4):1032–5. discussion 5–6
3. Ivey KM, White CE, Wallum TE, Aden JK, Cannon JW, Chung KK, et al. Thoracic injuries in US combat casualties: a 10-year review of Operation Enduring Freedom and Iraqi Freedom. J Trauma Acute Care Surg. 2012;73(6 Suppl 5):S514–9.
4. Keneally R, Szpisjak D. Thoracic trauma in Iraq and Afghanistan. J Trauma Acute Care Surg. 2013;74(5):1292–7.
5. Ritenour AE, Baskin TW. Primary blast injury: update on diagnosis and treatment. Crit Care Med. 2008;36(7 Suppl):S311–7.
6. de Ceballos JP, Turegano-Fuentes F, Perez-Diaz D, Sanz-Sanchez M, Martin-Llorente C, Guerrero-Sanz JE. 11 March 2004: the terrorist bomb explosions in Madrid, Spain–an analysis of the logistics, injuries sustained and clinical management of casualties treated at the closest hospital. Crit Care. 2005;9(1):104–11.
7. Smith JE. The epidemiology of blast lung injury during recent military conflicts: a retrospective database review of cases presenting to deployed military hospitals, 2003–2009. Philos Trans R Soc Lond Ser B Biol Sci. 2011;366(1562):291–4.
8. Argyros GJ. Management of primary blast injury. Toxicology. 1997;121(1):105–15.
9. Wightman JM, Gladish SL. Explosions and blast injuries. Ann Emerg Med. 2001;37(6):664–78.
10. Wolf SJ, Bebarta VS, Bonnett CJ, Pons PT, Cantrill SV. Blast injuries. Lancet. 2009;374(9687):405–15.
11. Hooker DR. Physiological effects of air concussion. Am J Phys (Legacy Content). 1924;67(2):219–74.
12. Zuckerman S. Experimental study of blast injuries to the lungs. Lancet. 1940;236(6104):219–24.
13. Shaham D, Sella T, Makori A, Appelbum L, Rivkind AI, Bar-Ziv J. The role of radiology in terror injuries. Isr Med Assoc J. 2002;4(7):564–7.
14. Sasser SM, Sattin RW, Hunt RC, Krohmer J. Blast lung injury. Prehosp Emerg Care. 2006;10(2):165–72.
15. Kirkman E, Watts S. Characterization of the response to primary blast injury. Philos Trans R Soc Lond Ser B Biol Sci. 2011;366(1562):286–90.
16. Mackenzie IM, Tunnicliffe B. Blast injuries to the lung: epidemiology and management. Philos Trans R Soc Lond Ser B Biol Sci. 2011;366(1562):295–9.
17. Avidan V, Hersch M, Armon Y, Spira R, Aharoni D, Reissman P, et al. Blast lung injury: clinical manifestations, treatment, and outcome. Am J Surg. 2005;190(6):927–31.
18. Phillips YY. Primary blast injuries. Ann Emerg Med. 1986;15(12):1446–50.
19. DePalma RG, Burris DG, Champion HR, Hodgson MJ. Blast injuries. N Engl J Med. 2005;352(13):1335–42.
20. Hirshberg B, Oppenheim-Eden A, Pizov R, Sklair-Levi M, Rivkin A, Bardach E, et al. Recovery from blast lung injury: one-year follow-up. Chest. 1999;116(6):1683–8.
21. Pizov R, Oppenheim-Eden A, Matot I, Weiss YG, Eidelman LA, Rivkind AI, et al. Blast lung injury from an explosion on a civilian bus. Chest. 1999;115(1):165–72.

22. Prat N, Rongieras F, Sarron JC, Miras A, Voiglio E. Contemporary body armor: technical data, injuries, and limits. Eur J Trauma Emerg Surg. 2012;38(2):95–105.
23. Mellor SG, Cooper GJ. Analysis of 828 servicemen killed or injured by explosion in Northern Ireland 1970-84: the Hostile Action Casualty System. Br J Surg. 1989;76(10):1006–10.
24. Kubodera T, Adachi YU, Hatano T, Ejima T, Numaguchi A, Matsuda N. Subcutaneous emphysema and ultrasound sonography. J Intensive Care. 2013;1(1):8.
25. Leinicke JA, Elmore L, Freeman BD, Colditz GA. Operative management of rib fractures in the setting of flail chest: a systematic review and meta-analysis. Ann Surg. 2013;258(6):914–21.
26. Slobogean GP, MacPherson CA, Sun T, Pelletier ME, Hameed SM. Surgical fixation vs nonoperative management of flail chest: a meta-analysis. J Am Coll Surg. 2013;216(2):302–11.e1.
27. Belenkiy SM, Buel AR, Cannon JW, Sine CR, Aden JK, Henderson JL, et al. Acute respiratory distress syndrome in wartime military burns: application of the Berlin criteria. J Trauma Acute Care Surg. 2014;76(3):821–7.
28. Pruitt BA Jr, Cioffi WG, Shimazu T, Ikeuchi H, Mason AD Jr. Evaluation and management of patients with inhalation injury. J Trauma (Injury, Infection and Crit Care). 1990;30(12):S63–S7.
29. Walker PF, Buehner MF, Wood LA, Boyer NL, Driscoll IR, Lundy JB, et al. Diagnosis and management of inhalation injury: an updated review. Crit Care. 2015;19:351.
30. Aboudara M, Mahoney PF, Hicks B, Cuadrado D. Primary blast lung injury at a NATO role 3 hospital. J R Army Med Corps. 2014;160(2):161–6.
31. Allan PF, Osborn EC, Bloom BB, Wanek S, Cannon JW. The introduction of extracorporeal membrane oxygenation to aeromedical evacuation. Mil Med. 2011;176(8):932–7.
32. Bickell WH, Wall MJ, Pepe PE, Martin RR, Ginger VF, Allen MK, et al. Immediate versus delayed fluid resuscitation for hypotensive patients with penetrating torso injuries. N Engl J Med. 1994;331(17):1105–9.
33. Garner J, Watts S, Parry C, Bird J, Cooper G, Kirkman E. Prolonged permissive hypotensive resuscitation is associated with poor outcome in primary blast injury with controlled hemorrhage. Ann Surg. 2010;251(6):1131–9.
34. Kasotakis G, Sideris A, Yang Y, de Moya M, Alam H, King DR, et al. Aggressive early crystalloid resuscitation adversely affects outcomes in adult blunt trauma patients: an analysis of the Glue Grant database. J Trauma Acute Care Surg. 2013;74(5):1215–21. discussion 21–2
35. Holcomb JB, Jenkins D, Rhee P, Johannigman J, Mahoney P, Mehta S, et al. Damage control resuscitation: directly addressing the early coagulopathy of trauma. J Trauma. 2007;62(2):307–10.
36. Holcomb JB, Tilley BC, Baraniuk S, Fox EE, Wade CE, Podbielski JM, et al. Transfusion of plasma, platelets, and red blood cells in a 1:1:1 vs a 1:1:2 ratio and mortality in patients with severe trauma: the PROPPR randomized clinical trial. JAMA. 2015;313(5):471–82.

Abdominal Trauma

Luke R. Johnston, Elliot M. Jessie, and Matthew J. Bradley

Introduction

The combination of blast injury, mostly due to improvised explosive devices (IEDs), and advancements in modern body armor has resulted in a change in injury patterns seen in the most recent US combat experience. Consequently, this has directly altered the management of abdominal trauma in combat casualties. While many of the general principles in the treatment of abdominal trauma remain the same, the severity of injuries to the perineum and pelvis, in particular, require adjustment to some of the standard strategies and even more extensive treatments in certain situations as compared to civilian abdominal trauma. Additionally, the widespread use of damage control laparotomy for the management of catastrophic intra-abdominal hemorrhage, severe contamination, and proximal vascular control of pelvic and junctional hemorrhage has unique applications in the management of dismounted complex blast injuries (DCBI). DCBI is defined by the US Army Institute of Surgical Research "as an injury caused by an explosion, occurring to a Service Member while dismounted in a combat theater that results in amputation of at least one lower extremity at the knee or above, with either amputation or severe injury to the opposite lower limb, combined with pelvic, abdominal, or urogenital injury" [1]. Despite the significant degree of injury sustained from complex blasts, advances in medical care have led to increased survival from the battlefield [2], and work is ongoing to continue to improve long-term functional outcomes [3].

Historical Perspective

Just over a century ago, penetrating torso injuries, including abdominal and perineal wounds, were nearly universally fatal. It was not until recent military conflicts that a significant reduction in mortality was seen following perineal and abdominal trauma [3].

During the United States Civil War, even those soldiers who survived long enough to reach surgical treatment were managed expectantly. While most surgeons at the time felt the delay from injury to an operation was far too great to overcome, a few actually felt that nonoperative management was the best treatment course [4, 5].

With medical and surgical progress, overall survival from blast injuries improved from the Civil War to World War I. However, mortality from colorectal injury remained as high as 77% [5]. During World War II, a noted increased survival in patients treated with diverting colostomy resulted in the surgeon general mandating this procedure for patients who suffered colorectal and severe perineal injury. In addition, the placement

L. R. Johnston (✉) · E. M. Jessie · M. J. Bradley
Uniformed Services University of the Health Sciences and Walter Reed National Military Medical Center, Bethesda, MD, USA
e-mail: luke.r.johnston.mil@mail.mil

of presacral drains, primary repair of extraperitoneal rectal injuries, and fecal diversion were credited with a reduction in mortality secondary to colorectal injuries to 37% [5, 6]. The use of rectal irrigation was also added to the management of severe rectal injuries and was thought to contribute to the continued improvements in mortality.

Further reductions in mortality associated with severe colorectal, perineal, and pelvic injury can be attributed to recent improvements in prehospital combat casualty care including the use of tourniquets and rapid evacuation from the battlefield. These innovations have made it possible for earlier advanced surgical interventions to take place on casualties who in previous conflicts would have died prior to reaching a surgeon [7]. This subsequently reduced mortality directly attributable to abdominal injuries to the low level it is today. In addition, while the mortality from close proximity high-energy DCBI has remained high, those that survive the initial trauma are unlikely to later succumb to their abdominal injuries [7].

Pathophysiology of Blast Injury

Abdominal trauma from blasts can result from several components (primary, secondary, or tertiary) of the blast mechanism. Primary blast injuries are direct injuries from a blast overpressure reaching an individual and transmitting forces directly onto the body. Secondary blast injuries are the result of debris or projectiles that are dispersed by the primary blast overpressure which can cause blunt or penetrating injury to the individual. Finally, tertiary blast injury is defined as an injury caused from a blast physically displacing an individual forcefully into another object [8].

The gastrointestinal system is at increased risk for injury from primary blast due to the presence of air-tissue interfaces within the hollow viscera. The colon and ileocecal region are most susceptible to these implosive forces, and bowel perforations are most likely to occur within these regions [9–12]. The proposed mechanism for bowel rupture involves a separation of the layers of the bowel wall from the implosive and shearing forces of the blast wave. This separation results in significant bowel wall edema with concomitant hemorrhage and thromboses. This combination of hemorrhage and thrombosis compromises perfusion and puts the bowel at risk for delayed perforation [11–13]. These mechanisms have been established in animal blast models where injury to hollow viscus organs is more common than to solid organs. Histopathologic examination of blast-injured intestine is consistent with the above explanations [10]. Compromise of mesenteric blood flow from either direct injury, shearing forces, or arterial air embolisms can also be consequences of the primary blast which can cause or worsen ischemia [8]. While combat DCBI injuries most commonly occur in an open-space environment, primary blast injury can have a much more pronounced effect in enclosed or underwater environments where abdominal injuries are two to four times more likely to occur [8, 10].

The abdominal viscera are additionally susceptible to secondary and tertiary blasts. These injuries are more similar to conventional blunt and penetrating mechanisms, albeit with potentially higher velocities and energies depending on the projectile and distance from the blast [14]. These latter two types of blast effects are the more likely cause of abdominal solid organ injury [14–16].

Demographics

Blast injury can occur from IEDs, which account for the majority of DCBI, rocket-propelled grenades, mortars, and any other exploding projectiles. This mechanism of injury (MOI) was responsible for 78% of combat casualties from the conflicts in Iraq and Afghanistan [17–20]. In general, blast injuries can be categorized into high and low energy and are associated with distinct injury patterns. Lower energy DCBI are associated with lower extremity wounds and fractures but are less likely to cause abdominal injury especially in the combatant wearing modern body armor. Conversely, intra-abdominal solid organ, hollow viscus injuries, pelvic fractures, and severe perineal injuries are often considered hallmark injuries associated with complex lower extremity wounds and amputations seen with high-energy DCBI [21].

While these associated injuries are distinctive to the DCBI pattern, the overall incidence of abdominal and perineal wounds within combat casualties is still relatively low. In fact, torso injuries overall were seen in only 8–10% of patients involved in IED blasts [20, 21]. Furthermore, in casualties with multi-extremity amputation due to DCBI, the incidence of abdominal injuries was only 4.7%, and the incidence of pelvis and perineal injuries was 5.6% [21]. However, in certain subsets of the most severely injured patients that require damage control laparotomy, multiple severe abdominal and pelvic injuries can be anticipated. A review by Authurs [7] discovered that of all patients managed with a damage control laparotomy at a single combat support hospital, small bowel, colon injuries, and rectal injuries were present in 68%, 54%, and 43% of casualties, respectively.

The DCBI pattern is very different from civilian blast injuries resulting from terrorist attacks or otherwise where the incidence of abdominal injury is more frequent (10–24%) than in combat casualties [13, 22]. In addition, penetrating injuries from the secondary blast effect appear to outnumber injuries from the primary blast with the colon and small bowel the most commonly injured intra-abdominal organs [23]. Whether primary or secondary blast effect causes the majority of DCBI has not been published.

It is important to note that the presence of abdominal injuries in the combat casualty following DCBI underscored the significance of the severity and lethality of injuries in these complex poly-trauma patients [24].

Assessment and Initial Evaluation

The initial assessment of abdominal trauma from DCBI follows the stepwise trauma evaluation of TCCC guidelines where catastrophic hemorrhage, airway, and then breathing are evaluated and addressed in order. This primary survey and initial management is usually conducted in the field by nonphysician medical providers, and any evaluation of the abdomen as part of a secondary survey is carried out by either a forward-deployed surgical team (Role II) or trauma team at a higher echelon in-theater treatment facility. In these settings the condition of the patient and the available technology often determine the algorithm followed in the search for intra-abdominal sites of injury [25]. The indications for abdominal surgery remain the same in DCBI relative to other traumatic mechanisms, and the management of the hemodynamically stable patient without penetrating injury is similar in evaluation and management to a patient suffering a blunt abdominal injury owing to the overall similar pathophysiology [15].

In any setting, physical exam remains central to the initial evaluation. Any evidence of penetrating injury will alter the early management. Due to the often significant perineal injuries, assessment for and the identification of a distal rectal or anal injury, which would alter operative management, must be carefully performed. In patients with any pelvic instability where a pelvic binder is placed, caution needs to be taken so as to not miss injuries obscured by the binder.

In the hemodynamically stable patient, and where available, CT scanning is the study of choice for evaluating for intra-abdominal injury. The contrast-enhanced CT scan can relatively quickly evaluate for injuries within the solid organs and has good sensitivity for more subtle injury to hollow viscus organs [15, 26]. The presence of intra-abdominal fluid should be taken in context with the clinical picture and warrants at least observation given the potential delayed manifestation of primary blast injury to the bowel [15].

However in high-energy DCBI, the presentation to the initial surgeon often includes a patient in hemorrhagic shock from one or more locations, with partially or completely amputated extremity(ies) and associated severe soft tissue injuries [2, 27]. A high suspicion should be maintained for abdominal and pelvic sources of bleeding in the hemodynamically unstable patient after peripheral sources of blood loss have been addressed with blood component resuscitation and early tourniquet application. A focused assessment with sonography for trauma (FAST) can be helpful in determining whether the abdomen is a source of hemorrhage and guide the evaluating surgeon toward laparotomy when other indications to explore the abdomen are absent or less emergent [8].

Examination for distal colorectal and anal injuries deserves special attention given the high mortality associated with these injuries when they are missed. Rolling the patient, abducting the legs (or residual limbs), and performing a digital rectal exam (DRE) for the assessment of anal tone and for the presence of hematochezia are imperative, albeit potentially difficult in the DCBI patient such as the patient shown in Fig. 10.1 [3]. When hematochezia is present, examination with rigid proctoscopy has a sensitivity of 90% for injuries and can be performed in the operating room to aid in decision-making in management [28]. Flexible endoscopy, if available, represents another option for rectal examination and allows for retroflexion to examine the distal rectum. Finally the addition of a small volume, 50–100 mL, of contrast per rectum, prior to CT scan, can aid in the diagnosis of occult rectal injuries, where extravasation of contrast or gas into the perirectal tissues can make the diagnosis [3].

Surgical Management

While the overriding principles of surgical management of trauma remain in place, the severe nature of injuries associated with DCBI and the often austere locations where initial surgical intervention takes place require changes in certain aspects of management. Among these is an increased focus on early damage control surgery with control of hemorrhage and gross contamination, an emphasis on second-look abdominal exploration to reduce missed injuries and lower threshold for fecal diversion via ostomy creation.

Damage Control

The term damage control has its origins in US Naval management of a vessel under duress where the ship's crew followed certain protocols to quickly address critical systems to keep the vessel afloat [25]. Damage control surgery, a term first coined by Rotondo et al. (1993) [29] for the management of severe abdominal trauma, is defined as the initial control of hemorrhage and contamination, followed by intraperitoneal packing and expedited abdominal closure to allow for further resuscitation and correction of coagulopathy, acidosis, and hypothermia. Bringing this concept full circle and back onto the battlefield, Blackbourne (2008) described the distinguishing features of combat damage control surgery. Combat damage control is unique in its staging of the care of injuries across various physical locations from the battlefield to forward surgical teams, to in-theater combat support hospitals, and eventually out of theater to the continental United States (CONUS)-based military treatment facilities.

While not unique to DCBI, the potential for severe intra-abdominal, pelvic, or otherwise non-compressible torso hemorrhage that can occur

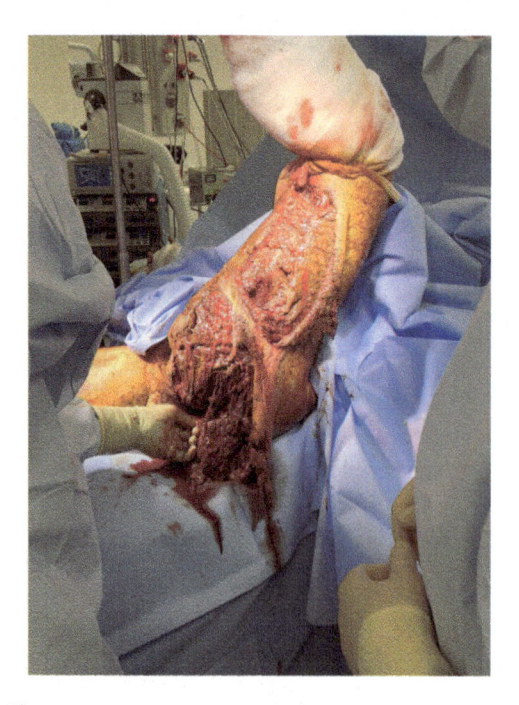

Fig. 10.1 Image shows an individual with severe perineal wounds from a DCBI. This patient will require ostomy formation both for distal rectal injuries and for wound care [38, 41]

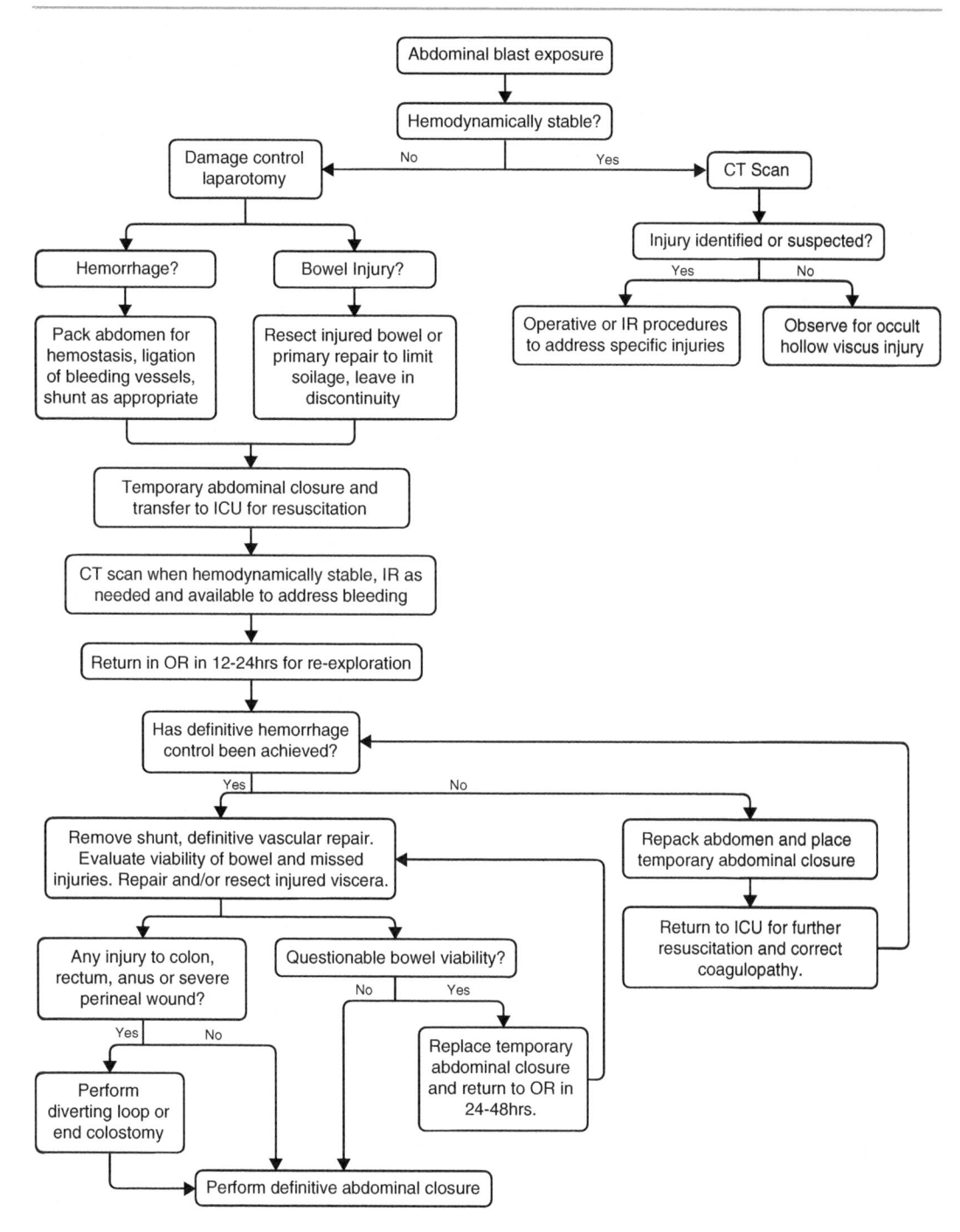

Fig. 10.2 Proposed algorithm for management of a patient with blast exposure to the abdomen. IR—interventional radiology

from blast injury makes damage control laparotomy particularly relevant in the overall management of abdominal DCBI. See Fig. 10.2 for a basic algorithm of damage control surgery for intra-abdominal injury.

When intra-abdominal hemorrhage is encountered, the first step in hemostasis is packing of the abdominal quadrants to tamponade bleeding. Injuries to the bowel with gross spillage should be managed in a quick and temporizing fashion, by either oversewing or stapling, and left in discontinuity. Mesenteric bleeding can be controlled with metal clips or suture ligation and is usually well tolerated due to collateralization. Techniques to manage major disruption of solid organs with significant hemorrhage include quick resection where feasible such as splenectomy for splenic injuries. Hepatic injuries can be managed with a variety of techniques depending on the degree of injury with resectional debridement and nonanatomic resections utilizing vascular clamps or staplers and chromic suture ligation, thermal coagulation, and/or use of various hemostatic agents, if available. Initial maneuvers to gain control of hepatic bleeding include clamping of the porta hepatis, or Pringle maneuver, mobilization of the liver by taking down the coronary and triangular ligaments to allow for access to the posterior and lateral surfaces and IVC, and manual compression between the surgeon's hands in an attempt to tamponade bleeding [30]. Continued packing with hemostatic gauze and/or laparotomy pads is also an appropriate option especially in a damage control setting.

This first damage control operation often takes place in the limited setting of a forward surgical team, sometimes with illumination only from a headlight. Consequently, brevity and emphasis on evacuation to the next level of care are the overriding priorities. When these essential tasks are accomplished, the fascia should be left open and the abdomen temporarily covered. While the presence of intra-abdominal packing or bowel in discontinuity would mandate this alone, the potential for delayed manifestations of primary blast injuries in particular requires the reexamination of the bowel with better visualization afforded at a higher level of care to ensure injuries have not been missed or have not progressed [25].

A number of options are available and have been used to accomplish the task of temporary abdominal closure they include: the use of towel clamps on the skin, suturing saline bags to the skin as a silo over the abdominal contents, placement of Ioban™ incisional drapes over blue towels, and the placement of specialized temporary abdominal closure or improvised wound vacuum-assisted closure (VAC).

Supplemental techniques in damage control surgery when abdominal or lower extremity exsanguinating hemorrhage cannot be immediately addressed, or if vital signs are lost, include the use of resuscitative thoracotomy with aortic cross-clamping or the placement of a resuscitative endovascular balloon for occlusion of the aorta (REBOA) which both can be lifesaving adjuncts to provide additional time for definitive abdominal hemorrhage control. For junctional bleeding of the lower extremities or pelvic bleeding, intra-abdominal aortic control can also be obtained initially at the diaphragmatic hiatus or at the infra-renal aorta to limit hemorrhage until direct control of the sources of bleeding can be obtained [30]. Vascular clamps can then be "marched down" to isolate the specific location of bleed. Alternatively, direct control of the iliac arteries can be achieved via an intra-abdominal or retroperitoneal approach.

After successful completion of initial damage control at the forward combat setting, the next goal is evacuation and continued resuscitation. The majority of transport in Afghanistan took place via helicopter but evacuation largely depends on the tactical situation, terrain, weather, and available modes of transportation. Regardless of the method of transportation, each will have limited space and medical capabilities. Of particular importance in transporting casualties in critical condition with an open abdomen is trying to limit hypothermia during transport [31]. In addition to the use of space blankets and modified "body bags" fitted with chemical hot packs to keep patients warm, targeting a limited initial operative time and proceeding with evacuation in 90 min or less will help achieve this goal [25].

Second-Look Operations and Definitive Treatment

The open abdomen from the initial damage control laparotomy necessitates at least one follow-on operation. The timing of this surgery and whether it is to be a definitive operation depend on the patient's condition and injuries present. In any patient, the take-back surgeries should coincide with sufficient resuscitation to correct any underlying coagulopathy, acidosis, and hypothermia associated with severe hemorrhagic shock. The timing of surgery generally varies form 12–48 h following the initial operation and should not exceed 72 h as increased infectious complications have been noted when packs are left in place passed this point [32].

When definite control of hemorrhage is achieved and repacking not necessary, exceptional vigilance is mandated for several findings that are specific to blast injury. Consistent with the pathophysiology of primary blast injury, subserosal hemorrhage can be found throughout the gastrointestinal (GI) tract, most commonly on the anti-mesenteric border of the bowel and most frequently found on the colon and terminal ileum, though the entire GI tract is at risk. Careful and thorough examination of the bowel for these findings is essential, and any area of injury needs to be repaired, resected, or if equivocal reexamined. Figure 10.3 shows a patient with a segment of bowel found a second look on a patient who suffered a blast injury that will require resection.

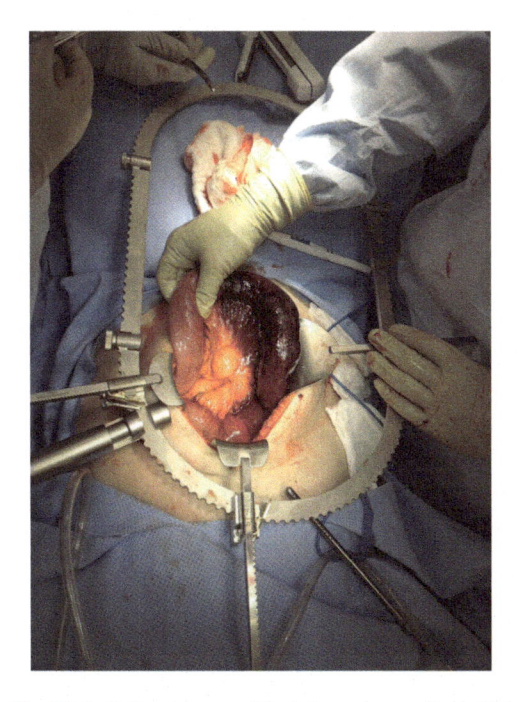

Fig. 10.3 Patient at second-look laparotomy after initial damage control laparotomy. A loop of clearly ischemic small bowel was identified and required resection

The natural history of blast induced small bowel hematomas ranges from uneventful resolution to frank perforation and leaves the surgeon with the difficult decision of deciding which areas require resection. When multiple segments are involved, this decision can become increasingly difficult [15]. Experimental animal models have found larger hematoma sizes to be predictive of delayed perforation (>1 cm in small bowel and >2 cm in colon) [12, 33]. Notable in these studies is the finding of delayed perforations seen as late as 14 days from the initial blast injury.

The management of the hemodynamically stable DCBI patient without penetrating abdominal trauma or other clinical or radiographic indications for laparotomy should include nonoperative observation with serial abdominal examination. In cases of indeterminate physical or radiographic findings, some surgeons have advocated for the use of diagnostic laparoscopy. In skilled hands this may be a valuable tool, though the limited availability especially in a deployed setting, potential to miss an injury when the entire bowel is at risk, and the increased physiologic demands on the pulmonary system in a patient who may also be suffering from blast lung injury have led many to discourage its use [15].

The duration of observation and serial abdominal examination in the patient without obvious abdominal injuries but with clear blast exposure to the abdomen remains an area of uncertainty. In animal models the majority of perforations occurred at the 3–5 days post blast. However, as previously mentioned, delayed perforation up to 14 days after blast exposure has occurred [34]. In the combat setting where a patient is to be medically evacuated out of theater, this question is at least partially obviated by the significant time the patient spends under medical supervision returning to CONUS medical treatment facilities. However, in practice the risk of a perforation or hemorrhage occurring during the prolonged air transports where no surgeon or operating room is available often resulted in any patient with concern for intra-abdominal injury undergoing exploratory laparotomy to definitively rule it out.

When this is not the case for whatever reason, a patient with evidence of blast exposure to the abdomen should be observed for 3–7 days while maintaining a low threshold for reimaging or surgical intervention should the patient develop any concerning abdominal symptoms [15, 35]. While the temptation to rely on CT scan or diagnostic peritoneal lavage to rule out intra-abdominal and specifically hollow viscus injury from DCBI is tempting, no study has evaluated the ability of either of these or any other modalities to definitively rule out injury caused by a blast. This leaves extrapolation from studies of blunt abdominal injury as the best proxy to inform decision-making and consequently requires increased caution and prolonged patient observation [15, 36].

Fecal Diversion

One area where the trend in the management of combat casualties has significantly differed from civilian trauma patient care is in the use of fecal diversion for colorectal and perineal injuries. Based in a history dating from World War II when the surgeon general mandated ostomy creation as part of the management of rectal injuries which saw a subsequent improvement in mortality [3], there has been a strong bias toward fecal diversion, usually involving the creation of a loop or end colostomy, in the management of colorectal injuries. However, in a trend beginning several decades ago, the current consensus in civilian rectal injuries is that primary repair of rectal injuries without fecal diversion is not only safe but associated with a reduction in overall complications [16].

Despite these findings in modern civilian research, numerous publications looking at combat colorectal trauma repeatedly show that failing to perform a fecal diversion procedure is not appropriate for what amounts to a categorically different degree of injury that occurs from DCBI to the distal colon and rectum [37, 38]. Fecal diversion performed for combat casualties in OIF and OEF sustaining colon and rectal injuries, from any MOI, was associated with a decrease in overall mortality from 10.8% to 3.7% [39]. Notably the patients who underwent fecal diversion in this group had higher injury severity

Table 10.1 Relative indications for fecal diversion in combat trauma

Destructive colon injury with tissue loss
Rectal injury
Anal sphincter injury
Severe perineal wounds with need for long-term wound care

scores. Additionally, fecal diversion has been associated with a decrease in leak rates in recent combat colorectal injuries [40, 41]. In summary, for combat-sustained colon or rectal injuries, a diverting procedure should be performed, and this most commonly involves creation of an end colostomy or an end or loop ileostomy. Table 10.1 lists the relative indications for fecal diversion in the combat trauma patient.

Ostomy formation can be performed at different points in patient management. For the patient undergoing damage control surgery where colorectal injuries have been identified, the initial goal is to control ongoing contamination. This can be accomplished by stapling and division proximal to the area of injury with either resection or primary repair of the individual injuries. Attempts to mature an ostomy are not necessary at this point in management, and leaving the patient in discontinuity is standard in the damage control setting.

Options for fecal diversion include loop colostomy, divided sigmoid colostomy, and end colostomy. While a loop colostomy has been recommended given the relative technical ease of eventual reversal, end colostomies made up 66% of the ostomies created for rectal injuries in recent military conflicts [38]. More proximal ileostomies, though sometimes required for the specific injury pattern, are not recommended given the significant length of colon remaining and potential for a large remnant fecal burden [3]. However, no published data has compared the outcomes of ileostomies versus colostomies or loop versus end colostomies.

Damage to the anus represents another injury that may require fecal diversion. Though a limited number of patients without concomitant abdominal injury did successfully undergo primary anal sphincter repair without fecal diversion, fecal diversion was still performed for 78%

of all anal injuries and 100% of patients with anal and rectal injuries in OIF and OEF [42]. Repair of the anal sphincter should not be performed in damage control surgery and should likely be delayed in all settings where significant contamination is present given reports from the recent military conflicts of two patients where attempted primary anal repair with definitive closure of a perineal wound developed severe pelvic sepsis and ultimately required abdominoperineal resection (APR) [42]. Techniques that are encouraged in the management of anal injuries include tagging the remnants of the damaged anal sphincter to facilitate future repair if possible, attempting to restore the perineal body to its correct anatomic location, and using local rotational flaps, such as a gluteal to prevent retraction of the anus and rectal tissues up into the pelvis [42, 43].

Trauma APR is rarely required in civilian trauma and was utilized in six reported cases in OIF and OEF with 100% survival. Trauma APR is indicated in cases of massive pelvi-perineal wounds with rectal destruction and pelvic necrosis resulting from massive ischemia [3]. In the reported cases, APR was reserved for the two cases of pelvic sepsis mentioned above and four additional cases of severe life-threatening hemorrhage where bilateral hypogastric artery ligation was required [42].

A final area where fecal diversion is indicated in DCBI is for severe perineal wounds with or without open pelvic fractures. While isolated severe perineal injury without anorectal involvement was less common than the combined presence of perineal soft tissue injury with anorectal injury, it did occur so surgeons need to be mindful of the overall management in these situations. In severe cases, in particular when an invasive fungal infection has been diagnosed or suspected and there is a need for extensive serial debridement with or without the application of negative pressure wound therapy, fecal diversion can be beneficial in preventing further perineal soilage and facilitating eventual wound closure [44].

The use of distal rectal irrigation following ostomy formation has been historically advocated. However, more recent studies of this practice have not supported it. The most recent military series published showed an association between rectal irrigation and intra-abdominal abscesses, though as the authors of this study admit, the evidence against distal rectal irrigation has been retrospective and could be confounded by only the most severely injured patients receiving the treatment [38]. Despite this, rectal irrigation is not advocated as there is no current data supporting its benefits. Presacral drainage for rectal injuries, another historically advocated practice, has similarly fallen out of favor due to a lack of more modern evidence supporting its benefit [45].

When to reverse ostomies created for DCBI is an area of ongoing research and debate. The majority, 70–86%, of patients who have had ostomies created for combat-related injury were able to have intestinal continuity restored, and the mean time for ostomy reversal has been 6–8 months from ostomy creation [38, 42]. While some civilian literature has suggested a shorter 1–2-week interval to reversal for those patients without destructive injuries to the colon, the more severe nature of DCBI has led military surgeons to recommend delayed reversal [46]. Little research has investigated the complications of and prognostic factors for uncomplicated colostomy reversal, though further research is forthcoming. At this point no factors associated with complications in reversal have been identified. The only predictor of having a permanent colostomy in the combat trauma population is the presence of additional abdominal injuries requiring laparotomy at the initial injury [38]. Interestingly open pelvic fractures, lower extremity amputations, and injury severity score do not predict the need for permanent ostomy [38, 42].

Prior to ostomy reversal, it is important to verify several clinical criteria to ensure a reasonable outcome. Among them are adequate functional status, including the ability to easily get to a restroom and transfer to a toilet, anal sphincter continence, and anorectal sensation. Common complications that need to be addressed prior to reversal include rectal stricture and distal anal stenosis. Basic testing to predict continence includes DRE and saline retention enema. Patients without control of sphincter tone on DRE or with inability to retain a saline enema should be further evaluated with anal manometry, pudendal nerve terminal motor latency testing, and endoanal ultrasound to evaluate if a surgical procedure, such as overlapping sphincteroplasty, or interventions such as biofeedback therapy could benefit the patient prior to reversal [3, 42]. Unfortunately, for some patients loss of anorectal function prevents ostomy reversal, and in a limited number of these patients, mucous leakage from the remnant rectum becomes troublesome enough that completion proctectomy is indicated [3].

Complications

Complications related to DCBI to the abdomen are in general not unique to the blast MOI. However, given the proportion of DCBI patients managed with an open abdomen or who had an ostomy as part of their care, complications related to these procedures are prevalent within this patient population. In fact, one study demonstrated that over half of patients evacuated to CONUS with an open abdomen were injured by a blast MOI [47].

The most prevalent and potentially difficult to manage complications related to damage control surgery and an open abdomen include ventral hernias and development of entero-cutaneous or entero-atmospheric fistulae. Little data focusing on combat trauma patients and absolute rates of these complications is available though, one series noted that only 18% of individuals evacuated to CONUS with an open abdomen were able to undergo primary fascial closure while 14% were treated with a planned ventral hernia or vacuum-assisted closure with AlloDerm® during their initial hospitalization [48]. Civilian literature reports a wide range of incidence (13–80%) of chronic ventral hernias complicating damage control surgery. Entero-cutaneous and the entero-atmospheric fistulae, a complication unique to the open abdomen, are the second most common complications related to damage control surgery, reported at rates of 5–19% in civilian literature, and can be devastating as the fistulae compromise the nutritional status of the patients trying to recover from their host of injuries [49].

Management of ventral hernia and enterocutaneous fistulae both require the optimization of the patient as part of overall management. Evidence to manage these complications begins with the initial resuscitation where a ratio-driven resuscitation of one unit of packed red blood cells to one unit fresh frozen plasma was found to independently predict early primary fascial closure in patients undergoing damage control laparotomy [50]. Further management includes maximizing patient nutrition via either enteral or parenteral means, providing local wound care to manage fistula output with wound VACs or modified ostomy appliances to prevent skin break down and allow for healing, and managing comorbid medical conditions. Inclusion of this host of management strategies has resulted in successful repair of even the most complex abdominal injuries [51].

Ventral hernia repair in DCBI patients can be confounded by a loss of abdominal wall components from the initial injury, consequently preventing the use of some of the more conventional techniques (Rives-Stoppa, component separation) to gain medial mobilization to perform a primary fascial closure. For fistulae, management is dictated by specific characteristics of the fistula such as output and location within the bowel. Many fistulae are able to be managed nonoperatively with local wound care and nutritional supplementation, though proximal high-output fistulae will often require surgical intervention [49].

Complications specific to ostomy creation include early complications such as leaks and ischemia and later complications including anorectal strictures, stomal hernias, and volvulus around the ostomy [38]. Early complications are often easily identified and can be addressed at interval laparotomies while the patient's abdomen is still open [37]. Delayed complication management is guided by conventional practices and a focus on future planned surgical intervention to reverse or maintain a permanent ostomy.

Future Advances in Care and Research

Advances in prehospital care on the battlefield have played one of the greatest roles in improving survival and allowing for more definitive operations to take place. Yet noncompressible torso hemorrhage remains an area for improvement. Currently in use in the hospital setting, REBOA is gaining increased acceptance as an excellent alternative to thoracotomy and aortic cross-clamping for temporary hemorrhage control. Efforts are underway to develop this device and enhance/increase the training of more individuals in the prehospital setting in order to bring this technology further downrange and closer to the battlefield. Control of catastrophic hemorrhage earlier in the course of patient care using this device may allow for further increases in survival especially in those combat casualties that died on the battlefield from potentially survival injuries.

Further research into long-term outcomes of anorectal trauma is being investigated in the J-STOMA database as well as the experimental use of sacral-nerve stimulation, magnetic sphincter augmentation, and pyloric valve transposition to try to allow for the reversal of ostomies in patients whose anal function currently is inadequate.

Conclusion

The management of abdomen trauma from DCBI has evolved significantly over the past century progressing from what was previously thought of as universally nonsurvivable injuries to injuries now considered completely survivable. While requiring highly individualized care given the vast possible intra-abdominal injuries that can occur, the basic principles of damage control surgery have allowed for a streamlining of early management decision-making that has resulted in a greater number of service members surviving. Further advances in down-range treatment options to address hemorrhage will only increase the number of patients surviving with abdominal injuries that will ultimately need surgical care.

Further research will be needed to guide the management of these complex and severely injured casualties.

Disclaimer The opinions or assertions contained herein are the private ones of the author/speaker and are not to be construed as official or reflecting the views of the Department of Defense, the Uniformed Services University of the Health Sciences or any other agency of the US Government.

Photo Disclaimer The appearance of US Department of Defense (DoD) visual information does not imply or constitute DoD endorsement.

References

1. Ficke JR, Eastridge BJ, Butler FK, Alvarez J, Brown T, Pasquina P, et al. Dismounted complex blast injury report of the army dismounted complex blast injury task force. J Trauma Acute Care Surg. 2012; 73(6):S520–S534.
2. Eastridge BJ, Mabry RL, Seguin P, Cantrell J, Tops T, Uribe P, et al. Death on the battlefield (2001–2011): implications for the future of combat casualty care. J Trauma Acute Care Surg. 2012;73(6):S431–S7.
3. Cannon JW, Hofmann LJ, Glasgow SC, Potter BK, Rodriguez CJ, Cancio LC, et al. Dismounted complex blast injuries: a comprehensive review of the modern combat experience. J Am Coll Surg. 2016;223(4):652–64. e8.
4. Blaisdell FW. Medical advances during the Civil War. Arch Surg (Chicago 1960). 123(9):1045–50.
5. Pruitt BA. Combat casualty care and surgical progress. Ann Surg. 243(6):715–29.
6. Lavenson GS, Cohen A. Management of rectal injuries. Am J Surg. 1971;122(2):226–30.
7. Arthurs Z, Kjorstad R, Mullenix P, Rush RM Jr, Sebesta J, Beekley A. The use of damage-control principles for penetrating pelvic battlefield trauma. Am J Surg. 2006;191(5):604–9.
8. Wolf SJ. Blast injuries. Lancet (British edition). 2009;374(9687):405–15.
9. Guy RJ, Kirkman E, Watkins PE, Cooper GJ. Physiologic responses to primary blast. J Trauma. 1998;45(6):983–7.
10. Mayorga MA. The pathology of primary blast overpressure injury. Toxicology. 1997;121(1):17–28.
11. Paran H, Neufeld D, Shwartz I, Kidron D, Susmallian S, Mayo A, et al. Perforation of the terminal ileum induced by blast injury: delayed diagnosis or delayed perforation? J Trauma. 1996;40(3):472–5.

12. Cripps NP, Cooper GJ. Risk of late perforation in intestinal contusions caused by explosive blast. Br J Surg. 1997;84(9):1298–303.
13. Katz E, Ofek B, Adler J, Abramowitz HB, Krausz MM. Primary blast injury after a bomb explosion in a civilian bus. Ann Surg. 1989;209(4):484–8.
14. Wightman JM, Gladish SL. Explosions and blast injuries. Ann Emerg Med. 2001;37(6):664–78.
15. Owers C, Morgan JL, Garner JP. Abdominal trauma in primary blast injury. Br J Surg. 2011;98(2):168–79.
16. Nelson TJ, Wall DB, Stedje-Larsen ET, Clark RT, Chambers LW, Bohman HR. Predictors of mortality in close proximity blast injuries during Operation Iraqi Freedom. J Am Coll Surg. 2006;202(3):418–22.
17. Owens BD, Kragh JF Jr, Wenke JC, Macaitis J, Wade CE, Holcomb JB. Combat wounds in operation Iraqi Freedom and operation Enduring Freedom. J Trauma. 2008;64(2):295–9.
18. Benfield RJ, Mamczak CN, Vo K-CT, Smith T, Osborne L, Sheppard FR, et al. Initial predictors associated with outcome in injured multiple traumatic limb amputations: a Kandahar-based combat hospital experience. Injury. 2012;43(10):1753–8.
19. Champion HR, Holcomb JB, Young LA. Injuries from explosions: physics, biophysics, pathology, and required research focus. J Trauma Acute Care Surg. 2009;66(5):1468–77.
20. Bird SM, Fairweather CB. Military fatality rates (by cause) in Afghanistan and Iraq: a measure of hostilities. Int J Epidemiol. 2007;36(4):841–6.
21. Eskridge SL, Macera CA, Galarneau MR, Holbrook TL, Woodruff SI, MacGregor AJ, et al. Injuries from combat explosions in Iraq: injury type, location, and severity. Injury. 2012;43(10):1678–82.
22. Martí M, Parrón M, Baudraxler F, Royo A, León NG, Álvarez-Sala R. Blast injuries from Madrid terrorist bombing attacks on March 11, 2004. Emerg Radiol. 2006;13(3):113–22.
23. Bala M, Rivkind AI, Zamir G, Hadar T, Gertsenshtein I, Mintz Y, et al. Abdominal trauma after terrorist bombing attacks exhibits a unique pattern of injury. Ann Surg. 2008;248(2):303–9.
24. Ramasamy A, Harrisson SE, Clasper JC, Stewart MP. Injuries from roadside improvised explosive devices. J Trauma. 2008;65(4):910–4.
25. Blackbourne LH. Combat damage control surgery. Crit Care Med. 2008;36(7 Suppl):S304–10.
26. Johnson EK, Judge T, Lundy J, Meyermann M. Diagnostic pelvic computed tomography in the rectal-injured combat casualty. Mil Med. 2008;173(3):293–9.
27. Jansen J, Thomas G, Adams S, Tai N, Russell R, Morrison J, et al. Early management of proximal traumatic lower extremity amputation and pelvic injury caused by improvised explosive devices (IEDs). Injury. 2012;43(7):976–9.
28. Mangiante E, Graham A, Fabian T. Rectal gunshot wounds. Management of civilian injuries. Am Surg. 1986;52(1):37–40.
29. Rotondo MF, Schwab CW, McGonigal MD, Phillips GR, Fruchterman TM, Kauder DR, et al. 'Damage control': an approach for improved survival in exsanguinating penetrating abdominal injury. J Trauma Acute Care Surg. 1993;35(3):375–83.
30. Morrison JJ, Rasmussen TE. Noncompressible torso hemorrhage: a review with contemporary definitions and management strategies. Surg Clin North Am. 2012;92(4):843–58, vii
31. Hirshberg A, Sheffer N, Barnea O. Computer simulation of hypothermia during "damage control" laparotomy. World J Surg. 1999;23(9):960–5.
32. Abikhaled JA, Granchi TS, Wall MJ, Hirshberg A, Mattox KL. Prolonged abdominal packing for trauma is associated with increased morbidity and mortality. Am Surg. 1997;63(12):1109.
33. Johansson L, Norrby K, Nyström P, Lennquist S. Intestinal intramural haemorrhage after abdominal missile trauma–clinical classification and prognosis. Acta Chir Scand. 1983;150(1):51–6.
34. Tatic V, Ignjatovic D, Jevtic M, Jovanovic M, Draskovic M, Durdevic D. Morphologic characteristics of primary nonperforative intestinal blast injuries in rats and their evolution to secondary perforations. J Trauma Acute Care Surg. 1996;40(3S):94S–9S.
35. Phillips Y, Zajtchuck JT. The management of primary blast injury. In: Bellamy RF, Zajtchuk R, editors. Textbook of military medicine. 5. Washington, DC: Office of the Surgeon General; 1991. p. 293–333.
36. Cripps N, Glover M, Guy R. The pathophysiology of primary blast injury and its implications for treatment. Part II: the auditory structures and abdomen. J R Nav Med Serv. 1998;85(1):13–24.
37. Cho SD, Kiraly LN, Flaherty SF, Herzig DO, Lu KC, Schreiber MA. Management of colonic injuries in the combat theater. Dis Colon Rectum. 2010;53(5):728–34.
38. O'Donnell MT, Greer LT, Nelson J, Shriver C, Vertrees A. Diversion remains the standard of care for modern management of war-related rectal injuries. Mil Med. 2014;179(7):778–82.
39. Glasgow SC, Steele SR, Duncan JE, Rasmussen TE. Epidemiology of modern battlefield colorectal trauma: a review of 977 coalition casualties. J Trauma Acute Care Surg. 2012;73(6 Suppl 5):S503–8.
40. Steele SR, Wolcott KE, Mullenix PS, Martin MJ, Sebesta JA, Azarow KS, et al. Colon and rectal injuries during Operation Iraqi Freedom: are there any changing trends in management or outcome? Dis Colon Rectum. 2007;50(6):870–7.
41. Duncan JE, Corwin CH, Sweeney WB, Dunne JR, Denobile JW, Perdue PW, et al. Management of colorectal injuries during Operation Iraqi Freedom: patterns of stoma usage. J Trauma. 2008;64(4):1043–7.
42. Glasgow SC, Heafner TA, Watson JD, Aden JK, Perry WB. Initial management and outcome of modern battlefield anal trauma. Dis Colon Rectum. 2014;57(8):1012–8.

43. Terrosu G, Rossetto A, Kocjancic E, Rossitti P, Bresadola V. Anal avulsion caused by abdominal crush injury. Tech Coloproctol. 2011;15(4):465–8.
44. Lundy JB, Driscoll IR. Experience with proctectomy to manage combat casualties sustaining catastrophic perineal blast injury complicated by invasive mucor soft-tissue infections. Mil Med. 2014;179(3):e347–e50.
45. Gonzalez RP. The role of presacral drainage in the management of penetrating rectal injuries. J Trauma. 1998;45(4):656–61.
46. Renz BM, Feliciano DV, Sherman R. Same admission colostomy closure (SACC). A new approach to rectal wounds: a prospective study. Ann Surg. 1993;218(3):279.
47. Vertrees A, Greer L, Pickett C, Nelson J, Wakefield M, Stojadinovic A, et al. Modern management of complex open abdominal wounds of war: a 5-year experience. J Am Coll Surg. 2008;207(6):801–9.
48. Vertrees A, Wakefield M, Pickett C, Greer L, Wilson A, Gillern S, et al. Outcomes of primary repair and primary anastomosis in war-related colon injuries. J Trauma. 2009;66(5):1286–91; discussion 91–3
49. Smith BP, Adams RC, Doraiswamy VA, Nagaraja V, Seamon MJ, Wisler J, et al. Review of abdominal damage control and open abdomens: focus on gastrointestinal complications. J Gastrointestin Liver Dis. 2010;19(4):425–35.
50. Glaser J, Vasquez M, Cardarelli C, Dunne J, Elster E, Hathaway E, et al. Ratio-driven resuscitation predicts early fascial closure in the combat wounded. J Trauma Acute Care Surg. 2015;79(4):S188–S92.
51. Glaser JJ, Sheppard FR, Gage FA, Kumar AR, Liston WA, Elster EA, et al. Warfare-related complex abdominal wall reconstruction using a bioprosthetic regenerate template and negative pressure therapy. Eplasty. 2009;9:e17.

Vascular Injuries

11

Timothy K. Williams and W. Darrin Clouse

Introduction

Blast injury has become increasingly commonplace in both military and civilian environments. The recent conflicts in Iraq and Afghanistan have marked a foundational shift in warfare and terrorist tactics, resulting in thousands of injured warfighters and civilians largely due to improvised explosive devices. Currently, blast injury represents the predominant cause of traumatic injury in modern military conflict, outnumbering wounds from conventional weaponry. Dismounted Complex Blast Injury (DCBI) in particular is characterized by unique and devastating injury patterns. The majority of patients sustain complex soft tissue, orthopedic, and genitourinary injuries, frequently sustaining immediate major limb amputation [1]. While vascular injury is inherent to any major amputation, rarely do these injuries offer the opportunity for repair, revascularization, or reconstruction. Nonetheless, blast injury accounts for the majority of vascular injuries in modern conflict. Furthermore, civilian injuries from terrorist attacks involving explosive devices are complicated by vascular injury in up to 10% of cases. Prompt and decisive action, to prevent loss of life and limb, is required and largely follows sound vascular injury management principles. In this chapter, we will explore the general approach to vascular injury management in the context of this unique and challenging patient population.

Epidemiology

Rates of vascular injury during military operations have been progressively increasing across military conflicts, from a rate of 0.96% in World War II to between 4% and 12% during the wars in Iraq and Afghanistan [2–4]. In modern conflict, approximately 70% of vascular injuries are attributable to explosive fragmentation [4, 5]. During Operation Iraqi Freedom, between the years of 2004 and 2006, there were 6800 documented casualties, with a total of 347 vascular injuries in 324 (4.8%) patients and an operative mortality rate of 4.3%. Extremity injuries accounted for 75% of vascular reconstructions performed, with an early amputation rate of 6.6% [6]. In a later report from the Joint Theater Trauma Registry (JTTR), between 2002 and 2009, there were 13,000 battle-related injuries in US troops, with a vascular injury rate of 12% [4]. Seventy-nine percent of these injuries occurred in the extremities,

T. K. Williams (✉)
Wake Forest Baptist Health,
Winston-Salem, NC, USA
e-mail: tkwillia@wakehealth.edu

W. D. Clouse
Harvard Medical School, Massachusetts General Hospital, Division of Vascular and Endovascular Surgery, Boston, MA, USA

with only 12% involving the torso and 8% cervical. It is likely that this perceived increase in vascular injury rates over time is a product of our improved ability to stabilize patients at the point of injury and transport them quickly to a facility with surgical assets. Additionally, the widespread use of tourniquets that increased progressively throughout the recent armed conflicts has allowed patients with otherwise fatal vascular injuries to survive long enough to undergo definitive surgical management [6].

Amputation following blast injury, either immediate or delayed, is common. To underscore the lethality of injury mechanism, patients who sustain immediate primary amputation have a mortality rate of approximately 50%, owing in part to rapid exsanguination and associated severe concomitant injuries [7]. Frequently these amputations occur in the proximal thigh, resulting in junctional vascular injuries that are frequently not amenable to tourniquet application. Most blast-related vascular injuries are due to secondary and tertiary blast effects (81%). The need for secondary amputation follows the extent of surrounding soft tissue injury. Additionally, blast-induced extremity vascular injury with coexisting fracture is associated with approximately a 50% amputation rate where attempts at limb salvage are made and a 77% amputation rate overall [8].

Reports of blast-related vascular injury in Western nations are rare. The overwhelming majority of vascular injury involving the civilian population, particularly in the United States, occurs from conventional mechanisms. Irrespective of mechanism, one can glean useful information from experience with civilian vascular injury, particularly with respect to its effect on mortality. Overall, the rate of traumatic vascular injury is low, accounting for only 1–4% of injured patients [9, 10]. Extremity vascular injury predominates, accounting for 40–80% of arterial injuries across reported series, with roughly an equal distribution affecting the upper and lower extremities [9–11]. Mortality rates from extremity vascular injury approach 5–10%, but vary based on the vascular territory [12–17]. A recent report from the National Trauma Data Bank (NTDB), spanning from 2002 to 2005, identified nearly 700 isolated lower extremity vascular injuries, the majority of which were due to penetrating mechanisms. The overall mortality rate was 3%, with injuries to the common femoral artery resulting in the highest mortality rate (7%). Major amputation was required in 6.5% of this cohort, with popliteal injuries in the highest amputation rate (9%) [17]. Additional prognostic factors influencing the risk for major amputation include multiple arterial injuries (18% vs. 9%; OR 4.9), prolonged ischemic interval greater than 6 h (24% vs. 5%; OR 4.4), soft tissue injury (26% vs. 8%; OR 5.8), and compartment syndrome (28% vs. 6%; OR 5.1) [18].

The majority of our knowledge regarding the natural history of blast injury involving civilians still centers around local populations injured in the broader context of military conflict. It has been observed that the distribution of vascular injury differs between the military and civilian populations, with civilian populations incurring truncal injury more frequently (13% vs. 4%; $p < 0.01$). This is likely that the widespread use of body armor by military personnel accounts for this disparity [6].

Diagnosis

Irrespective of mechanism, the fundamental approach to assessing for vascular injury and limb ischemia holds true. Clinical examination should focus on identifying the hard signs of vascular injury, including absent pulses, active bleeding, expanding hematomas, and audible bruits or palpable thrills, with positive findings mandating expeditious exploration and intervention. The presence of the "soft" signs of vascular injury requires a more nuanced approach. These findings include asymmetric/diminished pulse exam, a non-expanding hematoma, a history of hemorrhage, neurologic deficits, or proximity of the injury to vascular structures. Continuous wave Doppler utilization with calculation of the ankle-brachial index (ABI) should be utilized routinely, with a value of less than 0.9 suggesting the presence of injury. As a screening tool, this test is highly reliable, with sensitivities of 80–97% to detect the presence of arterial injury. However, this test does suffer from a high false-positive rate, with a wide specificity ranging from 40% to 100% [19–22]. Additional noninvasive pressure-based assessments include calculation of an ankle-ankle index or brachial-brachial index, which are useful in instances where contralateral extremity injury is not suspected. Displaced fractures should be reduced prior to pulse exam and ABI, as limb shortening may result in mechanical compression or kinking of arteries with a loss of distal pulses, even in the absence of injury. For patients with absence of hard signs, but suspicion of injury exists based on the presence of soft signs, a detailed pulse examination with ABI measurement should be performed. When the ABI or other alternate extremity index is below 0.9, additional interrogation is mandatory. When normal, observation is appropriate. Some minor injuries may not manifest with an abnormal ABI such as focal dissection, limited intimal injury, or pseudoaneurysm. Yet these are generally rare, with only 1–2% ultimately undergoing operative exploration for occult injury [20–24]. Even when wounds exist in proximity to major vascular structures, where the clinical exam is otherwise normal, occult vessel injury is present in a mere 10–12%, with only about 1% of these patients requiring intervention [24].

When further vascular evaluation is indicated, duplex ultrasound (DUS) is considered the first-line diagnostic modality [25–27]. It is particularly useful in the diagnosis of extremity vascular injury and can readily identify areas of narrowing, pseudoaneurysm, occlusion, arteriovenous fistulae, and intimal disruption. It is also useful for point-of-care evaluation and can be utilized intraoperatively to evaluate the suitability of a repair. Additionally, it commonly is utilized for routine surveillance and can be employed to track for progression or resolution of minimal injuries being managed nonoperatively. However, it is user-dependent and can be limited in its ability to diagnose junctional or truncal vascular injury [28].

Computed tomographic angiography (CTA) is increasingly being employed in the diagnosis of both truncal, cervical, and extremity vascular injuries. It has largely supplanted the need for conventional catheter-based angiography, with sensitivity and specificity of greater than 90% [29, 30]. In addition to providing visualization of vascular structures, CT provides information regarding vessel morphology, including adjacent soft tissue and bony architecture. CT angiography allows for visualization of vessel occlusion, dissection, and disruption, manifesting with either pseudoaneurysm or free extravasation of contrast. However, it does require transport of a patient to a location where active resuscitation may not be feasible; thus, a certain degree of clinical stability is frequently required. Additionally, it is subject to certain technical limitations, including artifact from bone and metal, as well as the possibility of incorrect bolus timing leading to poor opacification of blood vessels.

The use of catheter-based angiography still plays a role in the diagnosis, particularly when urgent surgical exploration is required. This can readily be performed in conjunction with open surgery, particularly when a hybrid operating room exists. Angiography is also commonly utilized to assess the suitability of an open repair intraoperatively. It is also a useful diagnostic modality in the presence of multiple bony or metallic fragments that would obscure CT imaging, which is frequently the case with blast injury patterns. Finally, angiography is utilized as an obligate component of endovascular therapy, which is increasingly being utilized for trauma and in anatomic distributions where open surgical control is challenging.

Management Considerations

For patients who have sustained blast injury, the posture toward vascular injury management represents a balanced approach, reflecting the need to address concomitant injuries that often represent conflicting priorities. Additionally, given the propensity for collateral damage, management of soft tissue injury plays a dominant role in the care of this patient population and frequently dictates the course of limb salvage efforts. We will examine the strategies for the clinical management of vascular injury, emphasizing the unique challenges that blast injury manifests.

Tourniquet Use

The widespread application of tourniquets for extremity vascular injury has become a routine strategy in modern military conflict and has been demonstrated to prevent early death from exsanguinating hemorrhage [31]. Certainly many victims of blast injury will sustain injuries that are not amenable to tourniquet application; however, lesser degrees of extremity injury may perceive significant lifesaving benefit. In 2009, Kragh et al. reported on 232 patients undergoing emergency tourniquet application for extremity injury. There were 31 deaths (13%). Tourniquet use in this group was strongly associated with improved survival when shock was absent as opposed to when present (90% vs. 10%; $P < 0.001$). Additionally, the prehospital application of tourniquets compared to in-hospital application resulted in a strong trend toward reduced mortality (11% vs. 24%, $p = 0.06$). Importantly, the widespread use of tourniquet did not come at the expense of increased limb loss. These data strongly support liberal and expeditious application of tourniquets following extremity vascular injury with hemorrhage to prevent the onset of shock, given that mortality is significantly increased once shock has occurred.

It is nonetheless challenging to apply the experience in combat to the civilian trauma population. However, there is increasing support for the widespread use of tourniquets within the civilian trauma community. Increasingly, via the American College of Surgeons, STOP the BLEED campaign, tourniquets and hemorrhage control kits are becoming available in public venues, similar to the widespread availability of automated external defibrillators, recognizing that immediate access to these devices is important in preventing shock from exsanguination.

Temporary Vascular Shunting (TVS)

Temporary vascular shunts (TVS) allow for rapid reperfusion of ischemic limbs and are ideally suited to situations where definitive vascular reconstruction is not feasible (Fig. 11.1). This strategy can be employed for a variety of reasons including lack of clinical expertise facilitating interfacility transport without ongoing ischemia and the need to address more acutely life-threatening concomitant injuries and to provide an interval between initial resuscitative efforts and definitive management for severely physiologically deranged patients [32]. Recent military conflicts have amassed a wealth of experience with the use of shunts [33–35]. The management priorities that have led to routine use of shunts in military conflict largely translate to civilian injuries as well.

The impact of TVS on limb salvage from military experience in Operation Enduring Freedom and Operation Iraqi Freedom has been well characterized. Chambers et al. reported the use of 27 temporary vascular shunts during OIF to facilitate transport to a higher echelon of care. A full 88% of shunts remained patent during transport, and shunt thrombosis was not associated with early limb loss [33]. Other reports have demonstrated even higher patency rates (96%), with 100% early limb salvage following a mean transport time of 5 h 48 min [35]. It does appear that

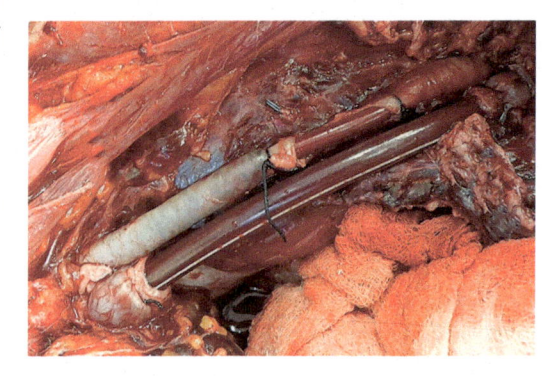

Fig. 11.1 Combined arterial and venous injury of the superficial femoral artery and femoral vein. Due to concomitant injuries in the blast-injured patient, shunts have been placed in the artery and vein to facilitate delayed repair

proximally placed shunts (proximal to the knee or elbow) have greater patency than distal shunts (86% vs. 12%); however, shunt thrombosis did not lead to decreased limb viability [34]. Shunts become dislodged in less than 5% of instances during transport, further supporting their safety [36]. While the use of shunts for venous injuries has been described, outcomes data are lacking. However, given the speed and ease of insertion, with minimal theoretical risk, it is a rational to consider [37, 38].

Common devices used to perform shunting include commercially available Argyle, Sundt, and Javid carotid shunts. Detailed descriptions of the technique of temporary vascular shunting can be found elsewhere [33]. Anticoagulation is not required to maintain shunt patency based on clinical and experimental data [33, 39]. Recent clinical reports have described the use of self-expanding stent grafts as temporary vascular shunts, suggesting that the increased luminal diameter creates improved flow characteristics that may further minimize limb ischemia and the risk of thrombosis [40].

Ultimately, the liberal use of shunts poses minimal risk and should be routinely employed. Even in instances when an isolated vascular injury is encountered with the resources to perform repair, the authors find initial shunt placement can be quite useful, providing additional time for improved case planning and hemodynamic optimization. Utilizing this posture toward vascular injury management can create an environment for a more precise and durable revascularization with improved limb outcomes.

Vein Repair

The management of venous injury, either isolated or with concomitant arterial injury, remains obscure. However, the routine repair of venous injuries has been supported by thought leaders in the field (Fig. 11.2). Rich et al. reported his experience with venous repair from the Vietnam Vascular Registry, where 124/377 (32.9%) venous injuries underwent repair [41]. While

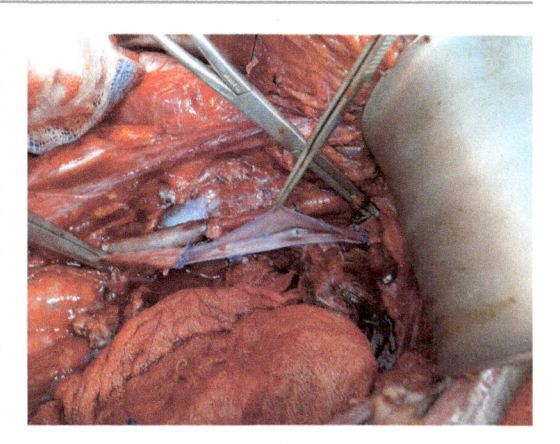

Fig. 11.2 Repair of a femoral vein injury using autologous contralateral saphenous vein, utilizing a panel graft technique

most repairs involved simple direct repair with a lateral suture technique ($n = 106$), a small number of patients underwent more complex repair with an end-to-end anastomosis ($n = 10$), vein patch graft ($n = 3$), and vein interposition grafting ($n = 5$). It was suggested that venous repair may play an important role in limb salvage by promoting improved arterial flow as well and durability following concomitant arterial reconstruction. While many venous repairs fail early, a major proportion of these may later recanalize [42, 43]. Concerns about the potential for thromboembolic complications following repair have been voiced; however, these complications have not manifested.

In more contemporary military experience, venous repair has been noted to be independently protective against amputation (RR = 0.2; 95% CI [0.04–0.99], $P = 0.05$) [44]. With respect to civilian trauma, conclusions regarding the utility of venous repair have been mixed, speaking to the wide variability in civilian extremity trauma severity, mechanism, and techniques [37, 45, 46].

For patients in extremis, ligation of named extremity veins can be performed, particularly when expertise in the conduct of vein repair is lacking. However, when a patient's physiology supports more deliberate management of venous injury, repair should be entertained [6]. The authors have taken an aggressive posture toward routine vein repair, particularly for high-risk distributions such as in the proximal limb, at watershed regions, and vein confluences. The presence of duplicate venous systems is not uncommon and should be identified. When present, these collateral drainage pathways may temper the need to perform repair. For patients sustaining complex injury with significant soft tissue disruption due to blast and explosive mechanisms, where key collateral pathways are likely to be disrupted, vein repair should be strongly considered. Again, the use of shunting for venous injury can be considered for patients in extremis; however, the impact of this is not well characterized [38]. Fundamentally, the goals of venous repair are to provide acute decompression of the injured limb and minimize tissue edema, to enhance the durability of arterial repairs, and to minimize the risk for long-term chronic venous stasis changes. Taken in this context, vein repair should be considered a core strategy in the management of extremity vascular injury, especially when due to blast injury mechanisms.

Fasciotomy

Routine fasciotomy is a fundamental component of surgical management for patient with vascular injury. The common indications include prolonged ischemia (more than 4 h), crush injury, complex blast injury, or when patient transport may preclude careful examining of the limb and lead to delayed intervention for compartment syndrome. With respect to both civilian and military extremity vascular injuries, failure to appropriately perform fasciotomy in a timely fashion or performing inadequate fasciotomy is associated with increased risk of limb loss, longer length of stay, and higher mortality [47, 48]. Based on data from the National Trauma Data Bank, early fasciotomy use has been shown to significantly reduce the need for delayed amputation for patients who sustained arterial injury (9% vs. 25%, $P < 0.001$). To this point, fasciotomy is mandatory in military environments for patients sustaining confirmed vascular injury or for those with prolonged application of tourniquets for extremity injury.

The techniques of lower leg four compartment fasciotomy are well described elsewhere. In general, a two-incision lower extremity compartment release is recommended. Via a longitudinal incision posterior to the tibia in the medial aspect of the mid-calf, the superficial posterior compartment is opened. The fascia is widely incised using Metzenbaum scissors in both the cephalad and caudal directions. Access to the deep posterior compartment is entered by release of the tibial attachment of the soleus muscle and extended widely in either direction. The lateral incision is performed 2–3 fingerbreadths lateral to the tibial edge. The anterior compartment is widely opened by analogous fascial incision. The lateral compartment is either entered via separation of the intercompartmental septum as viewed in the anterior compartment or through a separate fascial incision posterior to the intermuscular septum adjoining the anterior and lateral compartments. Care should be taken to create generous skin and fascial incisions, as limited incisions can fail to adequately decompress the compartments and lead to ongoing muscle necrosis and potential limb loss [48].

Upper extremity fasciotomy is more complex and less familiar to most surgeons, as it is performed infrequently, most commonly being required in the forearm. There are three compartments in the forearm: volar, lateral, and dorsal. Performance of upper extremity fasciotomy begins medially in the proximal arm, becoming sinusoidal from medial to lateral in the mid forearm (Fig. 11.3). Extension of the incision must be sufficiently lateral to open the fascia over the lateral compartment (mobile wad). The fascia overlying the superficial volar muscles is opened along the length of the incision. Care must be taken to open the fascia enveloping the deep volar compartment muscles as well. To decompress the dorsal compartment, a linear incision performed on the dorsal surface of the arm and the fascia is opened widely. Controversy exists regarding the need to perform a concomitant carpal tunnel release but has been described.

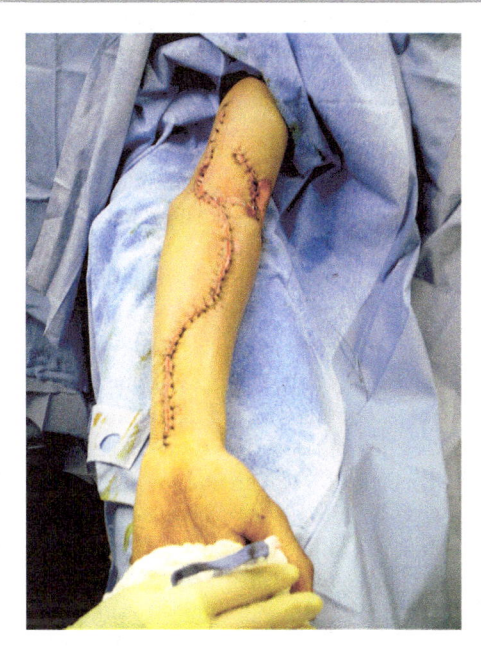

Fig. 11.3 Forearm fasciotomy incision closure involving the volar aspect of the forearm. Note the sinusoidal shape of the incision to facilitate decompression of both the volar and lateral compartments

Nonoperative Management

When isolated arterial injuries do not result in a diminution of distal perfusion, nonoperative management can be entertained. Lesions that can frequently be observed include intimal flaps, small pseudoaneurysms, arteriovenous fistulae, and nonspecific vessel narrowing. There is a growing body of data to support this approach for minimal intimal injury, suggesting freedom from intervention is achievable in over 90% of cases [49–51]. Experimental evidence suggests that intimal flaps resulting in greater than 75% luminal compromise are prone to thrombosis [52]. In practical terms, luminal compromise greater than 30–50% should prompt consideration for repair at the discretion of the provider, with consideration toward resource constraints, local expertise, and patient disposition.

Low-dose aspirin should be routinely prescribed for minimal lesions and appears beneficial [53]. Systemic anticoagulation can be considered; however, this is commonly contraindicated in the context of the severely blast-injured trauma patient. Small pseudoaneurysms and arteriovenous fistulae (<5 mm) are likely to heal, but may fail to resolve or worsen in a minority of patients, thus prompting the need for intervention. In summary, initial surveillance for these minimal vascular injury patterns is appropriate; however, the ability to closely monitor patients for changes is an essential prerequisite to pursuing nonoperative management.

Operative Management

The approach to operative management of vascular injury in the blast-injured patient follows the same core principles of vascular surgery that guide the repair of any vascular injury pattern. Initial management is focused on the control of hemorrhage. This can be performed through dissection and direct vessel control proximal and distal to the site of injury. However, certain instances mandate alternative approaches to inflow control. The use of tourniquets in the operating theater is commonplace and can be applied when the operative field is obscured due to rapid ongoing bleeding. This facilitates more deliberate and meticulous dissection, such that additional injury is not incurred. However, proximal extremity or junctional vessel injuries frequently are not amenable to tourniquet application, mandating alternate approaches. Inflow control at the level of the aorta or iliac vessels can be obtained through a laparotomy or retroperitoneal incision. Alternatively, vascular inflow can be obtained by endoluminal balloon occlusion at any level. When applied to the aorta, this hemorrhage control adjunct is known as Resuscitative Endovascular Balloon Occlusion of the Aorta (REBOA) [54]. Increasingly, this technique is applied as a less invasive means to control noncompressible torso hemorrhage (Fig. 11.4) but can also be used to gain control for junction injuries. This is commonly performed from the extremity contralateral to the injury and is described elsewhere in detail.

Once hemorrhage control is established, the injured vessel is widely exposed. Clamps or vessel loop control should then be limited to injured

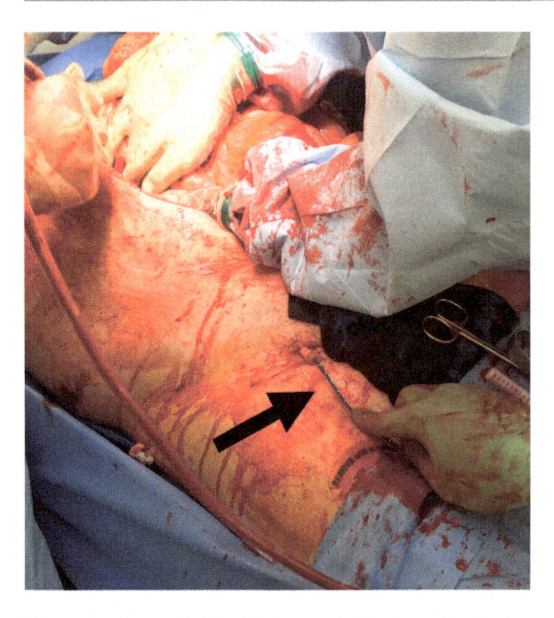

Fig. 11.4 Resuscitative Endovascular Balloon Occlusion of the Aorta. Aortic inflow control at the level of the supraceliac aorta was performed to prevent complete cardiovascular collapse from exsanguinating truncal hemorrhage from penetrating abdominal trauma. Arrow indicates the balloon catheter inserted through a 7 French introducer sheath

segment, with expeditious release of proximal balloons or tourniquets to minimize the global ischemic burden. Debridement and shunting should ensue, based on the physiologic state of the patient. When direct repair is being considered, it is important to resect the vessel back to a healthy, uninjured segment. While somewhat subjective, it is the author's stance to utilize the color of the vessel in order to determine viability. The adventitial surface should possess red vasa vasorum, indicating continued perfusion. The intima should be free from dissection of disruption and tan in color. Contused, hemorrhagic, or gray coloration implies vessel injury and warrants further debridement. Assessment of the vein follows a similar approach.

Systemic anticoagulation should be utilized when associated injuries do not preclude its use. When contraindications exist, the local administration of heparinized saline above and below the injury should be utilized at minimum. Effort should be undertaken to clear thrombus from the vessels proximally and distally using a Fogarty balloon catheter. Ideally, one should restore inflow from the proximal segment and back-bleeding from the distal segment prior to repair of the injury. Vasospasm is common, particularly in young trauma patients. This can be treated with the administration of vasodilators such as nitroglycerine and papaverine. Alternatively, gentle, judicious use of vascular dilators can be considered.

With rare exception, blast injuries preclude the opportunity for direct repair. If there is a short segment of disrupted vessel, an end-to-end anastomosis can be considered provided there is minimal tension. More commonly, interposition grafting is required. As such, wide preparation of the patient should be performed in anticipation of the need for conduit harvest.

Autogenous vein with little exception remains the gold standard conduit, especially with respect to traumatic injury [6]. In general, this should be obtained from an uninjured extremity, typically the contralateral great saphenous vein, so as to not further impair venous return. However, blast injury frequently results in bilateral lower extremity injury, thus potentially negating this as a viable option. In such instances, upper extremity arm vein represents the next best option. However, when the extent of arterial injury is limited without significant soft tissue disruption and in the absence of axial venous injury, a short segment of ipsilateral vein from the affected extremities can be considered. When multiple extremity injuries exist, autogenous vein from the least injured extremity represents the best option, albeit less than ideal. Rarely, deep vein conduit such as the femoral vein, hypogastric artery, or internal jugular vein may be considered but is technically more demanding and time consuming.

The utilization of prosthetic grafts for vascular reconstruction in military-related vascular trauma, particularly the highly contained wounds created with blast injury, has been consistently discouraged [55, 56]. To emphasize the commitment to this policy, only approximately 3–15% of vascular injuries during recent conflicts in Iraq and Afghanistan were repaired using prosthetic grafts [6, 56]. However, instances occur when the use of prosthetic graft may be the initial best option, particularly when reconstruction with autologous conduit is not an option or outstrips the capabilities of the local surgical assets. In these cases, the use of a prosthetic graft as a temporizing solution has been employed. Vertrees and colleagues reported a high percentage (80%) of prosthetic grafts ultimately undergoing explantation and reconstruction with autologous conduit. Factors influencing this decision included the intended use of prosthetic graft as a temporizing solution with a plan for delayed definitive repair; however, a few grafts required removal due to obvious graft infection or graft thrombosis. Importantly, this approach did not lead to any instances of graft blowout, nor did it result in amputation due to graft thrombosis [56]. The authors concluded that for complex repairs, when autologous conduit is limited, a temporary prosthetic graft followed by staged, definitive autogenous reconstruction may be a reasonable option [56]. In certain anatomic distributions, such as the carotid and subclavian territory, expanded polytetrafluoroethylene (ePTFE) grafts performed equal to vein over long-term follow-up. However, the use of prosthetics in the extremity resulted in a higher need for reintervention with long-term follow-up compared to autologous vein (69% vs. 23%; $p = 0.04$) [57].

Civilian literature also has a pessimistic view regarding the use of ePTFE for trauma, with exception given to large vessels in the junctional or truncal distribution [58, 59]. Patency of these grafts for extremity vascular injury has not been encouraging. Additionally, a 2015 meta-analysis showed an nearly twofold higher risk of secondary amputation (OR 1.88; CI 0.55–5.83, $p = 0.88$); however, this did not reach statistical significance [18]. Overall, autologous conduit remains the most durable option in the long term with less concern regarding graft infection or other complications such as stenosis or occlusion that likely mandate reintervention.

Following repair, the use of low-dose antiplatelet therapy is routine, unless otherwise contraindicated. Every effort to obtain soft tissue coverage of the repair should be taken, to avoid disruption or desiccation of the repaired segment. In certain instances, the extent of soft tissue injury precludes complete soft tissue coverage. Furthermore, wound closure may not be desirable in situations with significant wound contamination. The use of closed suction negative pressure dressings in this context has become instrumental for the management of complex wounds.

When considering repair of venous injuries, it is useful to perform Esmarch exsanguination of the elevated limb. This allows for full access to the vessel lumen without ongoing hemorrhage, as well as the ability to freely pass Fogarty catheters to clear thrombus from the vessel. It is reasonable to perform simple lateral suture repair of the vessel when the residual lumen will be at least 50% of its native diameter. Otherwise, repair using patch angioplasty, panel grafting, spiral grafting, or interposition grafting should be considered. When the vessel is transected, direct end-to-end repair can be performed when undo tension is not required.

When combined arterial and venous injuries exist, it is a matter of debate as to the ideal sequence of repair (Fig. 11.5). In certain instances, it is the author's preference to repair venous injury prior to arterial repair. These include scenarios where a temporary vascular shunt is utilized for the arterial injury and normalization of distal perfusion is established, the extremity injury is isolated and the extent of concomitant injuries is minimal, autogenous conduit

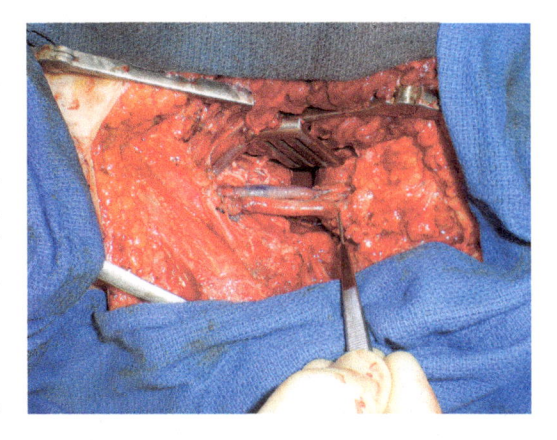

Fig. 11.5 Interposition graft repair of a combined arterial and venous injury utilizing autologous contralateral saphenous vein

is abundant, and significant surrounding soft tissue injury exists, where collateral venous pathways are likely obliterated. This strategy serves to improve arterial flow, minimize tissue edema, and minimize venous bleeding from injured collateral venous pathways.

Specific Injuries

Lower Extremity

Femoral Artery Injuries

The femoral artery, specifically the superficial femoral artery, is the most common site for vascular injury, accounting for approximately 25–50% in both civilian and military series. Obtaining vascular inflow control varies by the specific location of the injury. Common femoral artery (CFA) injuries typically require control at the level of the external iliac artery, either through a retroperitoneal or transabdominal approach. The retroperitoneal exposure, accomplished through an oblique lower abdominal incision parallel to the fibers of the external oblique (parallel to the inguinal ligament), is less familiar to most surgeons but provides excellent exposure. Further technical aspects of these exposures are available elsewhere.

When endovascular capabilities are available, direct endoluminal control can be obtained with a variety of balloon catheters. Alternatively, contralateral retrograde common femoral access can be obtained, through which an aortic occlusion balloon can be introduced to perform REBOA. The presence of collateral circulation may perpetuate some mild continued bleeding; however, this is typically manageable and does not preclude exploration of the injured vessel. Once inflow control is established, direct exposure of the injury should ensue promptly, typically via a longitudinal groin incision overlying the common femoral artery. When soft tissue injury from blast is extensive, detailed dissection may not be feasible or necessary, as the vessel may be already exposed.

Vascular repair will be dictated based on the extent of injury. Following appropriate vessel debridement, autogenous repair should be performed when physiology allows. Mobility of the vascular segment is minimal; therefore, opportunity for direct repair is limited. Patch angioplasty or interposition grafting with saphenous vein or alternative vein conduit is appropriate. It is important to restore luminal diameter to at least two-thirds the native luminal diameter; therefore, saphenous vein alone may be inadequate.

Disruption of the femoral bifurcation poses significant challenge and technical expertise for repair. Revascularization of both the superficial femoral artery (SFA) and profunda femoris artery (PFA) should be attempted when feasible. When complex injury has occurred, the planned temporary use of a bifurcated prosthetic graft can be entertained in lieu of a complex autologous repair. When a patient is in extremis, ligation of the PFA can be performed, as this vascular distribution typically receives collateral flow from the ipsilateral hypogastric artery. Alternatively, shunting of both the SFA and PFA can be performed when local resources are insufficient to perform such repairs.

Injuries to more distal segments of the SFA are more readily controlled. Inflow control can be established through a standard longitudinal groin incision. On occasion, inflow control can be obtained with the simple application of a high thigh tourniquet or blood pressure cuff. Tourniquets and blood pressure cuffs can also be used directly at the site of injury to staunch hemorrhage while proximal vascular control is obtained. Repair ensues as described above.

Popliteal Artery Injuries

The popliteal artery is the second most common location for lower extremity arterial injury and is frequently associated with concomitant venous injury in half of cases. Additionally, tibial nerve is not uncommon, occurring in approximately 10–30% of patients with vascular injury in this distribution. Due to these factors, injury to the popliteal artery accounts for the highest risk of requiring secondary extremity amputation.

Exposure is typically performed from a medial approach, with incisions above and below the knee. This provides access to the groin, abdomen, and chest, which is often mandatory following blast injuries with multiple sites of injury. The posterior approach is used rarely in the context of blast-injured patients and should be reserved for patients with isolated popliteal artery injury. Above the knee, a longitudinal incision is made at the anterior border of the sartorius muscle. Upon entry into the fascia, retraction of the sartorius posteriorly and the vastus lateralis anteriorly reveals an essentially avascular plane that leads directly to the distal SFA and suprageniculate popliteal artery in the region of the adductor hiatus. Below the knee, a longitudinal medial incision is made posterior to the tibia, being mindful to avoid injury to the great saphenous vein and nerve in this region. The gastrocnemius muscle is retracted posteriorly. Proximal tibial attachments of the soleus muscle can be divided to expose the origin of the anterior tibial artery, tibioperoneal trunk, and bifurcation. To gain more proximal exposure of the popliteal artery from the below-knee incision, division of the gracilis, semimembranosus, and semitendinosus tendons can be performed; however, attempts to reapproximate these muscle bands should be considered following repair. Often a small segment of vessel cannot be accessed from this approach, negating direct repair of injuries in this region. In such instances, ligation with bypass is performed. Again, consideration for the use of temporary vascular shunts of arterial and/or venous injuries is strongly encouraged in patients unfit for extensive repair.

Tibial Artery Injuries

Injury of the tibial vessels is not uncommon, but infrequently poses life-threatening hemorrhage in the absence of other injuries. Vascular control is typically performed with the application of a thigh tourniquet and Esmarch exsanguination of the leg. Extensive dissection of tibial vessels should be avoided, to prevent disruption of small caliber branch vessels. Exposure of the anterior tibial artery is performed through a lateral calf incision 2–3 fingerbreadths lateral to the anterior tibial edge. From a medial approach, the exposure is analogous to that of the popliteal artery, with a more distal extension of the incision based on the level of injury. The tibial attachments of the soleus muscle must be divided extensively to gain access to the tibioperoneal trunk, posterior tibial artery (PTA), and/or the peroneal artery.

Management of tibial injuries is typically performed with simple ligation given the rich collateral circulation frequently present, provided one of the three named tibial vessels remains intact. Confirmation of limb perfusion can be performed with intraoperative duplex or continuous wave Doppler. Alternatively, conventional angiography can be employed, particularly when it is being utilized simultaneously in the management of concomitant injuries. It is important to recognize that patients in shock may have objective evidence of poor extremity perfusion in the absence of vessel injury due to vasospasm, confounding the use of these diagnostic modalities. Sound clinical judgment must be employed based on the clinical context. Tibial reconstruction should rarely be entertained, based on a strong suspicion for profound limb ischemia. Again shunting can be considered even in the distal arteries, recognizing that patency is poor [34].

Upper Extremity

Axillosubclavian Artery Injury

Fortunately, subclavian artery injuries are rare, accounting for a mere 2% of all arterial injury, with axillary artery injuries occurring slightly more frequently. Detailed description of vascular exposures can be found elsewhere. In brief, the right subclavian artery is typically approached via a median sternotomy. Supraclavicular extension of the incision can be helpful, with or without resection of the clavicle or retraction (splitting the manubrium). The left subclavian artery poses more of a challenge given its more posterior location and is typically exposed via a left anterolateral thoracotomy. However, control can be obtained from an anterior approach and is aided by supraclavicular or cervical extension. Rarely, a trap door approach can be performed, but is morbid and should be utilized as a last resort. More distal exposure of the subclavian arteries can be accomplished via combined supraclavicular and infraclavicular incisions, with consideration for clavicular resection when needed. The need for clavicular reconstruction is controversial and is beyond the scope of this chapter.

To expose the axillary artery bilaterally, an infraclavicular incision is utilized, two fingerbreadths below the clavicle. A scapular/shoulder roll should be utilized to aid in exposure. Division of the pectoralis minor muscle can be performed to gain additional exposure. Care should be taken during these exposures to avoid injury to the dense surrounding nervous and lymphatic structures in these regions, particularly the brachial plexus, phrenic nerves, and thoracic duct (on the left).

Repair of the axillary and subclavian arteries should proceed in the general conduct of arterial repair previously discussed. However, a tension-free repair is particularly important, given the delicate nature of this vessel. Prosthetic materials have been more frequently utilized in this distribution when contamination is minimal given the larger vessel caliber; however, autologous conduit remains preferable when feasible. In more extensive injuries, ligation with or without revascularization using bypass can be considered, particularly when collaterals to the subclavian and axillary arteries remain preserved. Alternatively, ligation with extra-anatomic bypass can be considered.

Brachial Artery Injuries
Proximal control is easily accomplished with a tourniquet, blood pressure cuff, or manual compression. Exposure is achieved with a longitudinal medial arm incision in the groove between the biceps and triceps and can be extended as needed. Care should be taken to avoid injury to the median and ulnar nerves that are in close proximity. The basilic vein should be preserved when feasible to ensure adequate venous drainage of the arm. Below the elbow, division of the bicipital aponeurosis is performed to expose the brachial artery in this region and allows exposure of the brachial bifurcation.

Repair is based on the extent of injury and length of the disrupted segment. Mobilization and primary end-to-end anastomosis is occasionally feasible, provided tension is minimal. Otherwise interposition grafting with autologous conduit is preferred. When injuries occur distal to the profunda brachii, or in instances where a high brachial artery bifurcation exists, ligation may be considered due to the presence of these collateral pathways; however, shunting with a plan for delayed repair is preferable.

Radial and Ulnar Artery Injuries
Forearm vascular injuries are the most common upper extremity arterial injury pattern. Fortunately, these injuries rarely result in life-threatening hemorrhage and are easily controlled with a tourniquet, blood pressure cuff, or digital compression. Exposure in the upper forearm should begin by identifying the brachial artery with a typical antecubital exposure. More distally, an incision overlying the medial border of the brachioradialis muscle is performed to expose the radial artery. Exposure of the ulnar artery in the mid arm is more challenging, as it runs deep to the flexor muscle group. However, this artery can typically be traced along its length from the antecubital incision.

Management of radial and ulnar artery injuries is similar to that of the tibial vessels. Ligation of a single vessel is typically well tolerated. Again, the use of continuous wave Doppler is indispensable in this regard and should be employed routinely to assess distal perfusion. Direct end-to-end repair following spatulation of both segments is feasible. Interposition grafting is preferred for longer segment disruptions. Patch angioplasty for vessels of this caliber is typically not employed. For reconstructions at or beyond the wrist, assistance from a hand surgeon should be utilized when this resource is available.

Endovascular Therapies for Trauma

While endovascular interventions are increasingly commonplace, application in vascular trauma occurs in less than 8% of injuries [60]. However, particular injury patterns, typically in junctional or truncal regions, are ideally suited to these techniques. Perhaps the best example of this is the widespread use of thoracic stent grafts

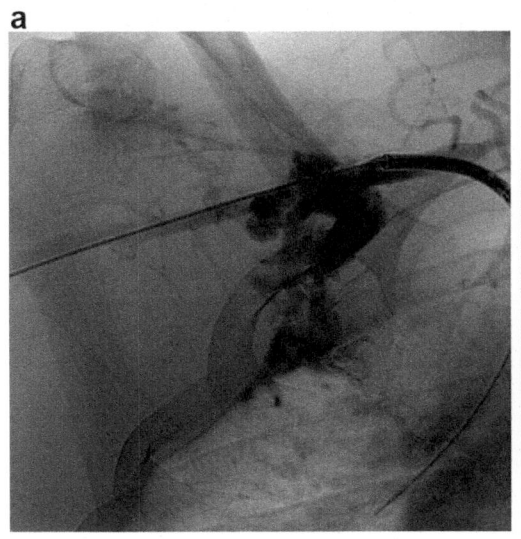

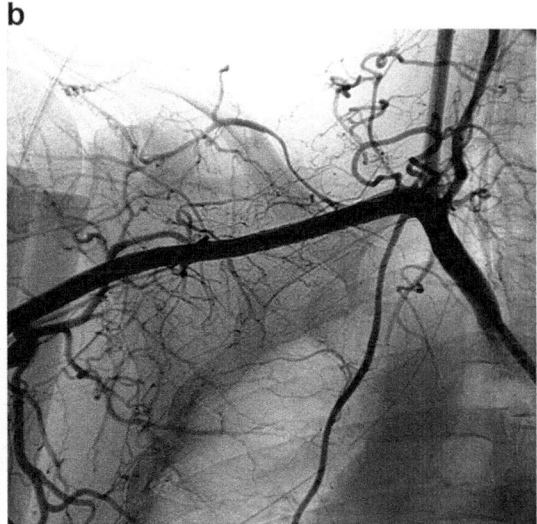

Fig. 11.6 Endovascular management of penetrating axillary artery injury. (**a**) Angiography demonstrates active contrast extravasation from the right axillary artery. (**b**) Following deployment of a self-expanding stent graft, repeat angiography demonstrates no residual contrast extravasation, with restoration of normal luminal diameter

for the repair of blunt aortic injury [61]. In both OIF and OEF, endovascular capability was established for role III surgical facilities and utilized in well over 100 cases of vascular injury [62].

Another common application for this technology is the use of covered stent grafts in the repair of penetrating axillosubclavian and innominate artery injury, with technical success rates exceeding 90% and low rates of morbidity and mortality [63, 64]. As mentioned, the technical challenges and morbidity associated with vascular exposure in this region make this an ideal injury pattern for endovascular repair.

Additional injury patterns amenable to catheter-based intervention include both blunt and penetrating solid organ or pelvic injuries, where imaging demonstrates the presence of contrast extravasation or pseudoaneurysm (Fig. 11.6) [40, 63, 65, 66]. Various techniques exist, including vessel embolization with coils or other embolic materials such as gel foam, as well as the use of covered stent grafts.

Even when hemodynamic instability exists, patients may benefit from endovascular intervention. Endovascular adjuncts such as REBOA can be employed as a temporizing measure to allow for a more calculated approach to vascular injury management and thereby providing the necessary time to mobilized endovascular assets. Additionally, the increasing availability of hybrid operating rooms can facilitate the fluid transition between open and endovascular techniques in real time or allowing both to proceed simultaneously, avoiding the need to physically move the patient to perform one or the other. It is reasonable to surmise the increased application of these techniques in the management of blast-injured trauma patients as the technologies continue to mature.

References

1. Ficke JR, Eastridge BJ, Butler FK, Alvarez J, Brown T, Pasquina P, et al. Dismounted complex blast injury report of the army dismounted complex blast injury task force. J Trauma Acute Care Surg. 2012;73(6):S520–S34.
2. DeBakey ME, Simeone FA. Battle injuries of the arteries in World War II: an analysis of 2,471 cases. Ann Surg. 1946;123(4):534.

3. Rich N, Baugh J, Hughes C. Acute arterial injuries in Vietnam: 1,000 cases. J Trauma. 1970;10(5):359.
4. White JM, Stannard A, Burkhardt GE, Eastridge BJ, Blackbourne LH, Rasmussen TE. The epidemiology of vascular injury in the wars in Iraq and Afghanistan. Ann Surg. 2011;253(6):1184–9.
5. Fox CJ, Patel B, Clouse WD. Update on wartime vascular injury. Perspect Vasc Surg Endovasc Ther. 2011;23(1):13–25.
6. Clouse WD, Rasmussen TE, Peck MA, Eliason JL, Cox MW, Bowser AN, et al. In-theater management of vascular injury: 2 years of the Balad Vascular Registry. J Am Coll Surg. 2007;204(4):625–32.
7. Ritenour AE, Baskin TW. Primary blast injury: update on diagnosis and treatment. Crit Care Med. 2008;36(7):S311–S7.
8. Gwinn DE, Tintle SM, Kumar AR, Andersen RC, Keeling JJ. Blast-induced lower extremity fractures with arterial injury: prevalence and risk factors for amputation after initial limb-preserving treatment. J Orthop Trauma. 2011;25(9):543–8.
9. Perkins Z, De'Ath H, Aylwin C, Brohi K, Walsh M, Tai N. Epidemiology and outcome of vascular trauma at a British Major Trauma Centre. Eur J Vasc Endovasc Surg. 2012;44(2):203–9.
10. Alam HB, DiMusto PD. Management of lower extremity vascular trauma. Curr Trauma Rep. 2015;1(1):61–8.
11. Barmparas G, Inaba K, Talving P, David J-S, Lam L, Plurad D, et al. Pediatric vs adult vascular trauma: a National Trauma Databank review. J Pediatr Surg. 2010;45(7):1404–12.
12. Tan T-W, Joglar FL, Hamburg NM, Eberhardt RT, Shaw PM, Rybin D, et al. Limb outcome and mortality in lower and upper extremity arterial injury a comparison using the National Trauma Data Bank. Vasc Endovasc Surg. 2011;45(7):592–7.
13. Franz RW, Shah KJ, Halaharvi D, Franz ET, Hartman JF, Wright ML. A 5-year review of management of lower extremity arterial injuries at an urban level I trauma center. J Vasc Surg. 2011;53(6):1604–10.
14. Asensio JA, Kuncir EJ, García-Núñez LM, Petrone P. Femoral vessel injuries: analysis of factors predictive of outcomes. J Am Coll Surg. 2006;203(4):512–20.
15. Mullenix PS, Steele SR, Andersen CA, Starnes BW, Salim A, Martin MJ. Limb salvage and outcomes among patients with traumatic popliteal vascular injury: an analysis of the National Trauma Data Bank. J Vasc Surg. 2006;44(1):94–100.
16. Dorlac WC, DeBakey ME, Holcomb JB, Fagan SP, Kwong KL, Dorlac GR, et al. Mortality from isolated civilian penetrating extremity injury. J Trauma Acute Care Surg. 2005;59(1):217–22.
17. Kauvar DS, Sarfati MR, Kraiss LW. National trauma databank analysis of mortality and limb loss in isolated lower extremity vascular trauma. J Vasc Surg. 2011;53(6):1598–603.
18. Perkins Z, Yet B, Glasgow S, Cole E, Marsh W, Brohi K, et al. Meta-analysis of prognostic factors for amputation following surgical repair of lower extremity vascular trauma. Br J Surg. 2015;102(5):436–50.
19. Weaver FA, Yellin AE, Bauer M, Oberg J, Ghalambor N, Emmanuel RP, et al. Is arterial proximity a valid indication for arteriography in penetrating extremity trauma?: a prospective analysis. Arch Surg. 1990;125(10):1256–60.
20. Schwartz MR, Weaver FA, Bauer M, Siegel A, Yellin AE. Refining the indications for arteriography in penetrating extremity trauma: a prospective analysis. J Vasc Surg. 1993;17(1):116–24.
21. Johansen K, Lynch K, Paun M, Copass M. Noninvasive vascular tests reliably exclude occult arterial trauma in injured extremities. J Trauma Acute Care Surg. 1991;31(4):515–22.
22. Nassoura ZE, Ivatury RR, Simon RJ, Jabbour N, Vinzons A, Stahl W. A reassessment of Doppler pressure indices in the detection of arterial lesions in proximity penetrating injuries of extremities: a prospective study. Am J Emerg Med. 1996;14(2):151–6.
23. Dennis JW, Frykberg ER, Crump JM, Vines FS, Alexander RH. New perspectives on the management of penetrating trauma in proximity to major limb arteries. J Vasc Surg. 1990;11(1):84–93.
24. Dennis JW, Frykberg ER, Veldenz HC, Huffman S, Menawat SS. Validation of nonoperative management of occult vascular injuries and accuracy of physical examination alone in penetrating extremity trauma: 5-to 10-year follow-up. J Trauma Acute Care Surg. 1998;44(2):243–53.
25. Knudson MM, Lewis FR, Atkinson K, Neuhaus A. The role of duplex ultrasound arterial imaging in patients with penetrating extremity trauma. Arch Surg. 1993;128(9):1033–8.
26. Fry WR, Smith RS, Sayers DV, Henderson VJ, Morabito DJ, Tsoi EK, et al. The success of duplex ultrasonographic scanning in diagnosis of extremity vascular proximity trauma. Arch Surg. 1993;128(12):1368–72.
27. Bynoe RP, Miles WS, Bell RM, Greenwold DR, Sessions G, Haynes JL, et al. Noninvasive diagnosis of vascular trauma by duplex ultrasonography. J Vasc Surg. 1991;14(3):346–52.
28. Bergstein JM, Blair J-F, Edwards J, Towne JB, Wittmann DH, Aprahamian C, et al. Pitfalls in the use of color-flow duplex ultrasound for screening of suspected arterial injuries in penetrated extremities. J Trauma Acute Care Surg. 1992;33(3):395–402.
29. Patterson B, Holt P, Cleanthis M, Tai N, Carrell T, Loosemore T. Imaging vascular trauma. Br J Surg. 2012;99(4):494–505.
30. Inaba K, Branco BC, Reddy S, Park JJ, Green D, Plurad D, et al. Prospective evaluation of multidetector computed tomography for extremity vascular trauma. J Trauma Acute Care Surg. 2011;70(4):808–15.
31. Kragh JF Jr, Walters TJ, Baer DG, Fox CJ, Wade CE, Salinas J, et al. Practical use of emergency tourniquets to stop bleeding in major limb trauma. J Trauma Acute Care Surg. 2008;64(2):S38–50.
32. Hancock H, Rasmussen TE, Walker AJ, Rich NM. History of temporary intravascular shunts in the management of vascular injury. J Vasc Surg. 2010;52(5):1405–9.

33. Chambers LW, Green DJ, Sample K, Gillingham BL, Rhee P, Brown C, et al. Tactical surgical intervention with temporary shunting of peripheral vascular trauma sustained during Operation Iraqi Freedom: one unit's experience. J Trauma Acute Care Surg. 2006;61(4):824–30.
34. Rasmussen TE, Clouse WD, Jenkins DH, Peck MA, Eliason JL, Smith DL. The use of temporary vascular shunts as a damage control adjunct in the management of wartime vascular injury. J Trauma Acute Care Surg. 2006;61(1):8–15.
35. Taller J, Kamdar JP, Greene JA, Morgan RA, Blankenship CL, Dabrowski P, et al. Temporary vascular shunts as initial treatment of proximal extremity vascular injuries during combat operations: the new standard of care at Echelon II facilities? J Trauma Acute Care Surg. 2008;65(3):595–603.
36. Woodward EB, Clouse WD, Eliason JL, Peck MA, Bowser AN, Cox MW, et al. Penetrating femoropopliteal injury during modern warfare: experience of the Balad Vascular Registry. J Vasc Surg. 2008;47(6):1259–65.
37. Williams TK, Clouse WD. Current concepts in repair of extremity venous injury. J Vasc Surg: Venous Lymphat Disord. 2016;4(2):238–47.
38. Marinho de Oliveira Góes Junior A, de Campos Vieira Abib S, de Seixas Alves MT, Venerando da Silva Ferreira PS, Carvalho de Andrade M. To shunt or not to shunt? An experimental study comparing temporary vascular shunts and venous ligation as damage control techniques for vascular trauma. Ann Vasc Surg. 2014;28(3):710–24.
39. Dawson DL, Putnam AT, Light JT, Ihnat DM, Kissinger DP, Rasmussen TE, et al. Temporary arterial shunts to maintain limb perfusion after arterial injury: an animal study. J Trauma Acute Care Surg. 1999;47(1):64–71.
40. Davidson AJ, Neff LP, DuBose JJ, Sampson JB, Abbot CM, Williams TK. Direct-site endovascular repair (DSER): a novel approach to vascular trauma. J Trauma Acute Care Surg. 2016;81(5):S138–S43.
41. Rich N, Hughes C, Baugh J. Management of venous injuries. Ann Surg. 1970;171(5):724–30.
42. Rich NM. Principles and indications for primary venous repair. Surgery. 1982;91(5):492–6.
43. Rich NM, Collins GJ Jr, Andersen CA, McDonald PT. Autogenous venous interposition grafts in repair of major venous injuries. J Trauma Acute Care Surg. 1977;17(7):512–20.
44. Gifford SM, Aidinian G, Clouse WD, Fox CJ, Porras CA, Jones WT, et al. Effect of temporary shunting on extremity vascular injury: an outcome analysis from the Global War on Terror vascular injury initiative. J Vasc Surg. 2009;50(3):549–56.
45. Meyer J, Walsh J, Schuler J, Barrett J, Durham J, Eldrup-Jorgensen J, et al. The early fate of venous repair after civilian vascular trauma. A clinical, hemodynamic, and venographic assessment. Ann Surg. 1987;206(4):458.
46. Nypaver TJ, Schuler JJ, McDonnell P, Ellenby MI, Montalvo J, Baraniewski H, et al. Long-term results of venous reconstruction after vascular trauma in civilian practice. J Vasc Surg. 1992;16(5):762–8.
47. Farber A, Tan T-W, Hamburg NM, Kalish JA, Joglar F, Onigman T, et al. Early fasciotomy in patients with extremity vascular injury is associated with decreased risk of adverse limb outcomes: a review of the National Trauma Data Bank. Injury. 2012;43(9):1486–91.
48. Ritenour AE, Dorlac WC, Fang R, Woods T, Jenkins DH, Flaherty SF, et al. Complications after fasciotomy revision and delayed compartment release in combat patients. J Trauma Acute Care Surg. 2008;64(2):S153–S62.
49. Stain SC, Yellin AE, Weaver FA, Pentecost MJ. Selective management of nonocclusive arterial injuries. Arch Surg. 1989;124(10):1136–41.
50. Frykberg E, Vines F, Alexander R. The natural history of clinically occult arterial injuries: a prospective evaluation. J Trauma. 1989;29(5):577.
51. Feliciano DV, Moore FA, Moore EE, West MA, Davis JW, Cocanour CS, et al. Evaluation and management of peripheral vascular injury. Part 1. Western Trauma Association/critical decisions in trauma. J Trauma Acute Care Surg. 2011;70(6):1551–6.
52. Neville R Jr, Hobson R 2nd, Watanabe B, Yasuhara H, Padberg F Jr, Duran W, et al. A prospective evaluation of arterial intimal injuries in an experimental model. J Trauma. 1991;31(5):669.
53. Hernández-Maldonado JJ, Padberg FT Jr, Teehan E, Neville R, DeFouw D, Durán WN, et al. Arterial intimal flaps: a comparison of primary repair, aspirin, and endovascular excision in an experimental model. J Trauma Acute Care Surg. 1993;34(4):565–70.
54. Stannard A, Eliason JL, Rasmussen TE. Resuscitative endovascular balloon occlusion of the aorta (REBOA) as an adjunct for hemorrhagic shock. J Trauma Acute Care Surg. 2011;71(6):1869–72.
55. Rich N, Hughes C. The fate of prosthetic material used to repair vascular injuries in contaminated wounds. J Trauma. 1972;12(6):459–67.
56. Vertrees A, Fox CJ, Quan RW, Cox MW, Adams ED, Gillespie DL. The use of prosthetic grafts in complex military vascular trauma: a limb salvage strategy for patients with severely limited autologous conduit. J Trauma Acute Care Surg. 2009;66(4):980–3.
57. Watson JDB, Houston R, Morrison JJ, Gifford SM, Rasmussen TE. A retrospective cohort comparison of expanded polytetrafluoroethylene to autologous vein for vascular reconstruction in modern combat casualty care. Ann Vasc Surg. 2015;29(4):822–9.
58. Feliciano D, Mattox K, Graham J, Bitondo C. Five-year experience with PTFE grafts in vascular wounds. J Trauma. 1985;25(1):71–82.
59. Shah DM, Leather RP, Corson JD, Karmody AM. Polytetrafluoroethylene grafts in the rapid reconstruction of acute contaminated peripheral vascular injuries. Am J Surg. 1984;148(2):229–33.

60. DuBose JJ, Savage SA, Fabian TC, Menaker J, Scalea T, Holcomb JB, et al. The American Association for the Surgery of Trauma PROspective Observational Vascular Injury Treatment (PROOVIT) registry: multicenter data on modern vascular injury diagnosis, management, and outcomes. J Trauma Acute Care Surg. 2015;78(2):215–23.
61. Lee WA, Matsumura JS, Mitchell RS, Farber MA, Greenberg RK, Azizzadeh A, et al. Endovascular repair of traumatic thoracic aortic injury: clinical practice guidelines of the Society for Vascular Surgery. J Vasc Surg. 2011;53(1):187–92.
62. Rasmussen TE, Clouse WD, Peck MA, Bowser AN, Eliason JL, Cox MW, et al. Development and implementation of endovascular capabilities in wartime. J Trauma Acute Care Surg. 2008;64(5):1169–76.
63. du Toit DF, Lambrechts AV, Stark H, Warren BL. Long-term results of stent graft treatment of subclavian artery injuries: management of choice for stable patients? J Vasc Surg. 2008;47(4):739–43.
64. Hershberger RC, Aulivola B, Murphy M, Luchette FA. Endovascular grafts for treatment of traumatic injury to the aortic arch and great vessels. J Trauma Acute Care Surg. 2009;67(3):660–71.
65. White R, Krajcer Z, Johnson M, Williams D, Bacharach M, O'Malley E. Results of a multicenter trial for the treatment of traumatic vascular injury with a covered stent. J Trauma Acute Care Surg. 2006;60(6):1189–96.
66. DuBose JJ, Rajani R, Gilani R, Arthurs ZA, Morrison JJ, Clouse WD, et al. Endovascular management of axillo-subclavian arterial injury: a review of published experience. Injury. 2012;43(11):1785–92.

Genitourinary Trauma

12

Matthew Banti and Jack Ryan Walter

Genitourinary Trauma

Operation Enduring Freedom (OEF) and Operation Iraqi Freedom (OIF) were the longest and most notable US military engagements of the early twenty-first century. The modern battlefield in these theaters witnessed a paradigm shift with the wide implementation of improvised explosive devices (IEDs) against coalition forces in Afghanistan and Iraq. Wartime trauma in the twentieth century can be largely attributed to high-velocity rounds from small arms as well as artillery explosive injury. The shift to IEDs in OEF and OIF changed this pattern and led to a significant amount of devastating trauma that has come to be known as dismounted complex blast injury [1]. Severe wounds to the lower extremities, pelvis, and external genitals are the hallmarks of IED injuries, and therefore the management of acute trauma to the genitourinary (GU) structures is of renewed importance on the modern battlefield. Modern combat lifesaving techniques and resuscitation efforts have led to increased survivability for casualties that in previous conflicts would have expired prior to transfer to higher echelons of care. As a consequence, patients with complex and severe genitourinary wounds will be encountered in combat medicine, and a working knowledge of the epidemiology, acute management, and strategies for GU reconstruction is essential not only to ensure proper care at the point of injury but also as a foundation for future reconstructive efforts.

Renal and Ureteral Injuries

The kidneys are paired structures that, in their orthotropic location, reside in the retroperitoneum and are bordered by the diaphragm superiorly; the ribs, quadratus lumborum, and aponeurosis of the transversus abdominis laterally; and the psoas major posteriorly. Anteriorly the right kidney is associated with the liver, duodenum, and colon, while the left kidney maintains close anatomic relation to the spleen, pancreatic tail, and colon. Enveloping the kidneys is a variable amount of perinephric fat contained within Gerota fascia. The protected location of the renal structures affords considerable resistance to injury, but even with these natural safeguards, the kidneys are susceptible to penetrating and deceleration injuries, with the latter being the primary mechanism in non-wartime civilian trauma [2].

In large-scale US military engagements in the early and mid-twentieth century, the kidney was the predominant genitourinary organ injury encountered among casualties. Penetrating abdominal trauma secondary to high-velocity munitions routinely caused severe damage to

M. Banti (✉) · J. R. Walter
Urology Service, Madigan Army Medical Center, Tacoma, WA, USA
e-mail: matthew.m.banti.mil@mail.mil; jack.r.walter.mil@mail.mil

major vascular, gastrointestinal, and genitourinary structures, with isolated renal involvement being exceedingly rare. Historical data on renal injury by Dr. Hugh Hampton Young in WWI is notable for a 50% mortality rate with nearly 40% of renal injuries involving a concomitant thoracic wound [3]. Flap-based renorrhaphy and other progress in renal surgery reduced some of the morbidity and mortality of these injuries, but advances in combat casualty care and rapid evacuation to definitive care via rotary-winged aircraft—especially during the Vietnam era—undoubtedly led to greater survivability. The use of Kevlar body armor in the first Gulf War is cited as the primary factor leading to the precipitous drop in penetrating injury to the kidneys and ureters seen in this wartime operation [4]. OEF and OIF have followed a similar trend, with Serkin et al. reporting kidney and ureteral injuries accounted for 281 (25.6%) of the 887 genitourinary injuries, a notable shift toward lower tract structure involvement [5]. Despite this decreased incidence, the life-threatening nature of renal and ureteral wounds necessitates prompt diagnosis and treatment when encountered in the combat wounded.

Management of Renal and Ureteral Trauma

Regardless of injury mechanism, renal injuries should be classified according to the American Association for the Surgery of Trauma (AAST) grading scale (Table 12.1) [6]. Traditionally,

Table 12.1 American Association for the Surgery of Trauma renal injury scale

Grade I	Contusion or nonexpanding subcapsular hematoma
Grade II	Nonexpanding perirenal hematoma, <1 cm cortical laceration without urinary extravasation
Grade III	Cortical laceration >1 cm without urinary extravasation
Grade IV	Laceration into collecting system or segmental renal artery or vein injury, contained hematoma
Grade V	Shattered kidney, renal pedicle avulsion

Adapted from [6]

combat-related kidney injuries were diagnosed during exploratory surgery, but availability of computed tomography (CT) has expanded significantly with only the most austere medical facilities lacking this capability. Blunt injury mechanisms account for 60–95% of renal trauma in the civilian experience but for only 2% in OEF and OIF [7, 8]. Nonetheless, blunt renal trauma must be considered in patients subjected to rapid deceleration or a direct blow to the flank, with rib fractures, flank ecchymosis, abrasions, and hematuria being indicative of an underlying kidney injury [9]. Abdominal and pelvic CT with immediate and delayed images should be obtained when gross or microscopic hematuria is present in a stable patient or when renal injury is suspected due to the aforementioned clinical signs or mechanism [2]. Regardless of AAST grading, hemodynamically stable patients can be initially managed with close observation and supportive care with the understanding that clinical deterioration of the patient due to ongoing blood loss, increasing flank pain, or abdominal distension should prompt immediate operative exploration as angioembolization of the kidney is unlikely to be available in forward casualty care facilities. Stable casualties with high-grade injuries (AAST IV–V) on observation warrant interval imaging to assess for urine leaks or urinomas that warrant drainage for proper healing.

Renal injury due to penetrating abdominal trauma is the most likely scenario to be present in battlefield casualties. Absolute indications for surgical exploration are life-threatening renal hemorrhage and avulsion of the ureteropelvic junction (UPJ) with the goal of renovascular control and kidney salvage. Damage control for ballistic injury to the hilar vessels will likely necessitate nephrectomy to control renal hemorrhage. Renal parenchymal injuries may be amenable to debridement and closure of the collecting system and parenchyma in layers with drain placement. In the absence of expanding or pulsatile retroperitoneal hemorrhage, renal exploration is not advocated. Opening of the retroperitoneal space can release the tamponade of a stable retroperitoneal hematoma. This results in a high rate of nephrectomy, as noted by the

63% nephrectomy rate reported by Hudak at the Balad Air Force Theater Hospital [10].

Management of ureteral injuries varies depending on the severity of injury and stability of the patient. The ultimate goal is diversion of urine to avoid leakage and urinoma formation, which carries a risk of sepsis, fistula, ileus, and abscess formation. Contusions may be managed with stent placement, while short defects in the abdominal ureter may be repaired with ureteroureterostomy over a stent with drain placement. Injuries to the pelvic ureter are routinely repaired with ureteral reimplant into the bladder. In the patient with extensive multisystem injuries, definitive reconstruction of the ureter should not be undertaken if the goal of exploration is damage control as this may compromise the intensive resuscitation required of these casualties. In these situations, the temporary diversion of urine can commonly be accomplished with ureteral ligation and percutaneous nephrostomy tube placement or externalization of the ureter to the skin surface. Both techniques are effective at controlling urine drainage although prompt nephrostomy tube placement by interventional radiology is required if the ureter is ligated. In the absence of this capability, the damaged ureter can be stented with a small catheter and brought to the skin surface to ensure urine diversion out of the peritoneal cavity. When utilizing this maneuver, excessive mobilization or tension can harm the delicate ureteral blood supply and lead to ischemic strictures or ureteral necrosis.

Bladder Injuries

Of Serkin's 887 reported genitourinary injuries in OEF and OIF, 189 (21.3%) involved the urinary bladder [5]. While the bladder's position within the bony pelvis affords considerable protection from traumatic injury, there is a strong association between bladder injury and pelvic fractures. Civilian urologic trauma experience notes 83–95% of bladder perforations occur with pelvic fractures, but only 10% of pelvic fractures involve bladder injury [11]. Similar to other genitourinary organs, bladder injury in wartime is overwhelmingly due to penetrating trauma, and thus in the majority of cases, exploratory surgery will occur. Bladder lacerations diagnosed operatively necessitate debridement of nonviable tissue and the closure, if possible, of the bladder mucosa and detrusor and serosa in a two-layer closure using absorbable suture. If additional bladder injuries are suspected, a transverse cystotomy can be made to further explore bladder integrity. Bladder decompression with a urethral catheter is mandatory, although devastating perineal blast injuries may warrant urinary diversion with suprapubic catheter drainage. Outside of immediate surgical exploration, traumatic bladder injuries may be assessed radiographically via cystography with instillation of intravesical contrast using fluoroscopy or plain films. Retrograde instillation of 300–350 mL of contrast (or until patient discomfort) ensures adequate bladder distension and is essential for visualization of an injury. Extraperitoneal ruptures will have a flame-like appearance and are likely to heal with catheter drainage alone, while intraperitoneal extravasation manifests as layering of contrast around the bowel. Intraperitoneal ruptures warrant operative exploration and closure with bladder drainage due to the risk for urine ascites. Eighty-nine (47%) of the extraperitoneal and intraperitoneal bladder injuries in Serkin's review were managed operatively [5]. Given the high rate of concomitant bony pelvis injuries, exploration by orthopedic surgeons for internal fixation can be combined with bladder repair for extraperitoneal ruptures, which may result in more rapid bladder healing than catheter drainage alone [12].

Penile Injuries

As was alluded to previously, implementation of IEDs in modern combat operations has shifted the pattern of genitourinary trauma away from penetrating injury to the kidneys, ureters, and bladder and instead toward involvement of the external genitalia. The predilection of penile, testiculoscrotal, and urethral trauma in OEF and OIF is certainly due to a multitude of factors. Unlike the privileged anatomic location of the upper urinary tract, the lower urinary tract structures lack natural shielding, and body armor available in the earlier stages of combat operations did not adequately protect the external genitals. As OEF and OIF transitioned into the insurgency stage, the wide implementation of IEDs resulted in a new devastating injury pattern that came to be known as dismounted complex blast injury. Blast injury from buried IEDs resulted in a spectrum of wounds to the external genitals, perineum, and lower extremities to dismounted service members, with a fivefold increase in genital injuries starting in 2010 compared to the years prior [13]. Countermeasures against these injuries included the introduction of Kevlar-reinforced "ballistic underwear" or "blast boxers" to service members in 2012, but to date, no studies have been published regarding their wartime efficacy.

The complexity of IED blasts encompasses shockwave (primary), penetrating fragments (secondary), deceleration (tertiary), and thermal (quaternary) injury patterns [14]. The predominant mechanism encountered among external genitalia injuries has been from penetrating fragments, which accounted for 75% of injuries in a 2015 review by Banti et al. Primary blast injuries were not noted in this review, and thermal involvement was rare at less than 1% [13].

As soft tissue structures, the penile and scrotal structures are susceptible to penetrating and tissue loss from penetrating injury, a reality that has significant impact on the patient's urinary, sexual, and psychological well-being. Given the primary mission of combat casualty care personnel and facilities, these issues are secondary to patient stabilization. That said, acute management of trauma to the external genitalia and urethra is of paramount importance for future function and reconstruction efforts, especially when severe injuries are sustained.

The penis is composed of deep structures—corpora cavernosa, corpus spongiosum, urethra—enveloped by Buck's fascia, the deep fascial layer of the penis. The walls of the erectile bodies are composed of tunica albuginea, a thick tissue layer with significant tensile strength. Superficial to Buck's fascia is the dartos layer

Table 12.2 American Association for the Surgery of Trauma penile injury scale

Grade I	Cutaneous laceration or contusion
Grade II	Buck's fascia (cavernosum) laceration without tissue loss
Grade III	Cutaneous avulsion, laceration through glans or meatus, cavernosal or urethral defect <2 cm
Grade IV	Partial penectomy
Grade V	Cavernosal or urethral defect ≥2 cm, total penectomy

Adapted from [6]

and penile skin. Approximately half of all traumatic penile injuries will be superficial penile lacerations or contusions graded as AAST I (Table 12.2) [12]. Management strategy in this case would mirror soft tissue injury to other organ systems with exploration, irrigation, and debridement, with immediate or delayed closure. With low-grade injuries encompassing the majority of patients with penile involvement, only 24% of cases required operative repair, and many minor injuries would be amenable to bedside treatment [5]. In contrast, AAST grade III–V penile wounds involve extensive penile tissue loss, fortunately with traumatic penectomy only noted in 1 of 501 patients in the Department of Defense Trauma Registry (DoDTR) [13]. Penile penetrating injury due to fragmentation or firearms should be explored operatively if the patient's hemodynamic status permits it, typically with degloving of the penis via a circumcising incision or direct exploration of the penetrating wound to adequately assess the deeper structures (Fig. 12.1). Meticulous irrigation and wound debridement are advocated, but extensive debridement should be avoided as tissue injury evolves following injury by high-speed projectiles [15]. When tissue viability cannot be adequately assessed, a staged approach with frequent returns to the operating room may result in a reduced need for aggressive debridement and loss of potentially viable tissue that is crucial for maintenance of penile function. Hudak noted approximately 45% of urologic surgeries in theater were reoperative in nature [10]. In severe cases with partial penile transection, salvage with reapproximation can be attempted, but the Balad

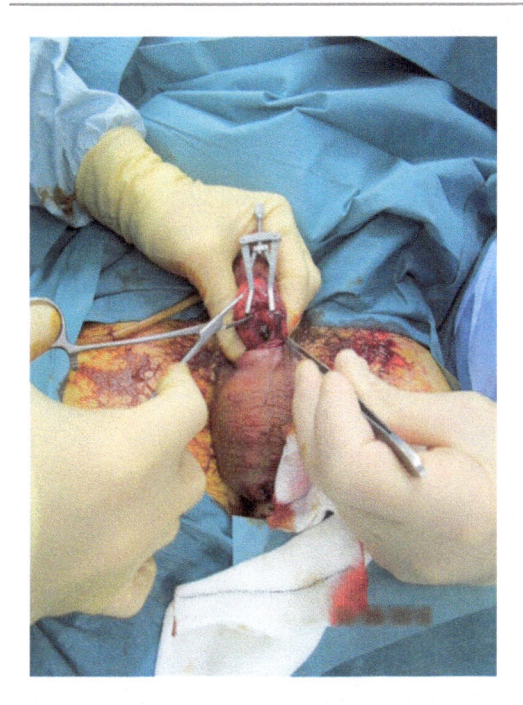

Fig. 12.1 Exploration of a penetrating penile injury from IED blast while on dismounted patrol

experience was notable for eventual partial penectomy in three patients due to necrosis [10]. Proximal skin disruption or avulsion leading to large cutaneous defects has also been encountered. Following initial debridement, these defects may be managed with local wound care or vacuum-assisted closure (VAC) devices to prepare for eventual coverage with split-thickness skin grafts during the reconstructive phase of the patient's care.

Urethral Injuries

The available literature from OEF and OIF describes 7 to 36 instances of urethral trauma accounting for 0.8–5% of genitourinary injuries encountered, respectively [5, 13]. Penetrating blast injury and gunshot wounds are cited as the primary mechanism—in contrast to civilian urethral trauma experience, which is overwhelmingly secondary to blunt pelvic fractures. Anatomically, the anterior urethra is composed of the fossa navicularis, pendulous, and bulbar segments with the posterior urethra encompassing the membranous and prostatic segments. The fossa navicularis and penile urethra are in the external portion of the phallus and thus are more vulnerable to penetrating trauma. The bulbar urethra travels in the perineum and is susceptible when this region is subject to blast or projectile injury as well as crushing during saddle trauma. Patients that sustain pelvic fractures are subject to pelvic fracture urethral injury (PFUI), seen in approximately 10% of cases, an injury that involves disruption of the membranous urethra due to shearing forces.

During the trauma survey of injured patients, the presence of blood at the urethral meatus should prompt further evaluation with retrograde urethrography. Blind passage of a urethral catheter is not advocated when blood is present owing to the risk of creating false passages and potentially worsening the urethral injury. Decompression and drainage of the urinary bladder is the most important objective when managing urethral trauma in the acute setting, and if a urethral catheter cannot be placed safely and expeditiously, the use of a suprapubic tube (SPT) is advised. Small bore percutaneous kits can be used to place a SPT using local anesthesia in the conscious patient. Alternatively, SPT drainage can be established in the operating room should urgent abdominal exploration or internal pelvic fixation be required. Endoscopic realignment is an additional option to establish urinary drainage and allow for urethral healing over a catheter, potentially obviating the need for formal urethroplasty in the future, although this is reported to be successful in only approximately 20–40% of patients [16, 17]. As this maneuver is performed using a cystoscope from a retrograde or combined antegrade approach, it is unlikely to be successful in the hands of inexperienced genitourinary endoscopists. Additionally, this approach can be time-consuming and should not be attempted if patient stability is in question.

Lacerations of the pendulous urethra should be explored operatively, typically through a subcoronal or circumcising incision. The tissue defect between the disrupted urethral ends should be assessed, and if it is a short defect (<1.5 cm), a primary anastomosis can be attempted to form a watertight, tension-free closure [18]. A primary repair using fine absorbable suture should always be performed over a 14–18 French Foley catheter. Meticulous closure of the corpus spongiosum and penile skin in layers over the repair can mitigate formation of fistulae. The Foley catheter should be maintained for 10–14 days, after which a pericatheter retrograde urethrogram or voiding cystourethrogram can be performed to ensure urethral integrity after the repair. Large segment defects are best managed with delayed reconstruction given the potential for chordee (abnormal penile curvature) when primary anastomosis is attempted. Patients with extensive urethral disruption are best managed with SPT placement and formal urethroplasty 3 months following their injury. Attempts to use tissue flaps or grafts for repair in the acute setting are not advised and have unacceptable rates of failure.

Scrotal and Testicular Injuries

Trauma to the scrotal structures has been the signature genitourinary injury of the overseas contingency operations (OCOs) to this point. The dependent anatomy, inconsistent armor shielding, and upward blast trajectory of IEDs when dismounted have resulted in the scrotum and testicles accounting for 75% of GU wartime wounds in OEF and OIF [13]. In contrast to the penile injuries encountered in theater, there has been a predominance of high-grade testicular trauma measured using the AAST grading scale (Table 12.3) [6]. Whereas 51% of penile injuries involved superficial skin lacerations or shrapnel peppering, 77% of testicular trauma involved tissue loss (Fig. 12.2) [13]. Total testicular destruction was noted in more than one-third of cases reviewed in the DoDTR. Additionally, as a paired structure, both testicles were affected in 42% of casualties [13]. With the demographic dominance of young males of reproductive age filling the ranks of the United States Armed Forces, high-grade trauma to the testicles has the potential to permanently inhibit future fertility and hormonal well-being among a large military population. The aforementioned implications reinforce the need to properly diagnose and treat scrotal and testicular trauma in the acute setting.

Table 12.3 American Association for the Surgery of Trauma testis injury scale

Grade I	Contusion or hematoma
Grade II	Subclinical tunica albuginea laceration
Grade III	Laceration of tunica albuginea with <50% parenchymal loss
Grade IV	Laceration of tunica albuginea with >50% parenchymal loss
Grade V	Total testicular avulsion or destruction

Adapted from [6]

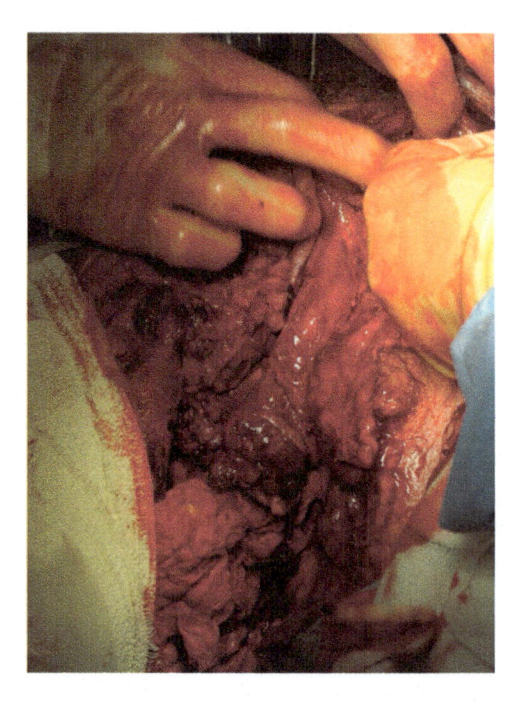

Fig. 12.2 Dismounted IED injury resulting in scrotal skin avulsion with major laceration of the tunica albuginea and exposure of the seminiferous tubules

Scrotal skin lacerations are commonly encountered in deployed environments and are amenable to simple washout and closure using fine absorbable suture or local wound care and healing with secondary intention advocated. This paradigm has been challenged in the current conflicts as a normal external appearance of the scrotum following IED blasts may belie underlying damage to the testicles. Hudak described high-grade injuries in casualties encountered in Balad with only small scrotal

Fig. 12.3 Combined penile and testicular laceration with primary closure of the tunica albuginea

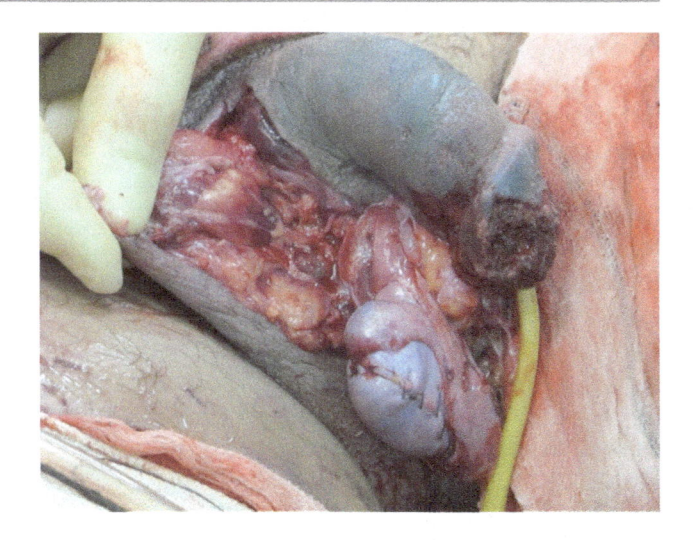

puncture wounds on initial assessment [10]. It has become routine practice to perform operative exploration and staging of scrotal trauma to ensure missed injuries are minimized. The scrotum can be explored via a transverse or midline raphe approach. Delivery of the testicles into the operative field allows for direct visualization of the tunica vaginalis, tunica albuginea, epididymis, and cord structures. Discovery of a hematocele on exploration or on ultrasound evaluation, if available, is highly suggestive of an underlying testicular wound and should be repaired. Hudak noted a 75% testicular salvage rate when only a scrotal injury was suspected and a 50% salvage rate when exploration was performed for a known testicular injury [10]. As is the norm in genital surgery, judicious debridement and closure are advocated. In the setting of grade III–IV testicular trauma, exposed seminiferous tubules should be debrided and the tunica albuginea closed primarily if feasible (Fig. 12.3). If the tunica is compromised and cannot be closed primarily, a patch of tunica vaginalis may be used for coverage. Additionally, should the testicle appear dusky with questionable viability, Doppler ultrasound or bleeding tissue may point to adequate flow, but given the routine nature of reoperative exploration in theater, tissue status can be reassessed at another session. Orchiectomy is an accepted aspect of damage control scrotal surgery, but clinical judgment is key when there is the potential to leave a patient anorchid. Grade IV–V involvement with contralateral testicular contusion would commonly be managed with completion orchiectomy and preservation of the testicle with low-grade injury. The presence of bilateral high-grade testicular wounds is uncommon, but preservation of any viable tissue is encouraged to maintain future reproductive and hormonal function (although there are no studies to confirm this accepted practice). The lax nature of scrotal skin and its usual redundancy result in the ability to close scrotal lacerations and skin loss in a primary fashion. Extensive skin loss will likely require skin grafting in the rehabilitation and reconstruction phase of patient care. In the acute setting, the use of VAC or moist dressings to minimize testicular desiccation may be employed to create a favorable wound bed for eventual grafting.

Conclusion

Colonel James C. Kimbrough, M.D., a veteran of WWI and WWII, is considered to be the father of US Army urology, and in 1956 he wrote: "Conservative treatment has proven efficient in renal damage. Early operation gives the best results in wounds of the ureter and bladder. Conservation of tissue is important in the treatment of wounds of the external genitals" [19]. These core principles were honed on the battlefields of the early twentieth century but continue to remain relevant in modern casualty care of urologic injuries. Expeditious management of the kidney, ureter, and bladder involvement in blunt and penetrating abdominal trauma will continue as a necessary skill of the military trauma surgeon in theater as compromise of these structures contributes significant morbidity and mortality risks. Blast injuries to the external genitals and urethra have become the signature urologic wounds of our modern military engagements. While trauma to these GU organs alone is rarely life threatening, the psychological, hormonal, reproductive, and functional aspects of external genital and urethral injuries should not be minimized. Rapid evaluation, operative management, and preservation of viable tissue will result in maximization of function and allow for further urologic reconstruction once the service member reaches higher echelons of care.

References

1. Dismounted Complex Blast Injury Task Force. Dismounted complex blast injury report of the army dismounted complex blast injury task force [Internet]. Fort Sam Houston: Army Medical Department; 2011. Available from: http://armymedicine.mil/Documents/DCBI-Task-Force-Report-Redacted-Final.pdf
2. Morey A, Brandes S, Dugi D, Armstrong J, Breyer B, Broghammer J, et al. Urotrauma: AUA guideline. J Urol. 2014;192(2):327–35.
3. Young H. Wounds of the urogenital tract in modern warfare. J Urol. 1942;47:59–108.
4. Hudak S, Morey A, Rozanski T, Fox C. Battlefield urogenital injuries: changing patterns during the past century. Urology. 2005;65(6):1041–6.
5. Serkin F, Soderdahl D, Hernandez J, Patterson M, Blackbourne L, Wade C. Combat urologic trauma in US military overseas contingency operations. J Trauma. 2010;69:S175–8.
6. Moore E, Malangoni M, Cogbill T, Peterson N, Champion H, Jurkovich G, et al. Organ injury scaling VII: cervical vascular, peripheral vascular, adrenal, penis, testis, and scrotum. J Trauma. 1996;41:523–4.
7. McAninch J. Genitourinary trauma. World J Urol. 1999;17(2):65.
8. Owens B, Kragh J, Wenke J, Macaitis J, Wade C, Holcomb J. Combat wounds in operation Iraqi Freedom and operation Enduring Freedom. J Trauma. 2008;64(2):295–9.
9. Serafetinides E, Kitrey N, Djakovic N, Kuehhas F, Lumen N, Sharma D, et al. Review of the current management of upper urinary tract injuries by the EAU Trauma Guidelines Panel. Eur Urol. 2005;67(5):930–6.
10. Hudak S, Hakim S. Operative management of wartime genitourinary injuries at Balad Air Force Theater Hospital, 2005 to 2008. J Urol. 2009;182:180–3.
11. Morey A, Iverson A, Swan A, Harmon W, Spore S, Bhayani S, et al. Bladder rupture after blunt trauma: guidelines for diagnostic imaging. J Trauma. 2001;51(4):683–6.
12. Elliott S, McAninch J. Extraperitoneal bladder trauma: delayed surgical management can lead to prolonged convalescence. J Trauma. 2009;66:274–5.
13. Banti M, Walter J, Hudak S, Soderdahl D. Improvised explosive device-related lower genitourinary trauma in current overseas combat operations. J Trauma Acute Care Surg. 2016;80:131–4.
14. Champion H, Holcomb J, Young L. Injuries from explosions: physics, biophysics, pathology, and required research focus. J Trauma. 2009;66:1468–77.
15. Santucci R, Chang Y. Ballistics for physicians: myths about wound ballistics and gunshot injuries. J Urol. 2004;171:1408–14.
16. Leddy L, Vanni A, Wessels H, Voelzke B. Outcomes of endoscopic realignment of pelvic fracture associated urethral injuries at a level 1 trauma center. J Urol. 2012;188(1):174–8.
17. Johnsen N, Dmochowski R, Mock S, Reynolds W, Miliam D, Kaufman M. Primary endoscopic realignment of urethral disruption injuries—a double edged sword? J Urol. 2015;194(4):1022–6.
18. Martinez-Pineiro L, Djakovic N, Plas E, Mor Y, Santucci R, Serafetinidis E, et al. EAU guidelines on urethral trauma. Eur Urol. 2010;57(5):791–803.
19. Kimbrough J. War wounds of the urogenital tract. J Urol. 1946;55:179–89.

Soft Tissue Injuries and Amputations

Gabriel J. Pavey and Benjamin K. Potter

Introduction

The wars in Iraq and Afghanistan represent the longest period of conflict in American history, with casualty numbers surpassing 59,000 [1] service members during the period following the terrorist attacks of September 11, 2001. Of these, musculoskeletal extremity wounds have been shown to comprise 50% of all combat-related wounds [2, 3] which often contain multidrug-resistant bacterial and fungal infection [3–7]. These wounds tend to be massive in nature and severity, given that nearly 75% are caused by an explosive blast, noted during two separate but consecutive reviews of the Joint Trauma Theater Registry (JTTR) done by Owens [8] in 2007 and Belmont [9] in 2013, a trend that steadily climbed during the twentieth century but peaked during the most recent conflict. The use of explosives, particularly in the form of improvised explosive devices (IEDs) or vehicle-borne IEDs (VBIEDs), coupled with improvements in body armor, point of injury tourniquet use, and expedited casualty evacuation to far forward advanced medical resources results in remarkable in increasing rates of survival, with survivors sustaining a characteristic combat injury pattern termed the dismounted complex blast injury (DCBI), a constellation of injuries increasingly encountered following a change in military strategy in Afghanistan [10–13]. In late 2009, the up-armored patrol vehicles utilized in Iraq and earlier in Operation Enduring Freedom were parked in favor of dismounted foot patrols in order to navigate the harsh mountainous terrain of Afghanistan and to permit troops to appear more approachable to the local Afghan populace.

Frequently, wounds from dismounted complex blasts are contaminated with foreign body debris and are at high risk for bacterial and fungal infection due to blast inoculation and relative immunosuppression during the course of treatment. Despite the devastating complexity of these injuries, with reports of as high as a 73% case fatality rate (CFR) of UK soldiers sustaining perineal and pelvic injury [10], remarkable rates of survival have been demonstrated, owing to improved resuscitation and stabilization efforts [14]. These successes, however, have ushered in the need for lengthy and often novel reconstructive techniques to allow for optimized function in the face of debilitating late complications. One specific challenge, the formation of heterotopic ossification in extremity wounds and residual limbs of combat wounded, can largely be attributed to our early efforts to preserve soft tissue and residual limb length. Given HO morbidity and recent findings of ubiquity within wounds associated with DCBI, HO represents a major focus of research for improving the quality of life for our wounded veterans and mitigating its effects in the future. In

G. J. Pavey · B. K. Potter (✉)
Uniformed Services University-Walter Reed Department of Surgery, Walter Reed National Military Medical Center, Bethesda, MD, USA
e-mail: Benjamin.K.Potter.mil@mail.mil

Table 13.1 Critical principles for DCBI and combat-related wound, fracture, and amputation management

In the emergency department/resuscitation bay
Emergent product-based resuscitation, ATLS assessment, antibiotics, and tetanus
Assess tourniquet placement, adequacy, and necessity
Assess need for pelvic binder or junctional tourniquet
In the operating room
Meticulous hemostasis and secure control of large/named vessels
Aggressive debridement of devitalized tissue and gross contamination; extend wounds longitudinally, keeping the eventual definitive reconstructive, flap coverage, or fixation needs in mind – *do not burn bridges*
Leave wounds and amputation wounds *open* with packing or negative pressure wound therapy dressing placement; consider antibiotic bead placement for open fractures and dilute Dakin's solution for severely contaminated wounds at risk for invasive fungal infection
Completion amputations should be managed in an open, length-preserving fashion – Salvage all viable soft tissue and bone; do not try to create definitive or "textbook" flaps during the index procedure(s)
Guillotine amputations are virtually never indicated and are not that much faster, and this antiquated technique sacrifices valuable viable tissue and eventual residual limb length
Long bone and pelvic fractures should be provisionally stabilized with external fixation, keeping half pins out of wounds and the exposure approaches for anticipated definitive fixation, when possible

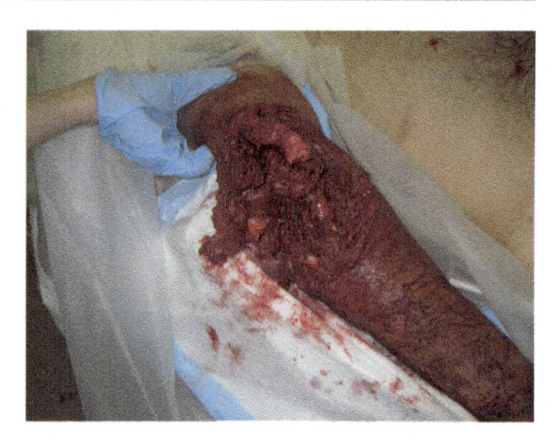

Fig. 13.1 Clinical photograph of a contaminated extremity wound. An open fracture of the right elbow with abundant gross contamination due to soil and foreign material, as is typical for combat- and blast-related wounds, is shown

this chapter, we will focus on soft tissue injury of extremities in limbs that have been successfully salvaged as well as the hallmark injury of DCBI – traumatic amputations. Key general principles for the management of combat-related soft tissue injuries, fractures, and amputations, in general, are listed in Table 13.1.

Soft Tissue Injury

Initial Management: Early Echelon Care

Early battlefield or prehospital care of complex soft tissue and bony injury, like other injuries with DCBI, focuses initially on controlling catastrophic bleeding. Once the service member is able to be transported to a higher level of care, the main goals become replacing circulating volume in a 1:1:1 ratio of plasma, packed red blood cells, and platelets, reversing acidemia and coagulopathy, and decreasing mortality [15]. If a pelvic fracture, amputation, or associated long bone fracture is suspected of contributing to blood loss, then "damage control orthopedics" or stabilization of these fractures with external fixation devices is performed alongside other resuscitative efforts, such as intrapelvic packing or vessel ligation to mitigate bleeding.

Following initial resuscitation and hemorrhage control, the surgical priorities of the orthopedic surgeon then turn to fracture stabilization of those fractures not previously addressed and debridement of grossly contaminated and/or visibly devitalized tissue (Fig. 13.1). Our discussion focuses on these orthopedic practices in the overall management of extremity soft tissue injury and amputations in the setting of DCBI. Initial management of DCBI typically requires multiple surgical teams working concurrently in order to minimize surgical time and prevent onset of the lethal triad of hypothermia, acidosis, and hypocoagulability. Traumatic extremity wounds characteristic of DCBI, often presenting as transfemoral amputations of varying lengths, require longitudinal extension of incisions to facilitate debridement of devitalized tissue and foreign debris that is driven proximally along tissue planes by the blast. Inspection of each muscle is performed, keeping the principles of debridement for evaluating its viability in mind, specifically; color, consistency, capacity to bleed/circulation, and contractility (testable with mechanical stimulation or electrocautery) are used for crude evaluation. Removal of the skin at this stage, despite anticipated amputation length, is limited to grossly nonviable tissue, as limb length preservation must also be considered during acute management to maximize functional outcomes. Isotonic warm irrigation fluid is copiously (at least 9 liters in large wounds) administered at low pressure via gravity or bulb syringe following sharp debridement, with intermuscular planes digitally explored for removal of hidden debris. A multicenter study (FLOW) comparing low-pressure versus high-pressure irrigation was finalized during the conflict that supported this technique in decreasing reoperation for infection [16].

Following a thorough inspection of wounds and tissue bed hemostasis, negative pressure wound therapy dressings are commonly applied in lieu of more conventional gauze dressings, although the latter remain a reasonable option in austere environments, to maintain an open wound. This achieves the goal of evacuating the inflammatory effluent from the wound and facilitates multiple evacuations to higher echelon of care that occur over the first few days following injury. In some cases, where wounds have large amounts of foreign debris, or in which fungal contamination is anticipated, the negative pressure devices can intermittently infuse the wound with sodium hypochlorite. Alternatively, gauze dressings can be soaked and placed in the wound bed, but this approach requires twice daily dressing changes or early serial debridements and becomes logistically more challenging. When choosing negative pressure wound therapy, care must be taken to ensure that neurovascular structures and tendon are protected from direct exposure to negative pressure and desiccation. Maintaining negative pressure can be difficult in larger wounds, and therefore a pressure of 125 mm Hg is widely used. Occasionally, a combination of negative pressure dressings and gauze dressings can be utilized for large wounds, or wounds that have difficulty holding the seal could be further augmented with the iodine-impregnated occlusive dressing (Ioban, 3 M).

In keeping with traditional open fracture care, stabilization of the all fractures should be performed in order to protect soft tissues from secondary injury and prevent or minimize secondary complications such as fat emboli and compartment syndrome. When possible, extremity soft tissue injuries without fractures should also be splinted to allow for soft tissue rest and contracture prevention, as these patients are subject to frequent transfers. Splinting of extremities should also consider contracture prevention, particularly avoidance of ankle equinus and digit contracture, as functional extremities will become vital in the service members' overall rehabilitation. Splints should be well padded and easily removable to permit wound inspection, compartment assessment, and neurovascular checks.

Definitive Management

Subacute management of DCBI-associated extremity soft tissue injury requires acute and astute clinical surveillance for assessing tissue that becomes overtly necrotic or declares itself as at risk. Retained nonviable tissue places the wound in danger of succumbing to infection from point of injury microorganisms as well as nosocomial infections commonly isolated in theater hospitals. Critical to soft tissue management in the setting of profound tissue injury and contamination is frequent serial debridement and irrigation which should be performed no less than every 72 h and more frequently for larger or more contaminated wounds. Initial re-debridement should occur within 48 and ideally 24 h of injury. If there is a large soft tissue deficit or wounds adjacent to a fracture or traumatic amputation, then antibiotic- and/or antifungal-impregnated beads are commonly placed on each debridement. Dilute sodium hypochlorite infusions using the Instill Wound VAC (KCI, San Antonio, TX) should be used for wounds that demonstrate evidence of or at high risk for invasive fungal infection (IFI), given the morbidity associated with IFI, with transfemoral amputations, and being dismounted at time of injury having been demonstrated to be independent predictors of IFI development [17–19]. Wound surveillance during serial debridements should balance the physiologic insult inflicted by serial surgical debridements and the importance of achieving a clean wound bed and the systemic insult of ongoing local inflammation. Wound beds can be considered clean when nearly all tissue is viable at the outset of the procedure during serial debridements.

Once wound beds are clean, a systematic approach to complex wound closure should minimize infections, maximize function, and limit morbidity of future procedures required for reconstruction. On some occasions, earlier closure or attempted closure may be necessary to avoid further repeated surgeries that obtain minimal gains for repeated physiologic insult. While closure of wounds prematurely may place the wound at risk of dehiscence, the constitutive elevation of serum inflammatory markers the body experiences during repeated surgery has also been shown to be a harbinger of wound dehiscence [20, 21]. If several wound beds exist, closure of a wound bed that is amenable to closure should not be delayed in favor of wounds that require more debridements. That is, all wounds should be left open initially, but wounds should be closed as soon thereafter as soon as patient physiologic status and gross wound appearance permit.

Closure of wounds often requires systematic and serial dermal mobilization to facilitate so-called delayed primary closure. Many novel techniques of delayed primary closure can be employed to achieve stable soft tissue coverage over small and intermediate wounds by leveraging biological creep, a biomechanical response of tissue tension that produces an overall increase in tissue mass. Mobilization of the skin can begin during the serial debridement phase of soft tissue management with the application of vessel loops in a "roman sandal" fashion secured by skin staples. Proprietary progressive wound closure devices may also be utilized for this purpose, although they are not necessary for most patients and wounds.

Optimally, these will be positioned in line with the proposed closure and overlying subdermal placement of a wound dressing, either VAC sponge or radiomarked gauze which can enhance stretch and decrease edema. Dermatotraction can be used when the tissue deficit is mostly circular in nature. Commonly used, Dermaclose (Dermaclose RC, Wound Care Tech., MN) allows for full-thickness soft tissue injury to be approximated by maintaining a constant inward radial tension force via a monofilament suture secured to the skin by stainless steel anchors placed at the periphery of wound. Conversion of type 3B open fractures to 3A open fractures is common, although only small studies have been done that demonstrate these successes [22, 23]. In the absence of these newer techniques, a #2 monofilament can be used as retention sutures as these are often readily available in austere environments. Given the tissue destruction that occurs in DCBI, many large wounds can be reduced to a stable wound that can be closed via secondary intention or granulation or be primarily closed in a delayed fashion using these techniques.

Reconstructive Ladder: Soft Tissue Injury Coverage

Larger soft tissue injuries involving profound volumetric tissue loss, particularly those associated with open fractures, cannot be reliably primarily closed and therefore require an escalation of the soft tissue reconstructive ladder. Planning for soft tissue coverage begins early in the debridement process and should ensure appropriate timing so that wounds appear clean, edema has decreased, and the patient is physiologically amenable to lengthier procedures and has realistic physiologic prospects for successful wound healing.

In our experience, associated fractures previously stabilized by external fixation are definitively covered at the time of definitive fixation, a process termed *fix and flap*. Patients undergoing these procedures are optimized by the multispecialty care team to ensure absence of infection and improved nutritional status. Despite these efforts, Sabino et al.'s review of flap coverage during a decade of war reported an overall complication rate of 30% with a significantly increased failure rates of muscle flaps (13%) versus fasciocutaneous flaps (6%) prompting the authors to preferentially choose fasciocutaneous flaps, when feasible [24]. Moreover, many of procedures in this study included flaps performed prior to the increase in DCBI patterned injury, a cohort of patients with more severe physiologic injury and at greater risk of thrombosis and flap failure. While a discussion of soft tissue injury is lacking without presenting flap coverage, a comprehensive review of our reconstructive experience is presented elsewhere in the text.

Often, orthopedic surgeons were responsible for the reconstructive decision-making and treatment of less severe extremity soft tissue deficits. When stable wound closure was not possible but major structures were adequately covered, then tissue adjuncts such as dermal regeneration template (DRT) were used to create a neodermis. Integra (Plainsboro, NJ), used extensively on wounds of nearly all sizes, is a bovine collagen bilayer matrix which provides a stable dermal layer with an overlying removable silicone bilayer that prevents insensible water loss and provides a protective barrier with an underlying collagen matrix that allows for tissue and capillary ingrowth. Application is performed in healthy wound beds without infection or at the time of provisional or definitive coverage. A NPWT dressing would be applied to mitigate shear forces on the integrating tissue and is changed every 3–5 days for 2 weeks at which time the wound is usually amenable to receive a split-thickness skin graft [25] (STSG). This approach led to successful coverage in 86% of all combat wounds [26] and 96% of upper extremity wounds [27]. Harvesting skin from the trunk was not uncommon given large areas of coverage needed and lack of lower extremity skin available.

For smaller wound beds, particularly those with exposed tendons (e.g., extensors of the hand, peroneal tendons), ACell (ACell, Columbia, MD), a porcine urinary bladder matrix, was used as coverage, which in either powder or sheet form provided an extracellular matrix of basement membrane without the complications of scar-producing contractures. Protocols varied but application was commonly done at the bedside or in the post-anesthesia care unit every other day. In a limited number of patients, typically with less severe injuries in a less affected limb, acute shortening [28] was performed to place tissues in approximation as to facilitate closure, but again these cases were infrequent in those that were injured via dismounted blast where more severe proximal injuries were typical.

Associated Fracture Management

Fractures associated with DCBI include pelvic, spine, and upper extremity fractures in multi-trauma patients with life-threatening injuries including extremity exsanguination, as well as visceral and intracranial injuries that preclude definitive management in favor of damage control orthopedics (DCO). As discussed briefly here, and in detail in Chap. 8, pelvic fractures which are concomitant in 40% of proximal bilateral lower extremity amputations [10] are managed emergently when thought to be contributing to intrapelvic hemorrhage and hemodynamic instability (Fig. 13.2). Closed reduction and external fixation is often performed without the aid of fluoroscopy in austere environments, so the use of anatomic landmarks and orientation is imperative [29].

After lifesaving intervention, open fractures, which make up 82% of all fractures in one study [8], require urgent debridement and irrigation followed by provisional external fixation of long bones for stabilization. External fixation placement provides acute fracture stabilization that limits secondary musculoskeletal injury, but also makes wound surveillance and serial debridement easier than splint immobilization. Principles of external fixation are similar to civilian trauma (i.e., stable construct, achieve bone apposition, and restore normal alignment); however, placement of half pins within the wound bed is discouraged as obtaining pneumatic seal following NPWT dressing placement becomes very difficult, obviating the advantage of those dressings.

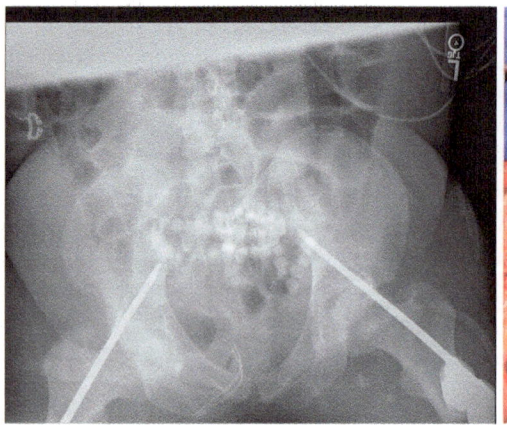

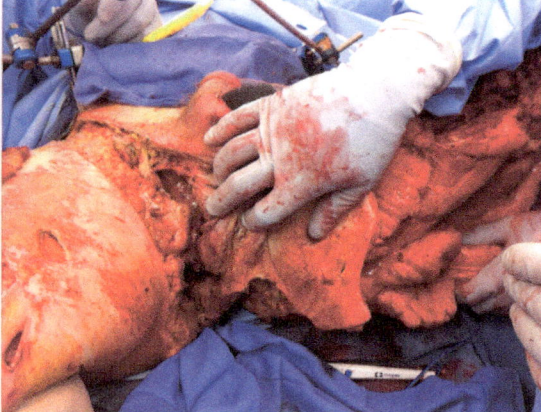

Fig. 13.2 Anterior-posterior radiograph (**a**) and clinical photograph (**b**) demonstrating an open book pelvic fracture with an associated open soft tissue injury in the groin crease. The fracture has been stabilized with an external fixator using supra-acetabular half pins, and antibiotic beads have been placed within the pelvis due to the open wound associated with this severe injury

When appropriate, fasciotomies are performed as increasing resuscitation volume and pressure changes during aeromedical evacuation in an intubated patient place extremities at risk for compartment syndrome. Definitive fracture fixation is beyond the scope of this text but will often be performed at higher echelons of care when the local soft tissue has stabilized and the patient is free of overt infection, which frequently coincides with planning for definitive soft tissue coverage or reconstructive soft tissue adjuncts previously discussed.

Complications of Soft Tissue Injury

Soft tissue trauma common to DCBI can be devastating, associated with open fractures, volumetric tissue loss, and injury to nerves and vessels which challenge the operative team during acute and subacute management. These challenges unfortunately do not subside once initial patient stabilization is achieved; complications such as infection, wound dehiscence, coverage failures, heterotopic ossification (HO), upper extremity contracture, and nerve injuries contribute to prolonged pain and disability and delay rehabilitation.

Complications of IFI (Fig. 13.3), the hallmark infection of DCBI [7], can be devastating as aggressive debridement in the acute period is performed as a lifesaving measure. Lewandowski

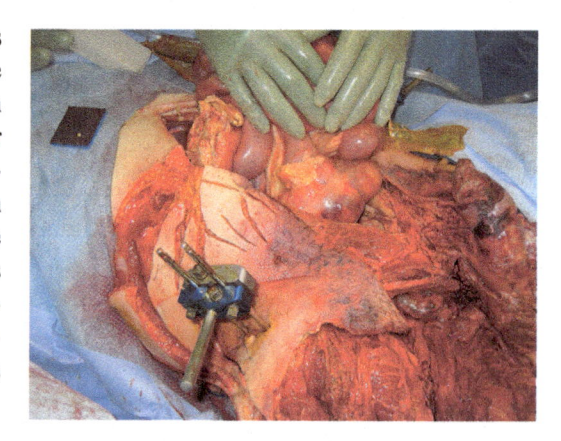

Fig. 13.3 Intraoperative photograph of the pelvis and lower abdomen of a DCBI patient with an open abdomen, open book pelvic fracture stabilized with a resuscitation (iliac wing) external fixator, and bilateral lower extremity amputations. The patient developed a devastating invasive fungal infection (IFI) while undergoing treatment and succumbed to the disease within 24 h of the photograph. Necrotic muscle, bowel, and abdominopelvic skin are evident due to the rapidly progressive infection

et al. compared patients with IFI to matched control trauma patients and showed more common revision to a proximal amputation level and higher requirement for skin grafts and dermal adjuncts. Later complications of IFI wounds include a 50% reoperation rate compared to 20% in controls and double the deep infection rate [19]. Late presentation of soft tissue infections can suggest osteomyelitis and, when they occur in residual limbs, require revision amputation. Revision amputation will be discussed further in this chapter, while DCBI infections will be discussed at length elsewhere in this text.

Soft tissue deficits are of specific challenge in DCBI, primarily because options are limited given broad soft tissue injury which can eliminate both skin graft and flap reconstructive options (Fig. 13.4). Transfer of large truncal muscles (e.g., latissimus dorsi, scapular, rectus abdominis) can weaken upper body control and present difficulties during core/truncal strength for rehabilitation. As discussed, flap complications, including overt necrosis and failure, can occur and are often predisposed by poor nutritional status and/or hypercoagulability. Sabino et al. reviewed 10 years of flap reconstruction in war wounded extremities and noted 30% complication rate in muscle flaps and 26% in fasciocutaneous flaps, most commonly due to infection [27].

In a study of predominantly blast-injured patients, flap coverage was noted to be particularly susceptible to HO formation, with a higher incidence among muscle versus fasciocutaneous flaps [30]. Predictably, HO that develops near joints results in stiffness and can profoundly affect function, as it has been shown to be an independent risk factor of decreased range of motion in the largest known study of open periarticular elbow fractures [31]. Early successes with the use of dermal regeneration templates [25], coupled with the shelf availability of these products, resulted in increased usage, with good results with regard to skin graft incorporation. However, while DRTs may be readily available, STSG donor sites are, by definition, sometimes limited. As a result, large wounds sometimes require coverage with STSG meshed to a 3:1 or 5:1 ratio, providing less than optimal durability, a concern paramount to prosthetic wear and therefore will be covered further in section on amputations.

In general, soft tissue transfers have been successful in maximizing function and in many cases facilitating limb salvage. However, some large wounds that do not necessarily require soft tissue coverage can create equally difficult challenges. Volumetric muscle loss (VML) refers to the traumatic or surgical loss of skeletal muscle that exceeds the capacity for self-regeneration. Specific to DCBI, VML is most problematic when it involves the quadriceps and hamstring muscle groups, but distal lower limb injury can also inhibit function as even small amounts of muscle loss (10–20%) can result in strength deficits that are disabling [32, 33]. Regenerative therapies offer some promise for VML [34]; extracellular matrix (ECM) scaffolds represent one evolving solution which seems to demonstrate regenerative potential when exposed to physiologic stress [35]. One case report of a combat-wounded marine sustaining VML underwent surgical application of a previously discussed ECM, ACell (Matristem; ACell Inc., Columbia, MD), to his vastus lateralis with early physiotherapy. The patient was able to demonstrate profound gains with the demonstration of tasks to include "hop-to" and "single-leg squat" [33]. Rehabilitative gains of patients with lower leg VML, and in many cases return to combat duty, have been demonstrated following training with the Intrepid Dynamic Exoskeletal Orthosis (IDEO) [36, 37]; however these patients do not represent the composite of injuries typical of DCBI and are outside the scope of this discussion [38, 39].

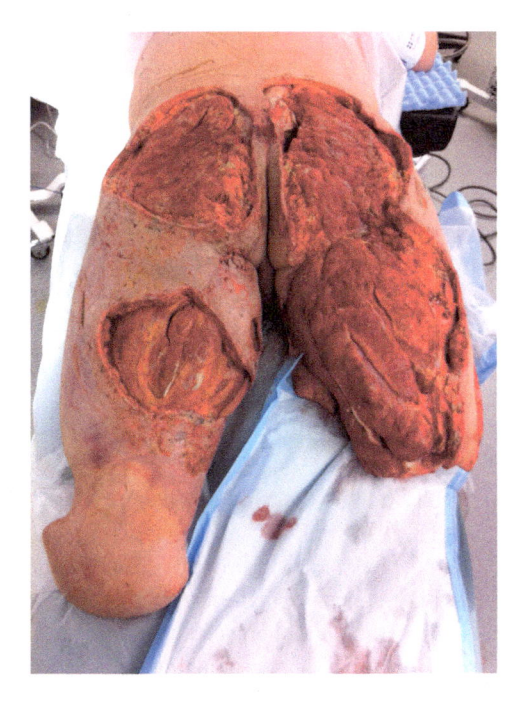

Fig. 13.4 Preoperative photograph of the buttocks and bilateral lower extremity amputations of a DCBI patient with severe associated degloving injury and skin loss

Inherent to large volume soft tissue loss is injury to nerves and vessels. In one study of combat wounds with nerve injury, 50 of 100 patients sustained profound tissue loss [40, 41], and of the 261 total nerve injuries (63% associated with blasts), a total of 55% were either axonotmesis or neurotmesis. Despite direct visualization of the injury, initial treatment of nerve injuries should be limited to tagging of nerve ends for future identification allowing for the large zone of injury to be declared. Treatment modalities include nerve repair, grafts or transfer, synthetic nerve conduits, or tendon transfers to restore or replace function. Studies showing superiority are not available, but the authors of the above study performed 46 operations which included 10 repairs and 32 grafts (25 early, 7 delayed). The long-term follow-up outcomes for grafts were mixed (8 good, 16 fair, 8 poor), with 7 of the 10 primary repairs reporting good outcomes.

As noted, high-energy blast injury of the dismounted soldier produces catastrophic injury patterns. Despite this, survivability is at an all-time high. Following lifesaving measures, initial management of the soft tissues focuses on performing adequate debridement to mitigate bacterial and fungal infection risk. What remains is often a reconstructive and rehabilitative challenge that requires a multidisciplinary, systematic approach for maximizing patient function. Flap coverage, dermal substitutes, and skin grafts seem to be endlessly at risk of failure and other complications which delay rehabilitation. Novel regenerative medicine developments offer hope for associated composite tissue loss and nerve injury but are in their infancy in clinical practice. All of these difficult challenges characteristic of traumatic soft tissue injury exist within the proximal traumatic amputation and therefore will be further explored in that context within the next section.

Amputations

Military trauma surgeons have been performing battlefield amputations for millennia with discussion of the procedure dating back to ancient times. Previously performed as a lifesaving measure in the treatment of combat open fractures and devitalized tissue, and as a consequence of tourniquet placement by Hippocrates, Pare, and Debakey, military surgeons in Iraq and Afghanistan have been presented with patients in large scale who had sustained *traumatic* amputations [42]. The use of IEDs by the enemy during these conflicts, coupled with advancements in protective equipment, point of injury tourniquet use, and rapid casualty evacuation, has produced over 2200 traumatic or trauma-related amputations in over 1700 surviving service members, with nearly half of those occurring between the fall of 2009 and the fall of 2014, a period that coincides with a strategic change in favor of dismounted patrols. As a result of these factors, bilateral proximal lower extremity amputations typify the characteristic injury pattern of DCBI, as 225 of 720 patients who sustained amputations between 2009 and 2012 sustained either double (191), triple [32], or quadruple [3] limb amputations [13]. Upper extremity trauma, when associated, more frequently occurs on the left as this tends to be the forward hand on the rifle of a patrolling soldier and more commonly affects the distal upper extremity [43]. Astonishingly, despite these injuries, 94% of severely wounded patients who sustained amputations admitted at a ROLE II/III facility survive and are successfully transferred to higher echelon of care [13], a testament to the successes of the initial management strategies discussed in this text. However, survival of these wounds introduces challenges of aftercare that can be wrought with complications that have hastened novel surgical treatments, innovative prostheses, and effective multidisciplinary psychosocial programs that enhance resiliency and offer promising outcomes after prolonged rehabilitation.

Initial Amputation Management

The initial care for severe lower extremity injury or true traumatic amputations occurs either by the service member themselves, others within their unit who have undergone combat lifesaver training, or the combat medics imbedded in the unit. Proximal amputations left untreated can be fatal in minutes as a result of exsanguination [2, 10, 14, 15, 44].

The employment of the Combat Application Tourniquet (CAT) at the point of injury is, in part, responsible for the improved survival rates of the recent conflicts. Rarely, when a CAT is unavailable or if the proximal nature of the injury precludes CAT application, then hasty tourniquets (rifle slings, cravats with sticks as a windlass, or belts) can be used to limit hemorrhage. More commonly hemorrhage control is performed by direct pressure by a "battle buddy" or medical personnel. In flight administration of blood products in a 1:1:1 ratio during helicopter evacuation, initiate early resuscitation efforts prior to arrival at the closest theater MTF. Pelvic binders, while available in some ROLE I forward aid stations, are typically applied by medical evacuation personnel and are effective in controlling intrapelvic bleeding for associated pelvic trauma.

Blast injury to extremities can result in wide ranging trauma with massive zones of injury, but efforts to preserve the limb or limb length are pursued except when immediate completion of a near amputation is obvious or attempted prolonged limb salvage places patient at risk of death. Hemorrhage control in the field hospital is tailored to the injury presentation and is of paramount importance. A review of the transfusion requirements of 720 DCBI patients from the JTTR showed an average of 18.6 units of packed red blood cells and 17.3 units of fresh frozen plasma despite tourniquet use in 80% of patients with increasing transfusion requirements coinciding with number of amputations [13]. In very proximal amputations, junctional tourniquets, those specifically focused on compression of major extremity vessels (femoral, axillary), can be used; however, efficacy is variable and therefore surgical hemostasis is often required. Visceral access is commonly required to control severe proximal lower extremity hemorrhage and includes intrapelvic iliac clamping in (less common) cases of unilateral injury, or laparotomy access in order to cross-clamp the infrarenal aorta in patients whom mortal exsanguination is imminent due to bilateral injuries [45]. If intrapelvic bleeding is suspected, external fixator application can be done at this time prior to removal of the pelvic binder and in consort with pelvic packing if supra-inguinal or pre-peritoneal access has been obtained [10, 12, 46].

During the initial surgery after lifesaving procedures, limb salvage is prioritized when possible (Fig. 13.5). Keeping these goals in mind, suggested initial indications for amputation are a grossly contaminated lower extremity with near traumatic amputation, a mangled extremity in a decompensating patient, or a crushed or dysvascular extremity with greater than 6 hours of warm ischemia time. Open, length- and tissue-preserving amputations are strongly recommended in an effort to preserve residual limb length and future reconstructive options [47, 48]. Guillotine amputations represent an antiquated technique that sacrifices valuable viable soft tissue and are not, in reality, that much faster than length-preserving techniques (Fig. 13.6). Therefore, guillotine amputations are avoided with the isolated exceptions of provisional disarticulations for which soft tissue status will not permit definitive closure at that level. The authors of the 2010 Current Concepts Review suggest that when possible, an intraoperative assessment made by at least two experienced surgeons to assess limb viability should be performed to confirm the necessity of amputation.

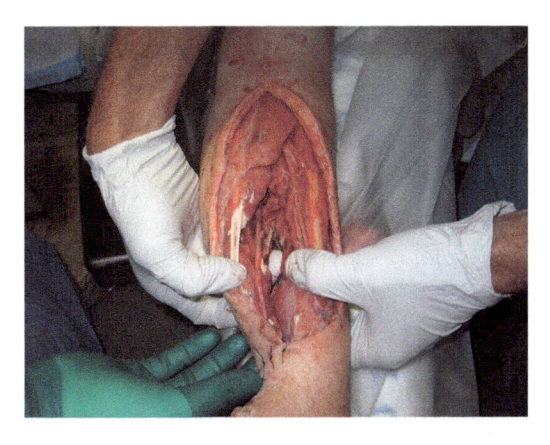

Fig. 13.5 Intraoperative photograph of the left upper extremity of a DCBI patient. Despite the severe nature of the wound with the evident "drive thru" sign in the distal forearm due to muscle loss, an open forearm fracture, and peripheral nerve injury, limb salvage is entirely feasible, and amputation is not indicated

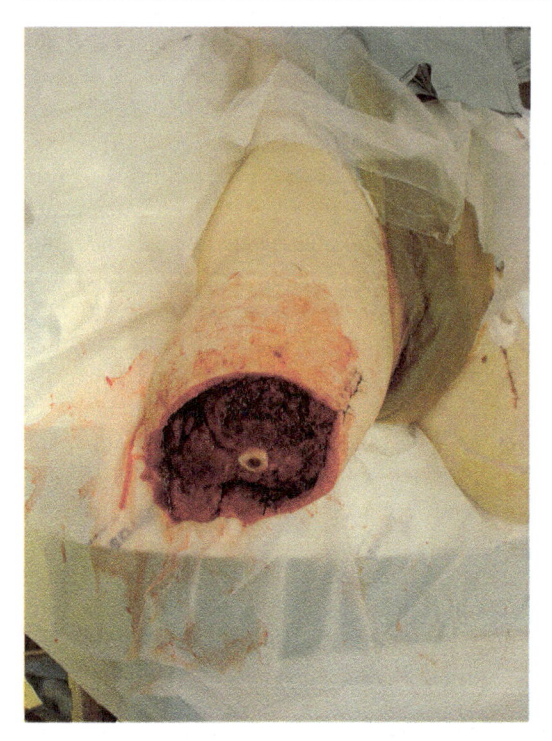

Fig. 13.6 Preoperative photograph of a guillotine amputation. This antiquate surgical technique is strongly discouraged due to the removal of valuable soft tissue which can be utilized to salvage additional residual limb length or even amputation levels. Do not perform guillotine amputations such as this

An aggressive debridement is vital to early wound management and should not be limited during initial surgical care since devitalized tissue, foreign body debris, and microorganism contamination can cause early systemic sepsis and/or late infection requiring future revision amputations. Therefore, an initial minimalist approach may not achieve preservation of ultimate limb length. That having been said, it is equally important to take a systematic approach in deciding what not to debride. Assessing the viability of tissue using the 4 C's described above is important in performing prudent debridements that will leave viable tissue for future coverage and/or reconstruction to facilitate limb length preservation. Predicting actual limb length during this stage is inappropriate; muscle debulking, crafting of skin flaps, and performing proximal neurectomies should be avoided and left to the surgeon responsible for definitive amputation closure. Fractures proximal to the amputation should not dictate revision to a more proximal level. After debridement is performed, the wound should be irrigated copiously, vessels ligated, and nerves and tendons tagged for future identification. Residual limbs are covered in a negative pressure wound dressing or gauze packing often with the placement of antibiotic-impregnated polymethylmethacrylate beads following careful electrocautery hemostasis.

Wounds that have high clinical suspicion of fungal contamination should be treated with Dakin's treated gauze or negative pressure wound dressing with Dakin's infusion capabilities. Parenteral antibiotics during these initial surgeries should be re-dosed often as much of the circulating volume present initially is either lost or diluted during resuscitation efforts. Topical antibiotic powder has also recently gained favor in mitigating and preventing orthopedic infections [49–53]. When used in combat-related traumatic amputations at a ROLE IV hospital, soon to be published data suggests a statistically significant risk reduction (13%) of late infection with application of antibiotic powder in residual limbs and a potentially added benefit of HO severity reduction. Published data of powder vancomycin application in a validated animal model of blast trauma inoculated with MRSA suggests that the greatest benefit of decreasing infection and mitigating HO was achieved with *point of injury* application [54, 55]. However, the promise of these adjunct therapies does not obviate the need for a well-performed debridement and keen wound surveillance. Wound appearance during initial treatment should guide medevac decisions, and wounds that appeared grossly contaminated or with wide areas of necrosis should return to the operating room in 24 h (Fig. 13.7), whereas clean appearing residual limbs can return in 48–72 h.

Definitive Amputation Management

Many textbooks have been dedicated to the surgical technique of performing various levels of amputations. Unfortunately, those techniques are

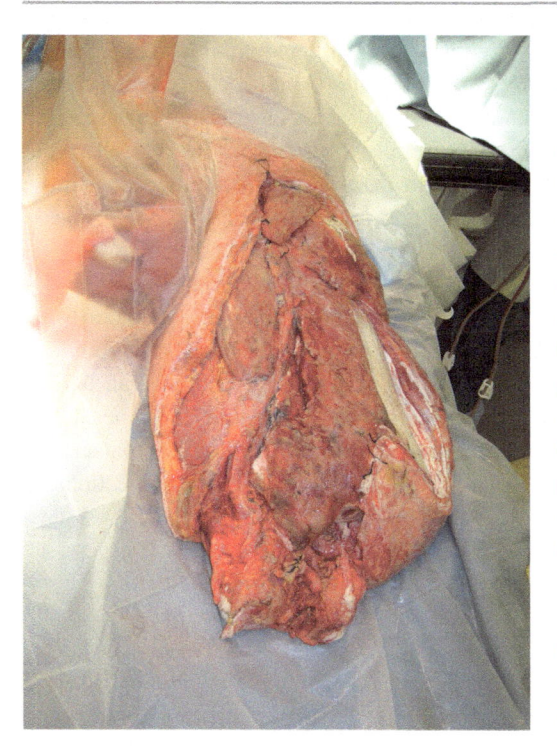

Fig. 13.7 Preoperative photograph of a left transfemoral amputation with persistent, recurrent tissue necrosis despite several prior debridements. Slow wound evolution with frequent loss of additional tissue during subsequent debridements is the rule rather than the exception for severe blast-related wounds such as this and highlights the importance of aggressive early debridements, serial wound examination, and delayed closure of open wounds and amputations, generally at level 4 or 5 facilities

only minimally helpful when performing amputations in patients who have sustained profound blast injury resulting in variable traumatic and iatrogenic tissue and bone loss. Furthermore, traumatic amputations in DCBI occur in young and previously active individuals who will not readily accept functional performance below their pre-injury level. Surgical goals aim to preserve limb length and maximize function, recognizing the anticipated complications when definitive amputations are performed within the zone of injury.

Management of the soft tissue envelope is critical in determining definitive limb length. The longest level possible is based on available soft tissues, highlighting the critical mistake of performing guillotine amputations, in which the bone will have to be significantly shortened to provide a stable soft tissue pad over the distal end of amputation. Bone length in favor of poor soft tissue coverage will be poorly tolerated during prosthetic rehabilitation. Durable soft tissue coverage in transfemoral amputations requires robust tissue, which reemphasizes the importance of aggressive but judicious debridement. Rarely in transfemoral amputations, unlike transtibial amputations, is debulking performed – all muscle bellies and fasciocutaneous flaps may serve a purpose. Myodesis is the attachment of muscle, or optimally its tendon, to the bone, through either bone tunnels or suturing to intact periosteum. Of particular importance is the adductor magnus myodesis which has been shown to be important biomechanically for realigning the limb and allowing functional muscle use during prosthetic gait training [56–58]. Myodeses also provide stability for the overlying myoplasty, a procedure which sutures antagonistic muscle groups together in order to create physiologic tension at the distal aspect of the residual limb and secure distal padding to avoid excessive motion with prosthetic loading. When performing a myoplasty, the adage of more is better is generally appropriate, as these muscles are subject to inevitable atrophy and a robust soft tissue pad typically decreases in thickness and volume over time.

The definitive limb length of a traumatic amputation and the patient's ultimate functional capacity are the sum result of the surgical decisions during each debridement. While most orthopedic surgeons recognize that gait energy expenditure is increased with more proximal amputations, it should not be a mantra that limb length should be inconsequentially preserved. In other words, a very long transfemoral amputation which has poor soft tissue coverage or a proximal transtibial amputation with a rigid knee joint does not necessarily impart improved function over more proximal levels. Thus, a more appropriate approach would be functional joint-level preservation, one which is free of contracture and supported by sufficient local musculature. That having been said, maximizing residual limb length for transfemoral amputees who have sufficient distal soft tissue padding allows for improved anchoring of donned prostheses and increased limb control with the presence of muscle groups proximal to the amputation.

Surgical solutions for saving residual limb length include the rotation and approximation of atypical skin flaps, harvesting spare parts from degloved tissue at early debridements, flap coverage, or staged application of biodermal substitutes prior to split-thickness skin grafting [59–65]. Fleming et al. term this variety of techniques used for preserving residual limb length as the "hybrid reconstructive ladder" and demonstrate these successes in their presentation of a case series of patients treated with contribution from each rung of the "ladder." A recent study comparing the use of STSG to delayed primary closure in residual limbs of combat amputees showed that in all cases where STSG was used the amputation level was salvaged [66]. However, the study was unable to determine whether the STSG involved the terminal end of the residual limb where poor durability has been a previous concern or offer conclusions with regard to prosthetic tolerance in light of these previous concerns. Kent et al., however, did address prosthetic ambulation in a case series of civilian amputees, wherein all nine amputees who received STSG for the terminal residual limb were ambulating independently in their prostheses. Of note, eight of these residual limbs were at the transtibial level [67] and do not fully represent the more proximal amputation levels more common to the focus of this text. Limb function also remains heavily dependent on the stability of the joint proximal to the residual limb. Free flap transfers to preserve amputation levels have been used extensively in the civilian literature [59, 68–70], but only case reports exist for their use in the lower extremities of combat blast injuries [65], and reporting on periarticular flaps in particular is limited to discussions of HO formation in whole limb salvage attempts. In the upper extremity, flap coverage is more commonly utilized, as each progressive joint preserved provides enhanced ability to position the terminal extremity and provide increasingly complex tasks [43]. Occasionally, revision of free tissue transfers near the distal residual limb is required in both the upper and lower extremity. In the lower extremity, delays in rehabilitation occur to allow for proper healing owing to the direct pressure and shear forces across the transferred tissue. The upper extremity tends to have the opposite problem in that robust or irregularly shaped coverage can create fitting difficulty for prosthesis. Ultimately, while often successful, an attempt to salvage an amputation level that is plagued by unstable wounds, pain, and poor prosthetic tolerance does not achieve the goals of promoting limb function. These complications can be reasons for revision amputation and negatively impact the outcomes of military amputees and will be discussed in detail in the next sections.

Early Amputation Complications

The residual limb(s) of combat-wounded patients have high rates of complication owing to the practice of zone of injury amputations, shown to be performed as frequently as 79% in the lower extremity [71–74]. Unequivocally, the most common, complex, and morbid early complication of proximal lower extremity amputations and associated upper extremity amputations is infection, occurring in 63% of soldiers sustaining blast injury [10]. The bacteriology of wounds isolated from point of injury wounds include relatively easily treatable *Pseudomonas aeruginosa* and *Staphylococcus aureus* [75]; however, an increasing infective trend of nosocomially acquired multidrug-resistant gram-negative infections, notably *Acinetobacter baumannii*, required the use of antimicrobials decades out of use due to their toxicity [5, 76–78]. In many cases, antimicrobial treatment alone did not adequately treat infections, with infections after attempted definitive closure necessitating reoperation in 27% and 13% of lower extremity and upper extremity residual limbs, respectively [76]. Deep infection of residual limbs typically requires multiple return trips to the operating room for serial debridement, and the 13% of upper extremity residual limb infections accounted for 51% of operating room returns. Despite serial procedures to clear deep infection, loss of amputation level due to these infections is fortunately uncommon

(3%), and limb shortening did not affect long-term outcomes of rehabilitation [73, 79].

Given the morbidity of deep infection, surveillance should be keen. Limbs which are painful, have wound breakdown and/or drainage, or are erythematous particularly in the setting of fever, leukocytosis, or elevated inflammatory markers require work-up. Fluid collections are common in residual limbs in the acute postoperative period (55%), and this finding alone is not an indication for revision surgery as the rate of deep infection is no different between patients who do and do not have a fluid collection [80]. Deep infection was more common when clinical signs of infection to include erythema or drainage were coupled with fluid collection; however, these clinical signs would typically initiate irrigation and debridement and possible amputation revision irrespective of CT findings.

Invasive fungal infections (IFI) occur commonly in patients sustaining blast injury where the presence of a traumatic amputation was found to be an independent risk factor for IFI [18]. Patients are suspected of deep fungal infection when they have high spiking fevers associated with profound leukocytosis (>20 K WBCs), particularly in the setting of recurrent or rapidly progressive wound necrosis. Typically, confirmation occurs well before the histopathology has been finalized as the tissue tends to have a characteristic appearance. Mucormycosis is characterized by black patches of tissue that is often recurrent or appears in previously healthy tissue, whereas *Aspergillus* mold infections typically have an orange-brown appearance. Surgical debridement is often performed on the 24–48 h cycle as opposed to 48–72 standards for bacterial infections or major open wounds, in general. These practices, while absolutely necessary, exacerbate the problem as patients are often undernourished due to frequent periods of perioperative and intraoperative fasting or holding of tube feeds. As a result, IFI wounds had a significantly higher number of operative procedures, a longer duration to wound closure, and increased risk in loss of an amputation level [19]. In a review of 14 traumatic hemipelvectomies (13 patients), the largest series to date, a fungal wound infection was associated with 12 of the 14 extremities [81, 82]. Unfortunately, despite earlier diagnosis and initiation of antifungal therapy and aggressive surgical debridement, proximal amputations (hip disarticulation and above) and mortality remain high [17]. In an effort to predict fungal infection in combat wounds, the Surgical Critical Care Initiative has developed a validated model that will allow give surgeons a tool for performing early (initial) aggressive debridement of wounds. Risk factors to include dismounted blast injury; above the knee amputation; perineal, GU, and/or rectal injury; and massive transfusion (>25u PRBCs) are highly associated and suggest the treatment strategy outlined in the clinical practice guidelines (JTTR CPG on Treatment of Invasive Fungal Infection in War Wounds).

Late Amputation Complications

HO prevalence in the traumatic amputations of DCBI patients has increased substantially from its already high rate compared to civilian trauma [83] and earlier military retrospective studies [71, 72, 84, 85]. Reporting from the mid-conflict era reproducibly showed that nearly 2/3 of combat-related amputations developed HO. More recent, currently unpublished data from our institution reporting on a cohort of amputations almost exclusively resulting from blast injury suggest HO prevalence of >90% (Fig. 13.8). While not all HO formation causes symptoms or requires excision, patients choose to undergo surgical resection for ongoing pain, skin breakdown, and poor prosthetic tolerance not responding to conservative measures of pain management, activity modification, physical therapy, and prosthetic modification in up to 40% of cases [71–73, 83–87]. When surgeries to remove HO are performed, they are often successful when timing and technique are optimized; however, the excision surgeries have a high rate of complications [88]. The use of 3D resin models is a valuable asset given the distorted anatomy and topography which can provide an intraoperative guide to follow when navigating arborous HO beds [86]. Following HO resection patients are commonly

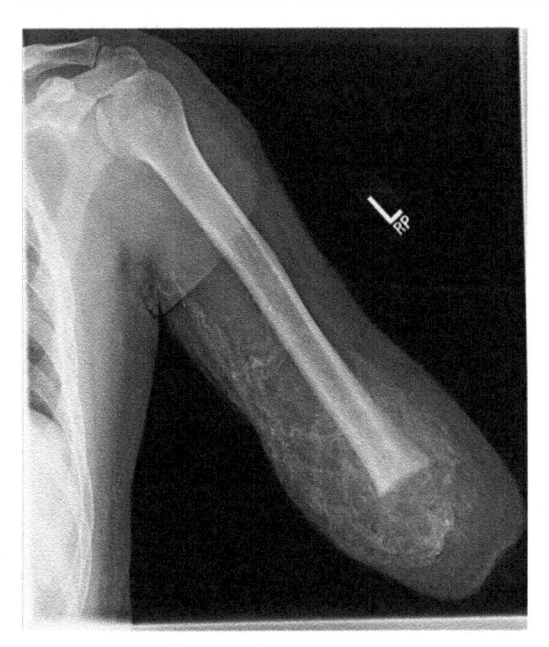

Fig. 13.8 Anterior-posterior radiograph of a left transhumeral amputation in a DCBI patient complicated by severe heterotopic ossification (HO). The HO caused pain with prosthesis wear as well as recurrent ulceration of the overlying split-thickness skin graft and required operative excision at approximately 9 months following injury

placed on a prophylactic COX-2 inhibitor for 2–6 weeks for recurrence prophylaxis; however, data remains inconclusive regarding the effectiveness or necessity of this prophylaxis.

Due to the morbidity associated with HO resection surgery and the delays in rehabilitation which often sets the service member back a number of months in their recovery, much research has gone into the early identification and prevention of HO formation. The development of HO has been associated with an elevated level of both circulating serum cytokines and those drawn from effluent of wound VAC cartridges (KCI, San Antonio) and may serve as a marker in the identification for patients at risk [20]. Similarly, the intraoperative use of Raman spectroscopy provides the surgeon a tool to identify and excise tissue (pre-HO) that has the potential for HO development [89, 90]. Since current prophylactic strategies can be harmful in a systemically injured patient (NSAIDs) or logistically not feasible in a forward deployed setting (radiotherapy), efforts have focused on identifying alternative potential prophylaxes. As a result, we developed a validated rodent model of blast-related traumatic HO [91, 92] which demonstrated a significant increase in HO formation when the traumatized residual limb was inoculated with MRSA [93]. Given the ubiquitous contamination of DCBI amputations, this offered local antibiotic powder as a potential treatment for not only limiting infection early but mitigating HO development risk [55]. Furthermore, other novel therapies such as palovarotene (Clementia Pharmaceuticals, Boston, MA), a retinoic-acid receptor γ-agonist that targets chondrogenesis, and rapamycin, an MTOR inhibitor, show profound efficacy in decreasing HO formation [93]. However, further studies are needed to determine the effects these drugs would have on wound and fracture healing of the multiply injured patient common to DCBI. Undoubtedly, increases in HO can be temporally associated with changing military strategies that have resulted in the proximal amputations characteristic of DCBI. As the conventional methods of warfare give way to those we now face, military and domestic terrorism trauma surgery must also evolve and demonstrate a pressing need for early identification of an applicable, safe, and effective method of HO prophylaxis for these patients.

In addition to symptomatic HO, neuromas, the formation of bursae, and redundant or deficient soft tissue can cause pain and poor fit and prosthesis tolerance decreasing function, a problem Tintle et al. termed persistently symptomatic residual limbs (PSRLs) [72]. In a study using ultrasound to diagnose abnormalities in the symptomatic residual limbs of physiologic and traumatic etiologies, 272 lesions were found in 136 residual limbs, of which neuromas were by far the most common [94]. A military study examining lower extremity reoperations found neuroma excision to be second only to HO resection as the elective reoperation sought out by patients with persistent pain [72]. Earlier work suggested that nearly 30% of residual limbs had symptomatic neuromata, but that study largely focused on transtibial amputations where nerve endings are more superficial and soft tissue is less robust and included many patients prior to the widespread practice of traction neurectomies [74]. Neuroma excision is largely successful in alleviating symptoms [95, 96] and has been shown in the combat amputee population to profoundly decrease reliance on both narcotic and neuropathic medications [73]. Alternatively, targeted muscle reinnervation, initially developed to augment the control of myoelectric upper extremity prostheses [97–99], offers an additional technique for managing symptomatic neuromata and will be discussed further later.

Other soft tissue complications can also be responsible for a PSRL and include myodesis failure, bursa formation, and scar revision to alleviate redundant soft tissue or removed adherent scars. When these surgeries can be performed without involving or revising the myodesis, less rehabilitative delay and decreased postoperative analgesic requirements are possible. Myodesis takedown, when performed, is typically accompanied by bone revision, however, and can more dramatically affect both pain and duration of non-weight bearing. While limb shortening is sometimes performed to accommodate a new soft tissue envelope or as a consequence of HO excision, neuroma excision or the strengthening revision of a failed myodesis, there is almost never a change in the amputation level [72]. The complications associated with proximal lower extremity amputations common to DCBI are mirrored by those encountered in the upper extremity amputations and include HO, wound dehiscence, symptomatic neuromas, and contracture development [73]. Overall, complications associated with traumatic amputations are high in both the civilian [100–102] and military populations; however, the sheer number of amputations resulting from blast injury, with many patients sustaining multiple amputations [13], has hastened the development of new surgical techniques and approaches in order to thwart the late complications inherent to the residual limb.

Many of the patients who sustained amputations early in the conflict have done surprisingly well and returned to a high level of function. However, many of these patients were unilateral or distal limb amputations whereas the DCBI amputee is proximal and often bilateral with associated upper extremity injury, with additional pelvic and perineal trauma. What will be the downstream health effects associated with these severe injury patterns? There is no true corollary in the medical literature to predict the physiologic outcomes on the horizon for the veteran care network and DCBI patients. In one study comparing traumatic amputees to nontraumatic amputees, those patients who had amputation secondary to trauma had lower coronary artery calcium scores and lower creatinine, but this is expected since vascular disease and poor kidney function are medical conditions that can result in amputation and are associated with overall poor health [103]. Modan et al. [104], in a 1998 *American Journal of Cardiology* article, compared Israeli military lower limb amputees ($n = 201$) to the general population and found that surviving traumatic amputees had increased mortality rates due to cardiovascular disease as well as hyperinsulinemia. However, their study found no differences with regard to obesity, stroke, hypertension, or lipid profiles. Although obesity was not shown to be associated in this study, decreased ambulation status is likely predictive of high BMI, but has not yet been clarified in the DCBI population. Osteoporosis, also a consequence of limiting weight bearing, is another concern with regard to patients with multiple proximal amputations, as proximal amputations were shown to be associated with low bone mineral density [105]. Therefore, appropriate counseling as well as pharmacologic supplementation should occur in order to prevent potentially debilitating fractures proximal to the residual limb. Undoubtedly, chronic low back pain, a common disability in the population as a whole, is common among proximal limb amputees (81%) compared to transtibial amputees, with alterations in gait kinematics found among both pain and pain-free groups [106]. Back pain was also more prevalent among amputees who experienced long-standing phantom limb pain, a suggestion that improved coping mechanisms may be protective. However, these studies are generally older and/or taken from civilian populations with pre-existing conditions, and therefore prospective research is necessary to determine whether the severity of the

DCBI injury pattern will more negatively affect overall health.

The residual limbs of patients who sustain traumatic amputations are wrought with late complications, such as heterotopic ossification and painful neuroma, as well as those developing complications for which we currently lack long-term data, such as osteoporosis, low back pain, obesity, and cardiovascular disease that can be attributed to the physiologic stress placed upon proximal level amputee. Despite these concerns, amputee outcomes among the combat-wounded population are surprisingly good and can be attributed to strong psychosocial frameworks, advances in prosthetics and rehabilitation, and novel approaches to amputation surgery which maximize function and decrease morbidity offering further promise and which will be the focus of the remaining discussion.

Amputee Outcomes

Previously much of our understanding of amputee outcomes was derived from the landmark Lower Extremity Assessment Project (LEAP) study which demonstrated high complication rates and generally poor functional independence among both patients undergoing limb salvage and trauma-related amputation [107–110]. In contrast, the Military Extremity Trauma Amputation versus Limb Salvage (METALS) study, a retrospective cohort of 324 service members who sustained severe lower extremity trauma, showed that amputees scored higher on the Short Musculoskeletal Function Assessment (SMFA), had lower rates of post-traumatic stress disorder, and performed vigorous activity at a higher rate than those undergoing limb salvage wherein the LEAP study scores were similar between groups. Authors of the study offer that these differences are likely attributed to the importance of established frameworks of rehabilitative and psychosocial support that exist for the amputee network. Initial amputee care, other injuries notwithstanding, allows for relatively early weight bearing, with access to state-of-the-art prostheses and incorporation within amputee rehabilitation centers where peer support is established early among rehabilitating service members [37]. Improved function between groups was noted despite similar reported rates of depression, inclusion of a high number of patients with proximal and/or bilateral amputations, and high reoperation rates. Tintle et al. reported that surgery for late complications improved patient satisfaction following interventions for PSRLs and in many cases resulted in a steep decrease in dependence on narcotic and neuropathic medications to alleviate pain [72, 73]. Members of the US Army Special Forces were also noted to have high rates of return to active duty (58%) compared to other service members, with no reported diagnoses of PTSD, and therefore absence of PTSD is thought to be protective. Therefore, while combat amputees from Iraq and Afghanistan have demonstrated better outcomes owing to resiliency and other non-injury factors than other severely injured military and civilian patients, disability is high and challenges abound as widely available prostheses are not always employed.

Upper extremity limb prostheses are historically not well accepted [73, 111]. Prosthesis rejection is attributed to increased weight of prostheses that offer limited functional utility and increases residual limb socket discomfort. Advances in prosthetic design as well as selective reoperation to alleviate debilitating symptoms have been shown increase regular wear rates from 19% to 87% of amputees undergoing revision procedures [73]. Acceptance gaps exist at a higher rate for more proximal upper extremity amputations, and therefore ongoing research continues in an effort to mitigate abandonment.

For patients who have high bilateral amputations or those that have sustained hip disarticulation or hemipelvectomy, prosthetic ambulation is less common. At final follow-up, none of the 12 hemipelvectomy patients who had contralateral lower extremity amputation were independently ambulating [82], whereas unilateral hemipelvectomy patients ambulate with prosthesis at a moderate rate [112, 113]. Reliance on wheelchair locomotion presents challenges largely related to the paucity of durable soft tissue available when closing these proximal amputations. As a result, decubitus ulcers and skin breakdown are common; however, heterotopic ossification has proved advantageous in some patients with selective partial resections providing a stable sitting platform.

Future Directions of Amputee Care

Two surgical techniques for improving residual limb acceptance of prostheses include targeted muscle reinnervation (TMR) and osseointegrated implants. TMR was developed by Drs. Todd Kuiken and Gregory Dumanian initially to gain improved intuitive control of myoelectric prosthetics in the upper extremity. Essentially, transected nerves that no longer function in a neuromuscular unit when distal muscles are lost are reassigned to power muscles that remain within the limb. These nerves can be "fired" to initiate movement of prosthesis by intuitive performance of the anatomic function of the transferred nerve, with the reinnervated muscle acting as a biologic amplifier of the nerve signal. While some outcomes have been reported [98, 114–116] following TMR with regard to prosthesis control, TMR is also being investigated as an additional treatment for neuroma pain in both the upper and lower extremity residual limb [117, 118] and is the focus of ongoing Department of Defense-funded study comparing neuroma pain in patients treated with neurectomy versus TMR.

Osseointegration refers to the direct skeletal attachment of prostheses to the residual limbs of amputees via a transcutaneous abutment. The use of osseointegrated implants has been around for decades, with its initial development by Branemark for dental prostheses. Indications for its use in amputees include patients who cannot tolerate socket-based prostheses due to problems with stability, comfort, or frequent skin irritation and breakdown. Good outcomes have been reported in limbs that previously did not accept donned prosthesis with high implant survival in some short-term follow-up studies [119, 120]. Skepticism remains, although frequent concerns regarding deep infection requiring implant removal are not founded [121]. Superficial infection rates of 18% have been reported, with the majority of these infections responding readily to a short course of oral antibiotics without further clinical sequelae [121]. Transhumeral osseointegrated implants have demonstrated similar promise [122] in part due to the poor acceptance of traditional prostheses by proximal upper extremity amputees. Given these promising results with regard to implant retention, prosthetic acceptance, and patient quality of life, a DoD sponsored study is ongoing in order to determine the role of osseointegrated implants for rehabilitating combat veterans.

Conclusion

DCBI has produced devastating but survivable injuries that require prolonged stabilization performed at multiple echelons of care, novel reconstructive techniques, and exhaustive rehabilitation that place great burden on the military healthcare system. The extremities have been particularly involved owing to improvements in body armor, and the military orthopedic team has encountered more proximal amputations with severe soft tissue loss contaminated with multidrug-resistant bacteria and invasive fungal infection. Despite aggressive debridement performed within the zone of injury, high rates of wound complications and near ubiquitous heterotopic ossification formation persist. Late surgeries to address symptomatic limbs are often successful in decreasing pain and improving prosthetic tolerance, but delay rehabilitation. Therefore, ongoing research focuses on early identification, prophylactic treatments, and accommodative limb prostheses that will decrease morbidity and enhance function. While these efforts build on our vast experience dealing with the combat injuries from Iraq and Afghanistan, their solutions have utility for civilian surgeons when challenged with the complex injury patterns associated with domestic terrorism and disaster intervention.

References

1. Fischer H. A Guide to U.S. Military Casualty Statistics: Operation Inherent Resolve, Operation New Dawn, Operation Iraqi Freedom, and Operation Enduring Freedom. Congressional Research Service Report November 20, 2014.
2. Belmont PJ, Owens BD, Schoenfeld AJ. Musculoskeletal injuries in Iraq and Afghanistan: epidemiology and outcomes following a decade of war. J Am Acad Orthop Surg. 2016;24(6):341–8.
3. Belmont PJ, Schoenfeld AJ, Goodman G. Epidemiology of combat wounds in Operation Iraqi Freedom and Operation Enduring Freedom: orthopaedic burden of disease. J Surg Orthop Adv. 2010;19(1):2–7.
4. Murray CK. Epidemiology of infections associated with combat-related injuries in Iraq and Afghanistan. J Trauma. 2008;64(3 Suppl):S232–8.
5. Calhoun JH, Murray CK, Manring M. Multidrug-resistant organisms in military wounds from Iraq and Afghanistan. Clin Orthop Relat Res. 2008;466:1356–62.
6. Hospenthal DR, Crouch HK, English JF, Leach F, Pool J, Conger NG, Whitman TJ, Wortmann GW, Robertson JL, Murray CK. Multidrug-resistant bacterial colonization of combat-injured personnel at admission to medical centers after evacuation from Afghanistan and Iraq. J Trauma Inj Infect Crit Care. 2011;71:S52–7.
7. Warkentien T, Rodriguez C, Lloyd B, et al. Invasive mold infections following combat-related injuries. Clin Infect Dis. 2012;55(11):1441–9.
8. Owens BD, Kragh JF Jr, Macaitis J, Svoboda SJ, Wenke JC. Characterization of extremity wounds in Operation Iraqi Freedom and Operation Enduring Freedom. J Orthop Trauma. 2007;21(4):254–7.
9. Belmont PJ Jr, McCriskin BJ, Hsiao MS, Burks R, Nelson KJ, Schoenfeld AJ. The nature and incidence of musculoskeletal combat wounds in Iraq and Afghanistan (2005–2009). J Orthop Trauma. 2013;27(5):e107–13.
10. Mossadegh S, Tai N, Midwinter M, Parker P. Improvised explosive device related pelvi-perineal trauma: anatomic injuries and surgical management. J Trauma Acute Care Surg. 2012;73(2 Suppl 1):S24–31.
11. Schoenfeld AJ, Dunn JC, Bader JO, Belmont PJ Jr. The nature and extent of war injuries sustained by combat specialty personnel killed and wounded in Afghanistan and Iraq, 2003–2011. J Trauma Acute Care Surg. 2013;75(2):287–91.
12. Cannon JW, Hofmann LJ, Glasgow SC, Potter BK, Rodriguez CJ, Cancio LC, Rasmussen TE, Fries CA, Davis MR, Jezior JR, Mullins RJ, Elster EA. Dismounted complex blast injuries: a comprehensive review of the modern combat experience. J Am Coll Surg. 2016;223(4):652–64.
13. Godfrey BW, Martin A, Chestovich PJ, Lee GH, Ingalls NK, Saldanha V. Patients with multiple traumatic amputations: an analysis of operation enduring freedom joint theatre trauma registry data. Injury. 2017;48(1):75–9.
14. Mamczak CN, Elster EA. Complex dismounted IED blast injuries: the initial management of bilateral lower extremity amputations with and without pelvic and perineal involvement. J Surg Orthop Adv. 2012;21(1):8–14.
15. Borgman MA, Spinella PC, Perkins JG, Grathwohl KW, Repine T, Beekley AC, Sebesta J, Jenkins D, Wade CE, Holcomb JB. The ratio of blood products transfused affects mortality in patients receiving massive transfusions at a combat support hospital. J Trauma. 2007;63(4):805–13.
16. Investigators FLOW, Petrisor B, Sun X, Bhandari M, Guyatt G, Jeray KJ, Sprague S, Tanner S, Schemitsch E, Sancheti P, Anglen J, Tornetta P, Bosse M, Liew S, Walter S. Fluid lavage of open wounds (FLOW): a multicenter, blinded, factorial pilot trial comparing alternative irrigating solutions and pressures in patients with open fractures. J Trauma. 2011;71(3):596–606.
17. Lloyd B, Weintrob AC, Rodriguez C, et al. Effect of early screening for invasive fungal infections in U.S. service members with explosive blast injuries. Surg Infect. 2014;15:619–26.
18. Rodriguez CJ, Weintrob AC, Shah J, Malone D, Dunne JR, Weisbrod AB, Lloyd BA, Warkentien TE, Murray CK, Wilkins K, Faraz S, Carson ML, Aggarwal D, Tribble DR, Infectious Disease Clinical Research Program Trauma Infectious Disease Outcomes Study Group. Risk factors associated with invasive fungal infections in combat trauma. Surg Infect. 2014;15(5):521–6.
19. Lewandowski LR, Weintrob AC, Tribble DR, Rodriguez CJ, Petfield J, Lloyd BA, Murray CK, Stinner D, Aggarwal D, Shaikh F, Potter BK, Infectious Disease Clinical Research Program Trauma Infectious Disease Outcomes Study Group. Early complications and outcomes in combat injury-related invasive fungal wound infections: a case-control analysis. J Orthop Trauma. 2016;30(3):e93–9.
20. Forsberg JA, Potter BK, Polfer EM, Safford SD, Elster EA. Do inflammatory markers portend heterotopic ossification and wound failure in combat wounds? Clin Orthop Relat Res. 2014;472(9):2845–54.
21. Forsberg JA, Elster EA, Andersen RC, Nylen E, Brown TS, Rose MW, Stojadinovic A, Becker KL, McGuigan FX. Correlation of procalcitonin and cytokine expression with dehiscence of wartime extremity wounds. J Bone Joint Surg Am. 2008;90(3):580–8.
22. Santiago GF, Bograd B, Basile PL, Howard RT, Fleming M, Valerio IL. Soft tissue injury management with a continuous external tissue expander. Ann Plast Surg. 2012;69(4):418–21.

23. Formby P, Flint J, Gordon WT, Fleming M, Andersen RC. Use of a continuous external tissue expander in the conversion of a type IIIB fracture to a type IIIA fracture. Orthopedics. 2013;36(2):e249–51.
24. Sabino J, Polfer E, Tintle S, Jessie E, Fleming M, Martin B, Shashikant M, Valerio IL. A decade of conflict: flap coverage options and outcomes in traumatic war-related extremity reconstruction. Plast Reconstr Surg. 2015;135(3):895–902.
25. Helgeson MD, Potter BK, Evans KN, Shawen SB. Bioartificial dermal substitute: a preliminary report on its use for the management of complex combat-related soft tissue wounds. J Orthop Trauma. 2007;21(6):394–9.
26. Seavey JG, Masters ZA, Balazs GC, Tintle SM, Sabino J, Fleming ME, Valerio IL. Use of a bioartificial dermal regeneration template for skin restoration in combat casualty injuries. Regen Med. 2016;11(1):81–90.
27. Valerio IL, Masters Z, Seavey JG, Balazs GC, Ipsen D, Tintle SM. Use of a dermal regeneration template wound dressing in the treatment of combat-related upper extremity soft tissue injuries. J Hand Surg Am. 2016;41(12):e453–60. https://doi.org/10.1016/j.jhsa.2016.08.015.
28. Hsu JR, Beltran MJ, Skeletal Trauma Research Consortium. Shortening and angulation for soft-tissue reconstruction of extremity wounds in a combat support hospital. Mil Med. 2009;174(8):838–42.
29. Gordon WT, Grijalva S, Potter BK. Damage control and austere environment external fixation: techniques for the civilian provider. J Surg Orthop Adv. 2012;21(1):22–31.
30. Wheatley BM, Hanley MG, Wong VW, Sabino JM, Potter BK, Tintle SM, Fleming ME, Valerio IL. Heterotopic ossification following tissue transfer for combat-casualty complex Periarticular injuries. Plast Reconstr Surg. 2015;136(6):808e–14e.
31. Dickens JF, Wilson KW, Tintle SM, Heckert R, Gordon WT, D'Alleyrand JC, Potter BK. Risk factors for decreased range of motion and poor outcomes in open periarticular elbow fractures. Injury. 2015;46(4):676–81. https://doi.org/10.1016/j.injury.2015.01.021.
32. Corona BT, Garg K, Ward CL, McDaniel JS, Walters TJ, Rathbone CR. Autologous minced muscle grafts: a tissue engineering therapy for the volumetric loss of skeletal muscle. Am J Physiol Cell Physiol. 2013;305(7):C761–75.
33. Corona BT, Rivera JC, Owens JG, Wenke JC, Rathbone CR. Volumetric muscle loss leads to permanent disability following extremity trauma. J Rehabil Res Dev. 2015;52(7):785–92.
34. Li MT, Willett NJ, Uhrig BA, Guldberg RE, Warren GL. Functional analysis of limb recovery following autograft treatment of volumetric muscle loss in the quadriceps femoris. J Biomech. 2014;47(9):2013–21.
35. Gentile NE, Stearns KM, Brown EH, Rubin JP, Boninger ML, Dearth CL, Ambrosio F, Badylak SF. Targeted rehabilitation after extracellular matrix scaffold transplantation for the treatment of volumetric muscle loss. Am J Phys Med Rehabil. 2014;93(11 Suppl 3):S79–87.
36. Patzkowski JC, Owens JG, Blanck RV, Kirk KL, Hsu JR, Skeletal Trauma Research Consortium (STReC). Deployment after limb salvage for high-energy lower-extremity trauma. J Trauma Acute Care Surg. 2012;73(2 Suppl 1):S112–5.
37. Doukas WC, Hayda RA, Frisch HM, Andersen RC, Mazurek MT, Ficke JR, Keeling JJ, Pasquina PF, Wain HJ, Carlini AR, MacKenzie EJ. The Military Extremity Trauma Amputation/Limb Salvage (METALS) study: outcomes of amputation versus limb salvage following major lower-extremity trauma. J Bone Joint Surg Am. 2013;95(2):138–45.
38. Blair JA, Patzkowski JC, Blanck RV, Owens JG, Hsu JR, Skeletal Trauma Research Consortium (STReC). Return to duty after integrated orthotic and rehabilitation initiative. J Orthop Trauma. 2014;28(4):e70–4.
39. Highsmith MJ, Nelson LM, Carbone NT, Klenow TD, Kahle JT, Hill OT, Maikos JT, Kartel MS, Randolph BJ. Outcomes associated with the Intrepid Dynamic Exoskeletal Orthosis (IDEO): a systematic review of the literature. Mil Med. 2016;181(S4):69–76.
40. Birch R, Misra P, Stewart MP, Eardley WG, Ramasamy A, Brown K, Shenoy R, Anand P, Clasper J, Dunn R, Etherington J. Nerve injuries sustained during warfare: Part I—epidemiology. J Bone Joint Surg Br. 2012;94(4):523–8.
41. Birch R, Misra P, Stewart MP, Eardley WG, Ramasamy A, Brown K, Shenoy R, Anand P, Clasper J, Dunn R, Etherington J. Nerve injuries sustained during warfare: Part II: outcomes. J Bone Joint Surg Br. 2012;94(4):529–35.
42. Stansbury LG, Branstetter JG, Lalliss SJ. Amputation in military trauma surgery. J Trauma. 2007;63(4):940–4.
43. Tintle SM, Baechler MF, Nanos GP 3rd, Forsberg JA, Potter BK. Traumatic and trauma-related amputations: Part II: upper extremity and future directions. J Bone Joint Surg Am. 2010;92(18):2934–45.
44. Jansen JO, Thomas GO, Adams SA, Tai NR, Russell R, Morrison J, Clasper J, Midwinter M. Early management of proximal traumatic lower extremity amputation and pelvic injury caused by improvised explosive devices (IEDs). Injury. 2012;43(7):976–9. https://doi.org/10.1016/j.injury.2011.08.027. Epub 2011 Sep 9.
45. Radowsky JS, Rodriguez CJ, Wind GG, Elster EA. A Surgeon's guide to obtaining hemorrhage control in combat-related dismounted lower extremity blast injuries. Mil Med. 2016;181(10):1300–4.
46. Banti M, Walter J, Hudak S, Soderdahl D. Improvised explosive device-related lower genitourinary trauma in current overseas combat operations. J Trauma Acute Care Surg. 2016;80(1):131–4.

47. Tintle SM, Keeling JJ, Shawen SB, Forsberg JA, Potter BK. Traumatic and trauma-related amputations: Part I: general principles and lower-extremity amputations. J Bone Joint Surg Am. 2010;92(17):2852–68.
48. Tintle SM, LeBrun C, Ficke JR, Potter BK. What is new in trauma-related amputations. J Orthop Trauma. 2016;30(Suppl 3):S16–20.
49. Kang DG, Holekamp TF, Wagner SC, Lehman RA Jr. Intrasite vancomycin powder for the prevention of surgical site infection in spine surgery: a systematic literature review. Spine J. 2015;15(4):762–70.
50. Khan NR, Thompson CJ, DeCuypere M, et al. A meta-analysis of spinal surgical site infection and vancomycin powder. J Neurosurg Spine. 2014;21(6):974–83.
51. Yan H, He J, Chen S, Yu S, Fan C. Intrawound application of vancomycin reduces wound infection after open release of post-traumatic stiff elbows: a retrospective comparative study. J Shoulder Elb Surg. 2014;23(5):686–92.
52. Zebala LP, Chuntarapas T, Kelly MP, Talcott M, Greco S, Riew KD. Intrawound vancomycin powder eradicates surgical wound contamination: an in vivo rabbit study. J Bone Joint Surg Am. 2014;96(1):46–51.
53. Caroom C, Tullar JM, Benton EG Jr, et al. Intrawound vancomycin powder reduces surgical site infections in posterior cervical fusion. Spine. 2013;38(14):1183.
54. Pavey GJ, Qureshi AT, Hope DN, Pavlicek RL, Potter BK, Forsberg JA, Davis TA. Bioburden increases heterotopic ossification formation in an established rat model. Clin Orthop Relat Res. 2015;473(9):2840–7.
55. Seavey JG, Wheatley BM, Pavey GJ, Tomasino AM, Hanson MA, Sanders EM, Potter BK, Forsberg JA, Qureshi AT, Davis TA. Early local delivery of Vancomycin significantly suppresses ectopic bone formation in a rat model of trauma-induced heterotopic ossification. J Orthop Res. 35(11):2397–406.
56. Gottschalk F. Transfemoral amputation. Biomechanics and surgery. Clin Orthop Relat Res. 1999;361:15–22.
57. Pinzur MS, Gottschalk F, Pinto MA, Smith DG. Controversies in lower extremity amputation. Instr Course Lect. 2008;57:663–72.
58. Jaegers SM, Arendzen JH, de Jongh HJ. An electromyographic study of the hip muscles of transfemoral amputees in walking. Clin Orthop Relat Res. 1996;328:119–28.
59. Kasabian AK, Colen SR, Shaw WW, et al. The role of microvascular free flaps in salvaging below-knee amputation stumps: a review of 22 cases. J Trauma. 1991;31:495–500.
60. Gallico GG III, Ehrlichman RJ, Jupiter J, May JW Jr. Free flaps to preserve below-knee amputation stumps: long-term evaluation. Plast Reconstr Surg. 1987;79:871–8.
61. Wood MR, Hunter GA, Millstein SG. The value of stump split skin grafting following amputation for trauma in adult upper and lower limb amputees. Prosthetics Orthot Int. 1987;11:71–4.
62. Yokota K, Nakanishi M, Sunagawa T, et al. Using full-thickness skin graft from amputated foot can provide a stump with durable skin. J Plast Reconstr Aesthet Surg. 2009;62(12):e667–9.
63. Anderson WD, Stewart KJ, Wilson Y, Quaba AA. Skin grafts for the salvage of degloved below-knee amputation stumps. Br J Plast Surg. 2002;55:320–3.
64. Parry IS, Mooney KN, Chau C, et al. Effects of skin grafting on successful prosthetic use in children with lower extremity amputation. J Burn Care Res. 2008;29:949–54.
65. Fleming ME, O'Daniel A, Bharmal H, Valerio I. Application of the orthoplastic reconstructive ladder to preserve lower extremity amputation length. Ann Plast Surg. 2014;73(2):183–9.
66. Polfer EM, Tintle SM, Forsberg JA, Potter BK. Skin grafts for residual limb coverage and preservation of amputation length. Plast Reconstr Surg. 2015;136(3):603–9.
67. Kent T, Yi C, Livermore M, Stahel PF. Skin grafts provide durable end-bearing coverage for lower-extremity amputations with critical soft tissue loss. Orthopedics. 2013;36(2):132–5.
68. Erdmann D, Sundin BM, Yasui K, Wong MS, Levin LS. Microsurgical free flap transfer to amputation sites: indications and results. Ann Plast Surg. 2002;48:167–72.
69. Bibbo C, Ehrlich D, Levin LS, Kovach SJ. Maintaining levels of lower extremity amputations. J Surg Orthop Adv. 2016;25(3):137–48. Review.
70. Baccarani A, Follmar KE, De Santis G, Adani R, Pinelli M, Innocenti M, Baumeister S, von Gregory H, Germann G, Erdmann D, Levin LS. Free vascularized tissue transfer to preserve upper extremity amputation levels. Plast Reconstr Surg. 2007;120(4):971–81.
71. Potter BK, Burns TC, Lacap AP, Granville RR, Gajewski DA. Heterotopic ossification following traumatic and combat-related amputations. Prevalence, risk factors, and preliminary results of excision. J Bone Joint Surg Am. 2007;89:476–86.
72. Tintle SM, Shawen SB, Forsberg JA, Gajewski DA, Keeling JJ, Andersen RC, Potter BK. Reoperation after combat-related major lower extremity amputations. J Orthop Trauma. 2014;28(4):232–7.
73. Tintle SM, Baechler MF, Nanos GP, Forsberg JA, Potter BK. Reoperations following combat-related upper-extremity amputations. J Bone Joint Surg Am. 2012;94(16):e1191–6.
74. Tintle SM, Keeling JJ, Shawen SB, et al. Operative complications of combat-related transtibial amputations: a comparison of the classic burges and modified Ertl tibiofibular synostosis techniques. J Bone Joint Surg Am. 2011;93:1016–21.

75. Murray CK, Roop SA, Hospenthal DR, Dooley DP, Wenner K, Hammock J, Taufen N, Gourdine E. Bacteriology of war wounds at the time of injury. Mil Med. 2006;171:826–9.
76. Hawley JS, Murray CK, Griffith ME, et al. Susceptibility of acinetobacter strains isolated from deployed U.S. military personnel. Antimicrob Agents Chemother. 2007;51:376–8.
77. Murray CK, Griffith ME, Mende K, Guymon CH, Ellis MW, Beckius M, Zera WC, Yu X, Co EM, Aldous W, Hospenthal DR. Methicillin-resistant Staphylococcus Aureus in wound cultures recovered from a combat support hospital in Iraq. J Trauma. 2010;69(Suppl 1):S102–8.
78. Murray CK, Wilkins K, Molter NC, Li F, Yu L, Spott MA, Eastridge B, Blackbourne LH, Hospenthal DR. Infections complicating the care of combat casualties during operations Iraqi Freedom and Enduring Freedom. J Trauma. 2011;71(1 Suppl):S62–73.
79. Penn-Barwell JG, Fries CA, Sargeant ID, Bennett PM, Porter K. Aggressive soft tissue infections and amputation in military trauma patients. J R Nav Med Serv. 2012;98(2):14–8.
80. Polfer EM, Hoyt BW, Senchak LT, Murphey MD, Forsberg JA, Potter BK. Fluid collections in amputations are not indicative or predictive of infection. Clin Orthop Relat Res. 2014;472(10):2978–83.
81. D'Alleyrand JC, Fleming M, Gordon WT, Andersen RC, Potter BK. Combat-related Hemipelvectomy. J Surg Orthop Adv. 2012;21(1):38–43. Review.
82. D'Alleyrand JC, Lewandowski LR, Forsberg JA, Gordon WT, Fleming ME, Mullis BH, Andersen RC, Potter BK. Combat-related Hemipelvectomy: 14 cases, a review of the literature and lessons learned. J Orthop Trauma. 2015;29(12):e493–8.
83. Matsumoto ME, Khan M, Jayabalan P, Ziebarth J, Munin MC. Heterotopic ossification in civilians with lower limb amputations. Arch Phys Med Rehabil. 2014;95(9):1710–3.
84. Forsberg JA, Pepek JM, Wagner S, Wilson K, Flint J, Andersen RC, Tadaki D, Gage FA, Stojadinovic A, Elster EA. Heterotopic ossification in high-energy wartime extremity injuries: prevalence and risk factors. J Bone Joint Surg Am. 2009;91:1084–91.
85. Forsberg JA, Potter BK. Heterotopic ossification in wartime wounds. J Surg Orthop Adv. 2010;19:54–61.
86. Potter BK, Forsberg JA, Davis TA, Evans KN, Hawksworth JS, Tadaki D, Brown TS, Crane NJ, Burns TC, O'Brien FP, Elster EA. Heterotopic ossification following combat-related trauma. J Bone Joint Surg Am. 2010;92(Suppl 2):74–89.
87. Polfer EM, Forsberg JA, Fleming ME, Potter BK. Neurovascular entrapment due to combat-related heterotopic ossification in the lower extremity. J Bone Joint Surg Am. 2013;95(24):e195(1–6).
88. Pavey GJ, Polfer EM, Nappo KE, Tintle SM, Forsberg JA, Potter BK. What risk factors predict recurrence of heterotopic ossification after excision in combat-related amputations? Clin Orthop Relat Res. 2015;473(9):2814–24.
89. Crane NJ, Polfer E, Elster EA, Potter BK, Forsberg JA. Raman spectroscopic analysis of combat-related heterotopic ossification development. Bone. 2013;57(2):335–42.
90. Harris M, Cilwa K, Elster EA, Potter BK, Forsberg JA, Crane NJ. Pilot study for detection of early changes in tissue associated with heterotopic ossification: moving toward clinical use of Raman spectroscopy. Connect Tissue Res. 2015;56(2):144–52.
91. Polfer EM, Hope DN, Elster EA, Qureshi AT, Davis TA, Golden D, Potter BK, Forsberg JA. The development of a rat model to investigate the formation of blast-related post-traumatic heterotopic ossification. Bone Joint J. 2015;97-B(4):572–6.
92. Qureshi AT, Crump EK, Pavey GJ, Hope DN, Forsberg JA, Davis TA. Early characterization of blast-related heterotopic ossification in a rat model. Clin Orthop Relat Res. 2015;473(9):2831–9.
93. Pavey GJ, Qureshi AT, Tomasino AM, Honnold CL, Bishop DK, Agarwal S, Loder S, Levi B, Pacifici M, Iwamoto M, Potter BK, Davis TA, Forsberg JA. Targeted stimulation of retinoic acid receptor-γ mitigates the formation of heterotopic ossification in an established blast-related traumatic injury model. Bone. 2016;90:159–67.
94. O'Reilly MA, O'Reilly PM, O'Reilly HM, Sullivan J, Sheahan J. High-resolution ultrasound findings in the symptomatic residual limbs of amputees. Mil Med. 2013;178(12):1291–7.
95. Ducic I, Mesbahi AN, Attinger CE, et al. The role of peripheral nerve surgery in the treatment of chronic pain associated with amputation stumps. Plast Reconstr Surg. 2008;121:908–14. discussion 915–7.
96. Sehirlioglu A, Ozturk C, Yazicioglu K, et al. Painful neuroma requiring surgical excision after lower limb amputation caused by landmine explosions. Int Orthop. 2009;33:533–6.
97. Kuiken TA, Dumanian GA, Lipschutz RD, et al. The use of targeted muscle reinnervation for improved myoelectric prosthesis control in a bilateral shoulder disarticulation amputee. Prosthetics Orthot Int. 2004;28:245–53.
98. Kuiken TA, Miller LA, Lipschutz RD, et al. Targeted reinnervation for enhanced prosthetic arm function in a woman with a proximal amputation: a case study. Lancet. 2007;369:371–80.
99. O'Shaughnessy KD, Dumanian GA, Lipschutz RD, et al. Targeted reinnervation to improve prosthesis control in transhumeral amputees. A report of three cases. J Bone Joint Surg Am. 2008;90:393–400.
100. MacKenzie EJ, Bosse MJ, Castillo RC, Smith DG, Webb LX, Kellam JF, Burgess AR, Swiontkowski MF, Sanders RW, Jones AL, McAndrew MP, Patterson BM, Travison TG, McCarthy ML. Functional outcomes following trauma-related lower extremity amputation. J Bone Joint Surg Am. 2004;86:1636–45.
101. Harris AM, Althausen PL, Kellam J, Bosse MJ, Castillo R, Lower Extremity Assessment Project (LEAP) Study Group. Complications following limb-threatening lower extremity trauma. J Orthop Trauma. 2009;23(1):1–6.

102. Pierce RO Jr, Kernek CB, Ambrose TA 2nd. The plight of the traumatic amputee. Orthopedics. 1993;16:793–7.
103. Nallegowda M, Lee E, Brandstater M, Kartono AB, Kumar G, Foster GP. Amputation and cardiac comorbidity: analysis of severity of cardiac risk. PM R. 2012;4(9):657–66.
104. Modan M, Peles E, Halkin H, Nitzan H, Azaria M, Gitel S, Dolfin D, Modan B. Increased cardiovascular disease mortality rates in traumatic lower limb amputees. Am J Cardiol. 1998;82(10):1242–7.
105. Flint JH, Wade AM, Stocker DJ, Pasquina PF, Howard RS, Potter BK. Bone mineral density loss after combat-related lower extremity amputation. J Orthop Trauma. 2014;28(4):238–44. https://doi.org/10.1097/BOT.0b013e3182a66a8a.
106. Kulkarni J, Gaine WJ, Buckley JG, Rankine JJ, Adams J. Chronic low back pain in traumatic lower limb amputees. Clin Rehabil. 2005;19(1):81–6.
107. Bosse MJ, MacKenzie EJ, Kellam JF, Burgess AR, Webb LX, Swiontkowski MF, Sanders RW, Jones AL, McAndrew MP, Patterson BM, McCarthy ML, Travison TG, Castillo RC. An analysis of outcomes of reconstruction or amputation after legthreatening injuries. N Engl J Med. 2002;347(24):1924–31.
108. MacKenzie EJ, Bosse MJ, Pollak AN, Webb LX, Swiontkowski MF, Kellam JF, Smith DG, Sanders RW, Jones AL, Starr AJ, McAndrew MP, Patterson BM, Burgess AR, Castillo RC. Long-term persistence of disability following severe lower-limb trauma. Results of a seven-year follow-up. J Bone Joint Surg Am. 2005;87(8):1801–9.
109. MacKenzie EJ, Bosse MJ. Factors influencing outcome following limb-threatening lower limb trauma: lessons learned from the Lower Extremity Assessment Project (LEAP). J Am Acad Orthop Surg. 2006;14(10):S205–10. Review.
110. McCarthy ML, MacKenzie EJ, Edwin D, Bosse MJ, Castillo RC, Starr A, LEAP Study Group. Psychological distress associated with severe lower-limb injury. J Bone Joint Surg Am. 2003;85(9):1689–97.
111. Resnik L, Meucci MR, Lieberman-Klinger S, Fantini C, Kelty DL, Disla R, Sasson N. Advanced upper limb prosthetic devices: implications for upper limb prosthetic rehabilitation. Arch Phys Med Rehabil. 2012;93(4):710–7.
112. Rieger H, Dietl K. Traumatic hemipelvectomy: an update. J Trauma. 1998;45:422–6.
113. Nowroozi F, Salvanelli ML, Gerber LH. Energy expenditure in hip disarticulation and hemipelvectomy amputees. Arch Phys Med Rehabil. 1983;64:300–3.
114. Miller LA, Stubblefield KA, Lipschutz RD, et al. Improved myoelectric prosthesis control using targeted reinnervation surgery: a case series. IEEE Trans Neural Syst Rehabil Eng. 2008;16:46–50.
115. Cheesborough J, Smith L, Kuiken T, et al. Targeted muscle reinnervation and advanced prosthetic arms. Semin Plast Surg. 2015;29:062–72.
116. Gart MS, Souza JM, Dumanian GA. Targeted muscle Reinnervation in the upper extremity amputee: a technical roadmap. J Hand Surg. 2015;40(9):1877–88.
117. Pet MA, Ko JH, Friedly JL, et al. Does targeted nerve implantation reduce neuroma pain in amputees? Clin Orthop Relat Res. 2014;472: 2991–3001.
118. Souza JM, Cheesborough JE, Ko JH, et al. Targeted muscle reinnervation: a novel approach to post-amputation neuroma pain. Clin Orthop Relat Res. 2014;472:2984–90.
119. Hagberg K, Häggström E, Uden M, et al. Socket versus bone-anchored trans-femoral prostheses: hip range of motion and sitting comfort. Prosthetics Orthot Int. 2005;29:153–63.
120. Brånemark R, Berlin O, Hagberg K, et al. A novel osseointegrated percutaneous prosthetic system for the treatment of patients with transfemoral amputation: a prospective study of 51 patients. Bone Joint J. 2014;96-B:106–13.
121. Tillander J, Hagberg K, Hagberg L, et al. Osseointegrated titanium implants for limb prostheses attachments: infectious complications. Clin Orthop Relat Res. 2010;468:2781–8.
122. Tsikandylakis G, Berlin Ö, Brånemark R. Implant survival, adverse events, and bone remodeling of osseointegrated percutaneous implants sfor transhumeral amputees. Clin Orthop Relat Res. 2014;472:2947–56.

Soft Tissue Infection

14

Jason Scott Radowsky and Debra L. Malone

Introduction

Blast injury is a common combat-related wounding mechanism. Initial tissue destruction is related to the blast waves, thermal and kinetic energy, as well as flying debris associated with the explosion. There is also potential for blunt trauma due to victim body and/or surrounding structure displacement. Blast injuries to service members who are on foot patrol (dismounted) represent an injury pattern being addressed with increased frequency because body armor allows warfighters to survive injuries that would have been lethal in the past. There are multiple novel sequelae associated with this type of injury including infection with a variety of pathogens which colonize and/or invade the casualty's soft tissue wounds. Unfortunately, these infections commonly complicate these wounds and may lead to loss of tissue secondary to necrosis and subsequent surgical debridement. This chapter seeks to familiarize the reader with this combat-related wound complication. In this chapter, we'll describe the presumed mechanism of these infections, the most common pathogens involved, and the diagnostic and treatment modalities that we specifically utilize to battle these serious infections. We will also describe in more detail some of the more serious and unique infections that we have encountered following these dismounted blast injuries. Our protocols are based upon scientific review of the literature as well as our personal experience in the care of these patients.

Infection in Combat-Related Wounds

Combat-related blast wounds are often associated with extensive soft tissue disruption (Fig. 14.1). This disruption commonly includes the skin, adipose tissue, muscle, tendon, and bones, most often of the extremities. Other body cavities (e.g., intra-abdominal, thoracic, spinal column, brain) are often injured as well. The soft tissue components involved are related to the position of the warrior at the time of the explosion and the directional energy associated with the explosion. Infection can and often does complicate these wounds. These infections may be related to the pathogens that inoculated the wound at the time of the blast from either agricultural or man-made structural environments. Other infections that may be encountered en route to the United States include hospital-associated multidrug-resistant organisms (MDRO) [1, 2]. Combat casualties are subject to infection via both modalities, potentially complicating treatment plans. Some of these soft tissue infections are infrequently seen in civilian settings, and so predetermined diagnostic and/or treatment paradigms were not available at

J. S. Radowsky
Blanchfield Army Community Hospital,
Fort Campbell, TN, USA

D. L. Malone (✉)
Department of Surgery, Walter Reed National Military Medical Center, Bethesda, MD, USA
e-mail: debra.l.malone.mil@mail.mil

Fig. 14.1 Initial presentation of dismounted blast wounds – not previously published per our knowledge

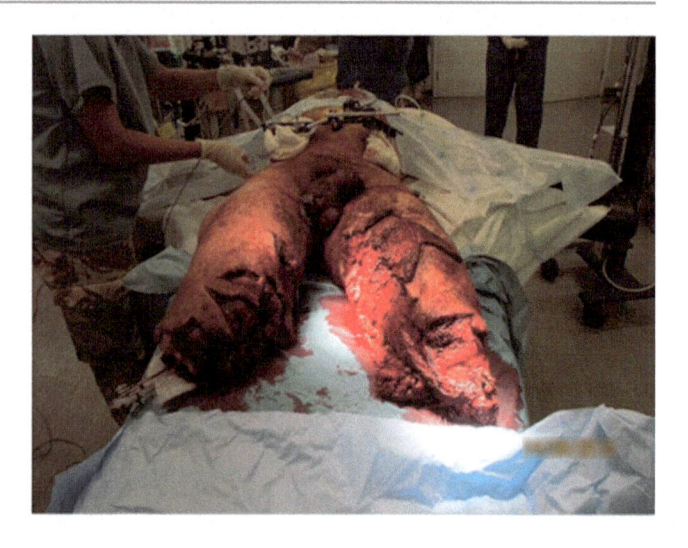

the start of the current wars. Thus, throughout the course of these conflicts, diagnostic and treatment strategies had to be developed to combat these unique infections.

Wounding due to the kinetic and thermal component of the blast contributes to the destruction of soft tissue. These wounds are typically complicated by some degree of ischemia as well. These effects can cause tissue necrosis that requires surgical debridement and subsequent further loss of tissue (e.g., loss of limb length/amputation). When fungal infection complicates these wounds, tissue loss can be even more profound. For example, our team determined that while there was no statistically significant difference in measured limb length, there was a much higher chance of revision to a higher level in those affected by IFI versus case matched controls. This included the progression of transfemoral amputations to hemipelvectomies or disarticulations [3].

Over the course of the wars in Iraq and Afghanistan, the military has encountered a multitude of infectious disease outbreaks [1, 4]. This situation led to investigations to determine the cause and best course of action to counteract the clinical complications associated with these outbreaks. One of the most concerning was the high prevalence of gram-negative MDRO colonization or infection (predominantly with MDR *Acinetobacter baumannii-calcoaceticus* complex and extended-spectrum b-lactamase (ESBL)-producing *Escherichia coli* and *Klebsiella pneumoniae*) in deployed patients in theater and in US military treatment facilities in the time frame between 2003 and 2009 [5]. Scott et al. determined that environmental contamination of field hospitals and infection transmission within healthcare facilities played a major role in this outbreak. Those investigators went on to note that novel strategies may be required to prevent the transmission of pathogens in combat field hospitals [1]. Zapor et al. discovered outbreaks of nosocomial infection with this pathogen in military treatment facilities in Europe and the United States as well [4].

Acinetobacter baumannii-calcoaceticus is a hardy organism endemic to the soil in theater and readily colonizes the skin, wounds, and artificial surfaces. However, its ubiquity is only part of the concern as it also becomes readily resistant to most conventional antibiotics and plays a significant role in increasing ICU and hospital length of stays. It has also affected many noncombat patients through nosocomial spread in hospital downrange and in the United States. On the basis of these findings, military healthcare providers set out to mitigate this problem. It was determined that maintaining infection control throughout the military healthcare system was critical. Guidelines for infection control practices were developed for deployed settings. Together with improved antibiotic stewardship, these efforts have led to a reduction of multidrug-resistant *Acinetobacter* [6, 7]. Interestingly, as the conflicts have progressed, other bacteria such as extended-spectrum beta-lactamase *E. coli* have become more prevalent.

Significant increases in focal and/or systemic invasive fungal infections (IFI) were first noticed in 2009 when improvised explosive devices began to be utilized more frequently in the Afghanistan conflict (Operation Enduring Freedom). This increase in fungal infections correlated with an increase in traumatic amputations as well [8]. These initial cases were diagnosed late in their course and often led to significant morbidity or death [9]. This led to a concerted effort to improve the efficacy of diagnosis and treatment and ultimately to encourage prevention of fungal infections. These initiatives included performance improvement efforts that involved documentation of clinical observations, cultures, and histopathology reports. Scrutiny of these observations elucidated patterns of clinical presentation and/or disease progression, and these observations led to clinical practice guidelines (CPG). These efforts began at the National Naval Medical Center in 2009 and have since become a global effort via the Joint Trauma System [10]. This global effort led to a CPG encompassing the entire continuum of care.

The rapid emergence of IFI led to efforts to fully characterize the extent of the problem. The Trauma Infectious Disease Outcomes Study Group (TIDOS) led these efforts and made the following initial observations:

1. 97% of IFI patients were injured by blast mechanism, the majority of which suffered critical and/or life-threatening injuries.
2. 80% of IFI patients were dismounted (foot patrol) when the explosion occurred.
3. 66% of these patients required mechanical ventilation.
4. Molds from the Mucorales order (e.g., Mucor, Saksenaea, and Apophysomyces spp.) and genus Aspergillus were the predominant molds identified on culture [11].

In an effort to categorize these infections for research and clinical predictive purposes, a system based off of the European Organization for Research and Treatment of Cancer/Invasive Fungal Infections Cooperative Group and the National Institute of Allergy and Infectious Diseases Mycoses Study Group (EORTC/MSG) classification system for IFI was created. This scheme utilizes histopathology and microbiology data to rank probability of disease as follows:

1. Proven – fungal element angioinvasion on histopathology
2. Probable – fungal elements on histopathology without angioinvasion
3. Possible – culture growth without histopathology [12]

In a 2016 report, TIDOS showed there have been 95 IFI patients. These patients have had 144 IFI wounds (1.5 IFI wounds per patient), including 57 proven, 49 probable, and 38 possible cases [11]. In order to guide IFI prevention strategies, Rodriguez et al. determined that suspicion of IFI is warranted in any patient who, in addition to surviving a dismounted blast injury, received massive blood product transfusion (>25 units at the time of initial resuscitation), has a traumatic above-knee amputation, and also has other truncal or pelvic injuries [13] (Table 14.1).

Initially, fungal infections were not suspected as a potential cause of the clinical deterioration of blast-wounded patients as this was a disease of the immunosuppressed, such as patients who were undergoing chemotherapy, have brittle diabetics, or with immunomodulating regimens following organ transplantation [14, 15, 16]. Following analysis of the initial cohort of patients, a theory of their susceptibility to invasive fungal infections was postulated. We believe that the mechanism of the injury itself and the subsequent large volume blood resuscitation, leads to a functional immunosuppression which renders the injured warfighter susceptible to invasive pathogens to which he would otherwise be resistant.

The blast mechanism drives organic material and debris deep into the wounds (Fig. 14.2). Indeed, there are geographical differences in invasive fungal infection rates. For example, combat trauma in agricultural southern Afghanistan is associated with significantly higher rates of fungal infections than similarly injured individuals in the more mountainous northern regions [17]. Traumatic amputations frequently occur in blasts

Table 14.1 Risk factors for developing invasive fungal infection

Potential risk factor	Univariate odds ratio (95% CI)	Multivariate odds ratio (95% CI)[a]
Injury circumstance		
Blast	11.6 (1.8–493.2)	5.7 (1.1–29.6)
Dismounted	5.3 (1.7–21.6)	8.5 (1.2–59.8)
Above the knee amputation	10.0 (4.2–29.1)	4.1 (1.3–12.7)
Associated injuries[b]	4.4 (2.2–9.4)	2.3 (0.8–6.3)
PRBC transfusions (>20 U in first 24 h)	47.1 (9.8–479.3)	7.0 (2.5–19.7)
Clinical characteristics in theater[c]		
Base deficit (‡ 10)	8.7 (3.0–31.8)	–
Shock index (>1)[d]	4.5 (2.2–10.4)	–

From Rodriguez et al. [13]
CI confidence interval, *PRBC* packed red blood cells
[a]Controls are matched to cases by injury date (− 3 months) and injury severity score (ISS; − 10). ISS was included in multivariate analysis to provide greater control of injury severity-based matching
[b]Includes perineal, genitourinary, and/or more severe pelvic/abdominal injuries
[c]Due to high correlation with PRBC, base deficit and shock index were not included in the multivariate analysis
[d]Shock index: heart rate/systolic blood pressure

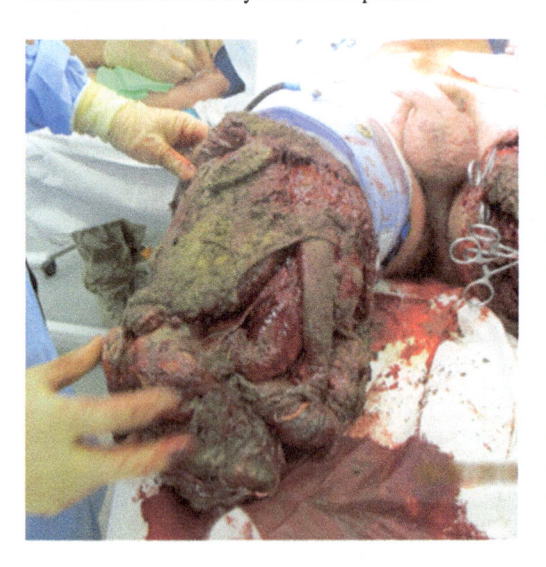

Fig. 14.2 Agricultural debris in wounds (From Tribble [33])

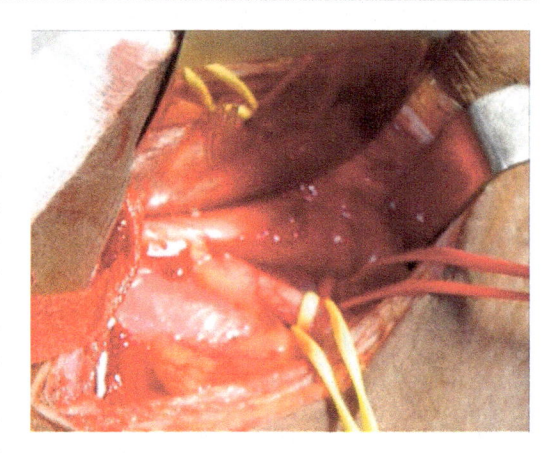

Fig. 14.3 Proximal vascular control

and are indicative of the large amount of the force applied to the casualty. The grievous wounds caused by blast may overstimulate the immune system which activates a systemic inflammatory state. If the burden of disease is extensive, and the immune system taxed, the patient may eventually have difficulty mounting appropriate responses to fungal and/or bacterial pathogens. Indeed, the rates of fungal infection increase with the number of limbs amputated and increased transfusion requirements [18].

Not only do massive transfusion requirements serve as a marker for the injury severity, but can lead to lead to immunosuppression [19]. The hemorrhage associated with traumatic limb amputations is controlled with tourniquets whenever possible or with direct cutdown with proximal control large vessels (Fig. 14.3). While cessation of blood flow is necessary to save a life, the resulting ischemia may provide an environment for enhanced opportunistic pathogen growth. Additionally, perineal wounds often involve soilage from a disrupted gastrointestinal tract which further contributes to the inoculation of ischemic tissue with bacterial and fungal pathogens. All of these factors combine to create a patient who can be challenging to treat.

Suspicion and/or Diagnosis

While most civilian patients' wounds are neither colonized nor infected upon presentation, 31% of wounds from the conflicts in Iraq and Afghanistan are, with *Acinetobacter* found in 22% of these wounds [20]. Multidrug-resistant bacteria are found in 13% of patients presenting to US hospitals from the war zone [21]. Therefore, all casualties arriving at medical facilities in the United States from Southwest Asia are swabbed for the presence of *Acinetobacter*, multidrug-resistant *Enterococcus*, and other bacteria which may be detrimental to wound healing and/or pose nosocomial problems for other patients. Groin swabs are obtained on all wounded warriors at the time of admission and wound cultures are obtained when there is suspicion for infection. Concern for pulmonary infection with *Acinetobacter*, which can be secondary to dust inhaled by the patient downrange, should be diagnosed with bronchoscopy and alveolar lavage.

The early initiation of systemic and local therapies is important for successful treatment of wound infection and is particularly imperative for invasive fungal infections. Therefore, when IFI is suspected, treatment should begin. Suspicion for infection should be high if new necrotic material is present on successive surgical debridements [22] (Fig. 14.4). In this scenario, the clinician should *not* wait for definitive diagnosis in order to begin focal and systemic antifungal therapy. This phenomenon will be described in greater detail below.

Microbial cultures are utilized to confirm clinical diagnosis and eventually focus pharmacological therapy. Bacterial, fungal, mycobacterial, and viral cultures are utilized in our wounded warrior population due to documented infection with these pathogens. Because fungal cultures may take 2–6 weeks to grow, we continue to monitor them for 6 weeks. Diagnosis of infection also includes the collection of intraoperative tissue for histopathology. The histopathology specimens are scrutinized for pathogens including fungal elements. We have created an intraoperative tissue collection protocol to guide this practice. We also developed a 24-hour (turnaround time) histopathology protocol in an effort to diagnose fungal disease as soon as possible.

Treatment

Once clinical suspicion has been established and wound cultures and tissue biopsies have been sent for analysis, aggressive multimodality therapy must be initiated in order to prevent further penetration of infection with associated progressive soft tissue loss and/or death. This approach involves surgical and medical treatment to ensure both local and systemic control. A multidisciplinary approach must be utilized to ensure proper implementation of available modalities. Excellent communication between members of the surgical, critical care, infectious disease, and wound care teams is essential.

Operative Exploration and Debridement

Local control of the infection is imperative for success, and this must start in the operating room with comprehensive exploration and aggressive debridement. At each operation, wounds must be examined closely in order to detect the presence of

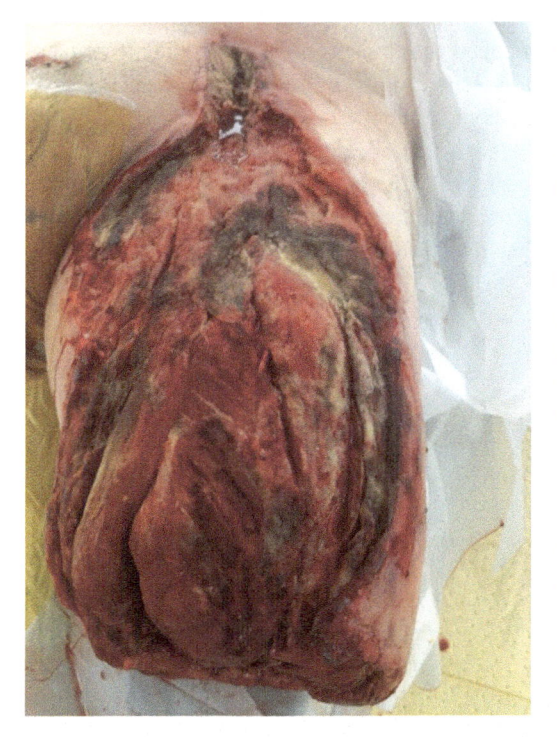

Fig. 14.4 Recurrent necrosis at subsequent operative exploration

infection, necrosis, and/or extension to the next extremity level or body region. The wounds and body cavities that incorporate the wounds must be examined very carefully for deep tissue involvement. For example, an infection involving thigh adductors may extend well into the pelvis. Delayed presentation of infection is not uncommon.

Prior to Operation Enduring Freedom in Afghanistan, surgical doctrine concerning invasive fungal infections typically recommended extremely aggressive local debridement with possible amputation [23]. Recently, this recommendation has tempered somewhat, but it is still crucial to debride back to healthy, bleeding tissue. Any remaining necrotic and/or infected tissue may act as a reservoir for penetration of the infection into deeper tissue planes and adjacent vital organs. Prevention of systemic dissemination may be impacted by the degree of debridement as well. Surgeons must also consider that angioinvasive fungal infections may create necrotic tissue by thrombosing vessels and thus render the distal tissue ischemic adding to the justification to debride aggressively. This thrombosis may also prevent systemic therapies from reaching the distal extremities to affect infection, further justifying the use of aggressive debridement to control additional spread [24].

Traumatic limb amputation might be considered a deterrent for debridement as it could deprive the patient of limb length or tissue coverage for future prosthetic fitting. However, the failure to adequately remove concerning tissue usually leads to even higher-level amputation later on as the disease progresses. Even with adequate debridements, "next"-level amputations, including joint disarticulations and hemipelvectomies/corpectomies, may be required if the infectious agent is aggressive (e.g., *mucormycosis*) [12]. The decision to perform these high-level amputations is difficult for the surgical teams and patients to make as the outcomes significantly affect the degree of disability and quality of life. Therefore, early aggressive debridement is critical to possible prevention of this horrific predicament.

Along those same lines, patients and/or family members should be made aware of the distinct possibility for significant tissue loss at each operation until the infection is controlled. It is not uncommon for patients who present with below-knee amputations to proceed to above-knee amputations or even more proximal revisions (Fig. 14.5). With the multimodality treatment that we prescribe, the surgeon should eventually be able to obtain and maintain clean surgical margins. Surgeons previously not experienced with this problem should be informed of this situation so as to minimize surgeon discouragement.

As stated above, infected wounds displaying necrotic tissue must be debrided. We debride wounds at least 4 cm into what appears to be healthy, viable tissue. Less than this has led to

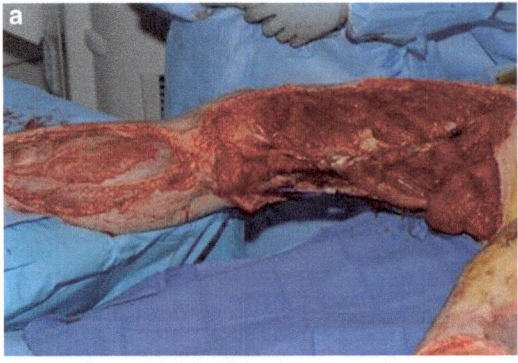

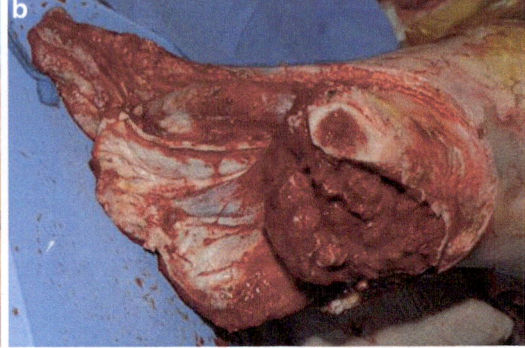

Fig. 14.5 (a) Progression of debridement leading to higher-level amputations. (b) Progression of debridement leading to higher-level amputations – not previously published per our knowledge

longer times to infection control per our experience. If a significant amount of wound necrosis is found in the operating room on any given day, the patient should be taken back to the operating room the next day; sooner if there is clinical decline. It is not uncommon for our patients with fungal infection to go to the operating room every day or every other day for the first 2 weeks of hospital admission. Once the wounds are clear of gross necrosis, the patients go to the operating room every second or third day until the wounds are either closed or definitively covered. We close wounds when wounds are clean and viable for at least two subsequent operations. Wounds that are not granulating and/or contracting are most likely still infected and/or contaminated and, if closed, are likely to become overtly infected and have to be reopened. These wounds may have a green/yellow sheen to them (Fig. 14.6). We have noticed that *Aspergillus* in particular has this appearance when a low-level infection remains. Experience has taught us that some tissue that looks overtly "sick," but not necrotic, can be saved. For example, muscle that is profoundly pale and/or edematous without the ability to contract may survive. This muscle should be observed on subsequent procedures, but only debrided if it becomes necrotic. This principle is critical for tissue associated with body components such as the forearm, hand, and other critical high-functioning zones.

Operative Management of Other Body Cavities

Mold in the abdominal cavity is quite remarkable (Figs. 14.7 and 14.8). The contents of the abdomen may take on a dusky appearance, and/or the surgeon can actually see the mold growing on the abdominal contents. *Aspergillus* appears as a light-medium green-colored sheen, while *Mucor* is gray-dark green and dull, for example. Involved bowel appears dry and excoriated.

When encountering intra-abdominal mold, we debride soft tissue structures such as associated fascia and adipose tissue. We do not debride or excise bowel, mesentery, or other intra-abdominal organs. If unable to close the abdominal fascia, we irrigate the abdominal cavity with an antimicrobial solution prior to placing a temporary abdominal closure. We combine amphotericin, 50 mg, with voriconazole, 200 mg, in 1 L of sterile water and then mix bacitracin, 1 gm, and gentamicin, 180 mg, in 1 L of NS. We then combine these two solutions in a bucket prior to pouring it into the abdomen. In our experience, perhaps the most important requirement is to get the abdominal fascia closed as soon as possible. Conceivably, this enables peritoneal fluid to bath critical excoriated structures, e.g., bowel, and may provide an avenue for systemic antifungal medications to get into the cavity.

Infection in the retroperitoneum can be difficult to treat as well due to the critical anatomical structures located there – e.g., major vascular

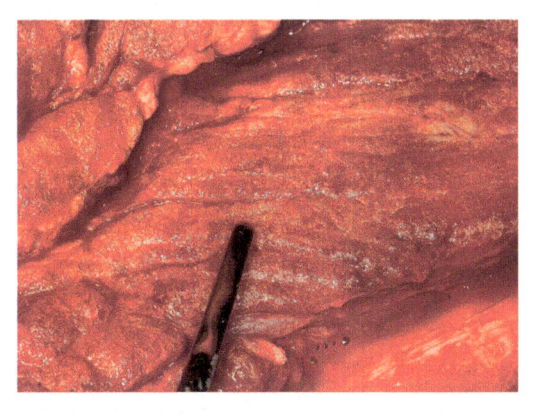

Fig. 14.6 Soft tissue sheen associated with ongoing infection

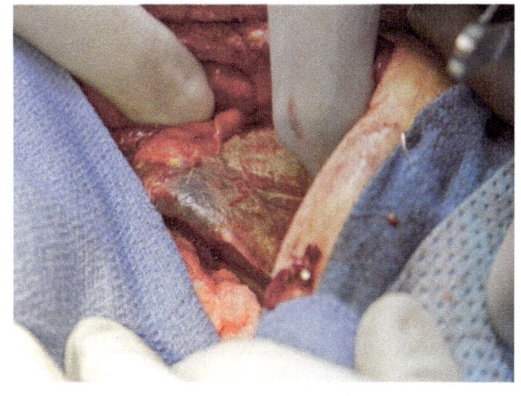

Fig. 14.7 Mold on the liver – not previously published per our knowledge

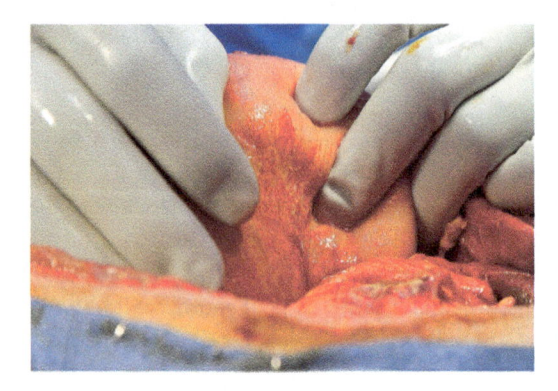

Fig. 14.8 Mold on the bowel and mesentary – not previously published per our knowledge

structures, urological organs, and rectum. In these circumstances we debride noncritical soft tissue such as adipose tissue and muscle, but maintain the other structures. When mold is seen in conjunction with these critical organs in the retroperitoneum, we add instillation vacuum therapy with 0.025% Dakin's solution as described below. Alternatively, antimicrobial bead therapy may be utilized (also described in more detail below).

Infection especially mold in the thorax including the lungs, heart, and pericardium can be daunting. The principle of debriding muscle if it pertains to the heart doesn't apply, of course. In situations involving the thorax, we close the cavities as soon as possible with the hope that systemic antifungal medications will bathe the infected organs via pulmonary or pericardial fluid and/or be delivered systemically via the vasculature as well.

Normal saline (NS) is most commonly utilized to wash wounds in the operating room. Our blast wounds are washed with a non-pressurized system – i.e., trickled as opposed to pressurized irrigation. After debridement and washes with NS, most of our surgeons will pour 0.05% chlorhexidine gluconate onto/into the infected wound and let it sit for 1 min prior to rinsing with NS. This is done in an effort to decrease pathogen burden. On occasion 0.025% Dakin's solution is utilized to rinse wounds as well.

The serial debridements are also a good time to assess the efficacy of the overall treatment regimen. If little or no new necrotic tissue is noted, then the regimen is likely working. However, should substantial nonviable tissue be found following removal of dressings, then there must be consideration of an alternative or more aggressive treatment approach such as broadening antimicrobial coverage or initiating different wound dressing strategies.

As mentioned above, our team has an OR tissue sampling protocol that we call "the Blast Protocol." This protocol is performed every time the patient with a current wound infection goes to the operating room. According to this protocol, tissue samples are obtained from soft tissue that is suspicious for infection. Compromised muscle and either adjacent or abnormal adipose tissue are sampled. We have found that *Aspergillus* has a predilection for adipose tissue, hence the reason to obtain this. Other sites sampled should be at the discretion of the operative surgeon. Specimens should be taken of necrotic tissue and from the junction of viable and necrotic tissue. Typically, this is the last piece of borderline-viable tissue that has been removed. For each necrotic body part, one specimen is sent for histopathological examination to evaluate for fungal elements. Another specimen is sent for fungal, aerobic, and anaerobic bacterial culture. We also send specimens for viral and mycobacterial culture. Histopathological specimens are stained with H&E and GMS, and PAS and the operative surgeon receives the final histopathology report within 24 h (Fig. 14.9).

Local Nonoperative Wound Care

Both old and new technologies are used for wound care in these patients. Between debridements, local/focal therapies should not stop. Early experience with using conventional dressings led to rapid deterioration of involved tissue necessitating higher-level amputations during the next operation. Dakin's soaked gauze was utilized with some success in some of the earliest patients; however, these large wounds required multiple daily dressing changes which were very manpower intensive as well as uncomfortable for the patients. Our current recommendations include utilizing a negative pressure dressing system. For wounds with severe necrosis on subsequent operations, we utilize the negative pressure dressing system in which 0.25%

Dakin's solution is instilled into the wound for 30 s, allowed to dwell for 4.5 min, and then suctioned for 55 min. This cycle continues until the dressing is taken down in the operating room. This system allows for constant pharmacological antimicrobial therapy while maintaining excellent exudate control. This system also encourages wound granulation and contraction [25]. Furthermore, there is evidence that negative pressure wound therapy is beneficial in terms of bacterial load reduction and granulation tissue production in large blast wounds over conventional dressing techniques [26].

Additional local therapies include inserting methyl methacrylate beads which have been impregnated with antimicrobial medications. The beads are made by mixing amphotericin, 500 mg; voriconazole, 200 mg; tobramycin, 1.2 gms; and vancomycin, 1 gm, with polymethyl methacrylate. Once formed, the beads are strung together to form chains. These chains are then placed into the wound in the areas most involved with disease and then covered with negative pressure dressings to allow for high-dose local dispensing of antifungal and antibacterial chemotherapy. This is obviously not an option at a small front-

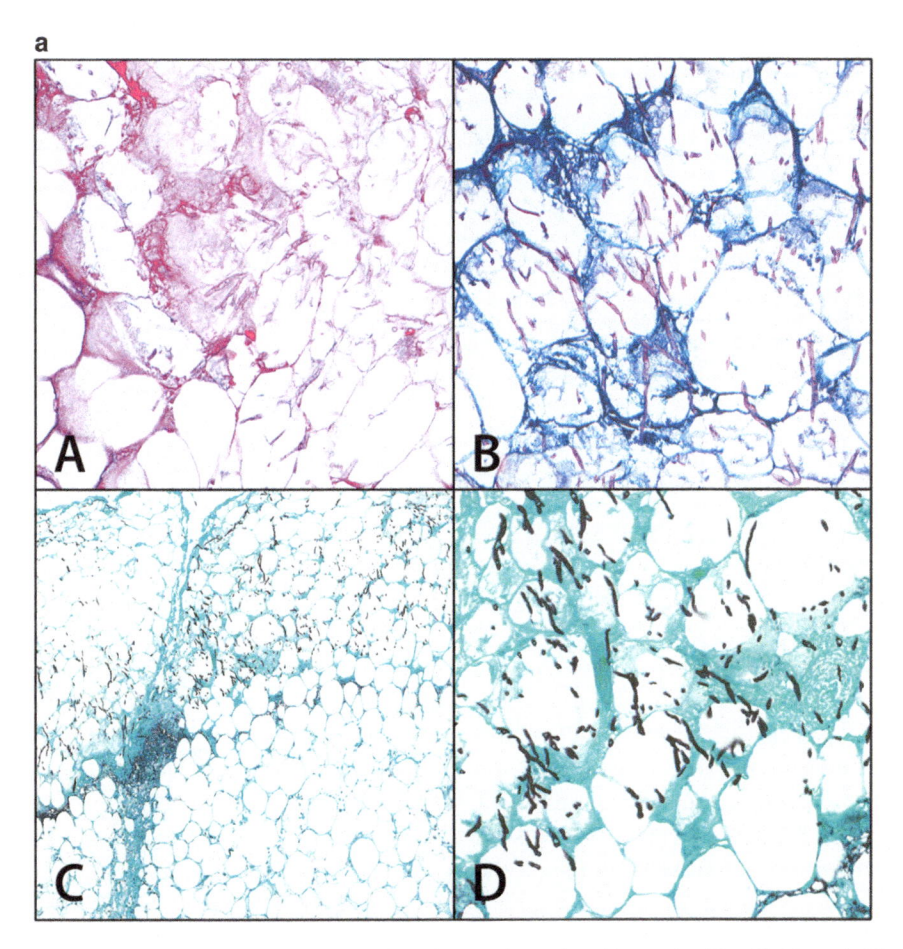

Fig. 14.9 (**a**) Necrotic fibroadipose tissue with fungal organisms consistent with *Aspergillus* spp. morphology (septate, acute angle branching). (A) Hematoxylin and eosin stain, 20×; (B) periodic acid-Schiff stain, 20×; (C) Gomori methenamine silver stain, 5×; (D) Gomori methenamine silver stain, 20×. (**b**) Necrotic fibroadipose tissue with fungal organisms consistent with aseptate zygomycete species (broad, ribbonlike hyphae). Angioinvasion can be seen in parts A and D (From Heaton et al. [34])

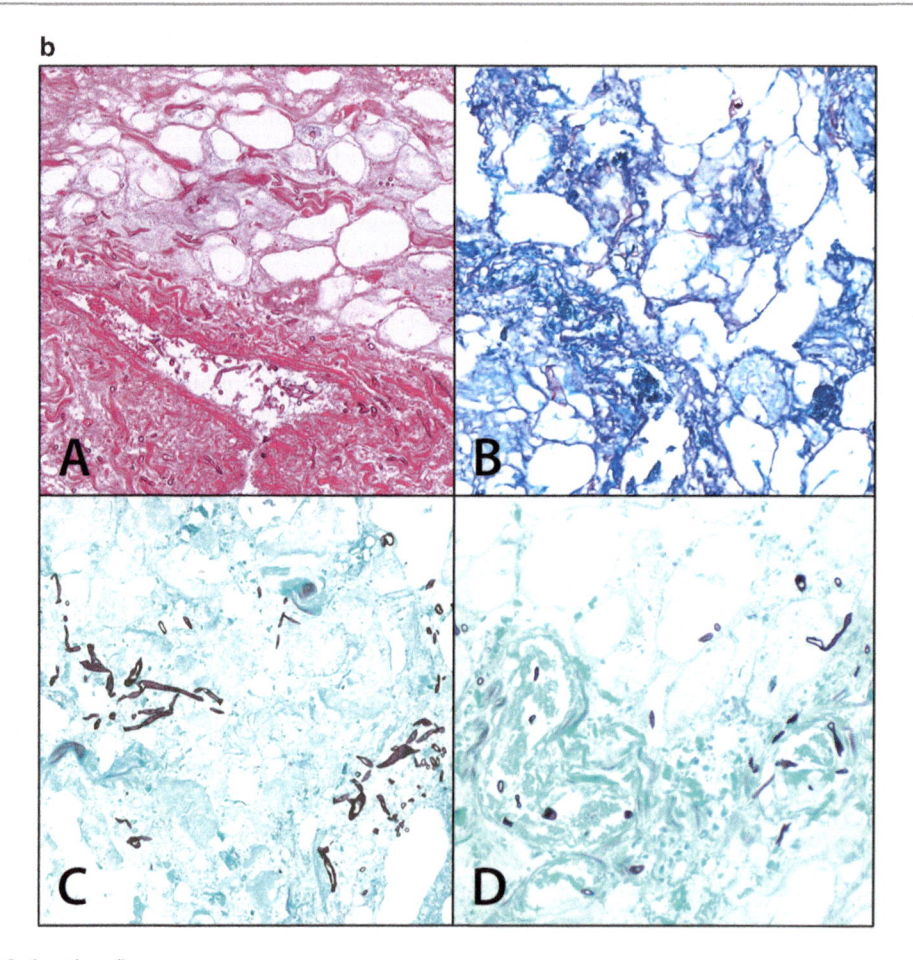

Fig. 14.9 (continued)

line facility in theater which likely will not have the requisite materials.

Timing of Wound Closure

Timing of wound closure is critical and a component of our protocol that took considerable time and experience before we felt comfortable creating a guideline. Wounds infected with fungus are either overtly necrotic, infected with fungus that is readily apparent visually, or slightly atypical – e.g., with a slimy film or sheen. Early attempts were made to close wounds during the atypical phase, but after having to reopen these wounds routinely, we learned to wait until this film or sheen disappeared. We realized that once a wound started to granulate and contract with amelioration of this atypical appearance, then it was time to close or cover definitively with a graft, flap, or primarily. These patients also tend to have profound anasarca in the early stages of the disease, and we typically wait for this to resolve prior to closure as well. We recommend continuing to monitor closed wounds for 6 weeks as they may become overtly infected again.

Reconstruction

Combat wounds can be devastating with extreme degrees of tissue loss and can take months to years to heal. Not uncommonly, patients require surgical reconstruction, and so our orthopedic

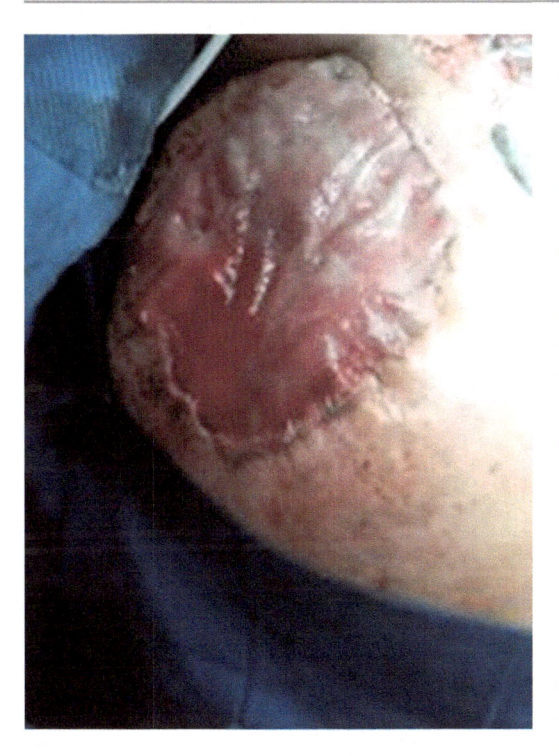

Fig. 14.10 Integra covering an amputation wound

and plastic surgery colleagues are extremely busy members of our team. Reconstructive procedures include, but are not limited to, rotational and free flaps, synthetic mesh, and utilization of tissue progenitor factors. In an effort to create a stronger pre-dermal wound base, we often place Integra™ (Integra LifeSciences, Plainsboro, NJ) over the wound prior to placing a skin graft (Fig. 14.10). Integra™ is a collagen-glycosaminoglycan biodegradable matrix. Our orthopedic surgeons in particular use Integra over wounds that will have to support a prosthetic. ACell® products (ACell Inc., Columbia, MD) contain an acellular extracellular matrix scaffold derived from pig bladder. This material allows for epithelial and progenitor cell attachment and proliferation. We often use ACell® to fill large, empty cavities.

Systemic Therapy

The use of multiple broad-spectrum antibiotics early in the war led to rapid drug resistance among multiple bacterial pathogens, especially *Acinetobacter*. A significant and unexpected number of patients with resistant *Acinetobacter* were noted, and guidelines were published to promote intelligent use of antibiotics to prevent its continued proliferation. Presently, we utilize the following guidelines: since most of these injuries include open fractures, empiric gram-positive coverage with Ancef or clindamycin are appropriate with broad-spectrum prophylaxis added should there be any abdominal and/or pelvic injury [27]. When found, the initial treatment of *Acinetobacter* should be with a carbapenem; though with such high rates of resistance, cultures should be checked frequently for sensitivities. Often rarely used antibiotics like colistin will be required.

Antimicrobial therapy is integral to combating soft tissue infections in blast casualties. As with surgical debridement, initiation must be aggressive and early to prevent establishment of severe focal infection and/or dissemination to distant organs. For example, surgery alone will not cure IFI. Systemic antifungal medications are required in order to eradicate mold. Furthermore, antimicrobial therapy may be the only method to treat infections in tissue that cannot be aggressively debrided such as the lungs, heart, brain, or major vascular structures, as mentioned above. Thus, should the patient meet criteria for infection, empiric initiation of systemic antimicrobials including antifungal medications is warranted. Antifungal medications are definitely started when there is tissue necrosis on two consecutive debridements, not including the first in-theater debridement.

When there is fungus in the wounds, there are usually bacteria as well [10]. Therefore, empiric antimicrobial therapy includes antibiotics as well as antifungals. Based upon the microbial profile of our patient population, this treatment involves the use of vancomycin, meropenem, voriconazole, and liposomal amphotericin B. Viral and mycobacterial pathogens can also cause wound infection in these patients requiring treatment. Our institutional experience has demonstrated that wound cultures growing mold of the order *Mucorales* will have a second non-*Mucorales* fungus present 30% of the time. We have also demonstrated that *Aspergillus* species takes longer to grow than order *Mucorales* and, therefore, may not be evident in the early stages of disease, but due to its virulence we empirically treat the patient. We have also documented cases of disseminated *Aspergillus* in this patient population. Therefore, dual use of voriconazole (to treat *Aspergillus*) and liposomal amphotericin B for *Mucorales* and *Rhizopus* is utilized for wounds infected with either or both of these fungi. If long-term treatment is required, the antifungal medications may be focused based on culture results once the cultures have had adequate time to grow.

We stop systemic and topical antifungal treatments when there is no evidence of IFI on histopathology or culture and when wounds have remained viable with no further evidence of infection for at least 2 weeks. However, if these patients have fungal infection in more than one body region (e.g., abdomen, extremity), long-term antifungal treatment may be indicated.

If cultures should return with growth of fungal isolates, in a wound that never demonstrated infection, this situation may represent colonization rather than infection.

Historically, there has been considerable trepidation concerning the use of amphotericin given its reported nephrotoxicity. However, with the newer liposomal formulation, this issue has been mitigated with few if any cases of renal impairment noted in this patient population and a general reduction in other patient populations [28]. Previously, voriconazole has been associated with liver and renal disease, and so hepatic and renal function tests are tracked, while these patients are receiving this medication. Our team has demonstrated that the utilization of liposomal amphotericin B and/or voriconazole is not associated with either renal or liver failure in this combat casualty patient population [29].

Posaconazole can be considered an alternative to voriconazole under certain circumstances. Initially most of these seriously injured patients are intubated, and ileus with the potential for bowel absorption issues complicates their clinical course. Therefore, intravenous options are preferred, and thus voriconazole is the initial choice. Once patients are well enough to be extubated or at least demonstrate normal bowel function, they may be switched to oral posaconazole for the completion of their antifungal therapy. However, if they are going to the operating room frequently and thus made NPO routinely, the IV formulation is recommended for continued use.

Rule Out Ischemia

Not uncommonly, major and minor vascular structures are damaged, ligated, and/or debrided in the process of wounding, hemorrhage control, and operative debridement. Proximal vascular control via retroperitoneal or transabdominal approaches is practiced routinely at the time of presentation after combat trauma. Most often vascular inflow is restored after surgeons gain control of more distal hemorrhage, but on occasion these major vascular structures are ligated. The potential ischemia associated with this patient history must be considered when the surgeon encounters relentless necrosis in the OR. Vascular studies (e.g., computed tomography angiography, CTA) may be considered in order to diagnose vascular insufficiency and evaluate for vascular reconstruction if needed to preserve tissue. Vascular outflow deficiencies due to major venous disruptions are a common occurrence in our patient population and can lead to considerable tissue loss. Therefore, significant efforts are made to preserve these veins.

Minimization of Immunosuppression

Generally, these patients are physiologically healthy prior to injury, but there are substantial physiological derangements which occur in these severely injured patients. Excellent critical care is required to ensure that there are no further physiological insults to the patient. These strategies include adequate nutrition in order to meet extraordinary and targeted caloric requirements for wound healing and tissue regeneration. Prevention and treatment of nosocomial infections and multiple organ dysfunctions is critical.

Minimization of immunosuppression is critical to getting control of soft tissue infection, and so blood product transfusion should follow present-day protocols including restrictive strategies (Hb of 7 g/dL or lower) unless the patient is in hemorrhagic shock. As these patients are often subjected to significant blood loss through operative debridement, and with loss of the hematopoietic regions of long bones due to amputation, phlebotomy should be minimized if possible.

As longer storage (older) blood may have deleterious effects on the immune system, only the most recently collected leukoreduced units are used in this patient population [30]. Additionally, there is a concern that spilt iron from breakdown products in these transfusions fuels fungal growth, further warranting judicious transfusion strategies [31].

Pain Control

Pain management is an acute and chronic problem in these patients and is often accompanied by post-traumatic stress. The etiology is multifactorial with contributions from disease, inflammation, and injury to multiple organ systems. In the acute setting, the goal is to reregulate pain (i.e., downregulate the central nervous system). Phantom pain in amputees begins within the first 2 weeks after amputation and can be challenging to control. The primary goal of chronic pain management is prevention to the extent possible.

Multimodality management includes pharmacological and non-pharmacological therapies. Pharmacological therapies include nonsteroidal anti-inflammatory drugs, gabapentinoids, acetaminophen, alpha-2 agonists, ketamine, and esmolol, with opioids utilized as rescue therapy. Transcutaneous electrical stimulation is utilized as a non-pharmacological therapy at times.

Pain management is very difficult and labor intensive in these patients. For that reason, we utilize an acute pain management service whose only responsibility is to keep these patients as comfortable as possible.

Infection Control

Acinetobacter and enterococcus, whether drug resistant or not, present a challenge for infection control. These bacteria, along with fungal organisms, present a significant threat to other immunocompromised patients in the hospital. Given that dismounted blast injury patients are generally in the intensive care unit for significant periods of time, this places other ill patients (combat trauma or otherwise) at risk. Preventive strategies must be utilized to prevent the spread of these pathogens from the wounded warrior to other patients.

Ongoing Investigations

Intense research continues in the quest to learn more about blast-related soft tissue wounds in an effort to improve patient outcomes. One such effort is the Combat-Related Extremity Wound Infection (CEWI) analysis. This consists of a 3-year retrospective study with plans to continue prospectively. To date, data has determined that 1409 patients had open extremity wounds and 354 (25%) were related to CEWI. Fifty-six percent of patients with amputations had infections. Independent risk factors in patients who incurred a CEWI in less than 30 days included traumatic amputations, IED/blast mechanism, first documented shock index of ≥ 0.80, ≥ 10 units of blood product transfusion within the first 24 h post-injury, and 4 wound sites. Interestingly, having a non-extremity infection ≥ 4 days prior to CEWI diagnosis was protective, suggesting that antibiotic exposure decreased CEWI events. Two hundred seventy-four patients with CEWI who received ≥ 3 days of antimicrobial treatment were reviewed to assess antimicrobial prescribing practice patterns. Findings included that patients frequently received ≥ 2 antimicrobials for directed CEWI treatment, those with osteomyelitis were most commonly treated with fluoroquinolones, and that meropenem and vancomycin were the most common therapy combination [32]. Many planned next steps include the examination of the microbial content of combat-related wounds with and without infection, determination of how infection disseminates locally and systemically, effect of aeromedical transport at altitude on soft tissue infection, refinement of variables for outcome analysis, and evaluation of the effectiveness of vancomycin/carbapenem combinations as empiric therapy among patients with deep soft tissue infections.

Conclusion

The novel infectious sequelae of blast injuries require both a high level of suspicion and aggressive treatment strategies. Both bacterial and fungal pathogens are generally found deep in the tissues of these casualties and are countered with systemic antibiotics and purposeful surgical debridement. Between operations, local wound care with negative pressure therapy and other adjuncts allows for preservation of soft tissue. Failure to initiate early interventions may result in unsalvageable disseminated infection or significantly increased morbidity.

Disclaimer The views expressed in this chapter are those of the author and do not reflect the official policy of the Department of Army, Navy, Air Force, Department of Defense, or US Government. The identification of specific products, scientific instrumentation, or organization is considered an integral part of the scientific endeavor and does not constitute endorsement or implied endorsement on the part of the author, DoD, or any component agency.

References

1. Scott P, Deye G, Srinivasan A, Murray C, Moran K, Hulten E, Fishbain J, Craft D, Riddell S, Linder L, Mancuso J, Milstrey E, Bautista CT, Patel J, Ewell A, Hamilton T, Gaddy C, Tenney M, Christopher G, Petersen K, Endy T, Petruccelli B. An outbreak of multidrug-resistant Acinetobacter baumannii-calcoaceticus complex infection in the US military health care system associated with military operations in Iraq. Clin Infect Dis. 2007;44(12):1577–84.
2. Kallen AJ, Hidron AI, Patel J, Srinivasan A. Multidrug resistance among gram-negative pathogens that caused healthcare-associated infections reported to the National Healthcare Safety Network, 2006–2008. Infect Control Hosp Epidemiol. 2010;31(5):528–31.
3. Lewandowski LR, Weintrob AC, Tribble DR, Rodriguez CJ, Petfield J, Lloyd BA, Murray CK, Stinner D, Aggarwal D, Shaikh F, Potter BK. Early complications and outcomes in combat injury-related invasive fungal wound infections: a case-control analysis. J Orthop Trauma. 2016;30(3):e93–9.
4. Zapor MJ, Moran KA. Infectious diseases during wartime. Curr Opin Infect Dis. 2005;18(5):395–9.
5. Weintrob AC, Roediger MP, Barber M, Summers A, Fieberg AM, Dunn J, Seldon V, Leach F, Huang XZ, Nikolich MP, Wortmann GW. Natural history of colonization with gram-negative multidrug-resistant organisms among hospitalized patients. Infect Control Hosp Epidemiol. 2010;31(4):330–7.
6. Hospenthal DR, Crouch CK, English JF, Leach F, Pool J, Conger NG, Whitman TJ, Wortmann GW, Murray CK, Cordts PR, Gamble WB. Response to infection control challenges in the deployed setting: Operations Iraqi and Enduring Freedom. J Trauma. 2010;69:S94–S101.
7. Crouch HK, Murray CK, Hospenthal DR. Development of a deployment infection control course. Mil Med. 2010;175:983–9.
8. Warkentien T, Rodriguez C, Lloyd B, Wells J, Weintrob A, Dunne JR, Ganesan A, Li P, Bradley W, Gaskins LJ, Seillier-Moisewitsch F, Wortmann GW, Landrum ML, Kortepeter MG, Tribble DR. Invasive mold infections following combat-related injuries. Clin Infect Dis. 2012;55(11):1221–9.
9. Radowsky JS, Strawn AA, Sherwood J, Braden A, Liston W. Invasive mucormycosis and aspergillosis in a healthy 22-year-old battle casualty: case report. Surg Infect. 2011;12(5):397–400.
10. Lloyd B, Weintrob AC, Rodriguez C, Dunne JR, Weisbrod AB, Hinkle M, Warkentien T, Murray CK, Oh J, Millar EV, Shah J, Gregg S, Lloyd G, Stevens J, Carson ML, Aggarwal D, Tribble DR. Effect of early screening for invasive fungal infections in U.S. service members with explosive blast injuries. Surg Infect. 2014;15(5):619–26.
11. Trauma-Related Infection Research Area/Infectious Disease Clinical research Program, Department of Preventive Medicine and Biostatistics, University of the Uniformed Services, 2016 Annual report.
12. Weintrob AC, Weisbrod AB, Dunne JR, Rodriguez CJ, Malone D, Lloyd BA, Warkentien TE, Wells J, Murray CK, Bradley W, Shaikh J, Aggarwal D, Carson ML, Tribble DR, Infectious Disease Clinical Research Program Trauma Infectious Disease Outcomes Study Group. Combat trauma-associated invasive fungal wound infections: epidemiology and clinical classification. Epidemiol Infect. 2015;143(1):214–24.
13. Rodriguez CJ, Weintrob AC, Shah J, Malone D, Dunne JR, Weisbrod AB, Lloyd BA, Warkentien TE, Murray CK, Wilkins K, Shaikh F, Carson ML, Aggarwal D, Tribble DR. Risk factors associated with invasive fungal infections in combat trauma. Surg Infect. 2014;15(5):521–6.

14. Radhakrishnan R, Donato ML, Prieto VG, Mays SR, Raad II, Kuerer HM. Invasive cutaneous fungal infections requiring radical resection in cancer patients undergoing chemotherapy. J Surg Oncol. 2004;88:21–6.
15. Mehrad B, Paciocco G, Martinez FJ, Ojo TC, Iannettoni MD, Lynch JP 3rd. Spectrum of aspergillus infection in lung transplant recipients: case series and review of the literature. Chest. 2001;119(1):169–75.
16. Muskett H, Shahin J, Eyres G, Harvey S, Rowan K, Harrison D. Risk factors for invasive fungal disease in critically ill patients: a systematic review. Crit Care. 2011;15(6):R287.
17. Tribble DR, Rodriguez CJ, Weintrob AC, Shaikh F, Aggarwal D, Carson ML, Murray CK, Masuoka P. Environmental factors related to fungal wound contamination after combat trauma in Afghanistan 2009–2011. Emerg Infect Dis. 2015;21(10):1759–69.
18. Godfrey BW, Martin A, Chestovich PJ, Lee GH, Ingalls NK, Saldanha V. Patients with multiple traumatic amputations: an analysis of operation enduring freedom joint theatre trauma registry data. Injury. 2017;48(1):75–9.
19. Torrance HD, Brohi K, Pearse RM, Mein CA, Wozniak E, Prowle JR, Hinds CJ, O'Dwyer MJ. Association between gene expression biomarkers of immunosuppression and blood transfusion in severely injured polytrauma patients. Ann Surg. 2015;26(14):751–9.
20. Sheppard FR, Keiser P, Craft DW, Gage F, Robson M, Brown TS, Petersen K, Sincock S, Kasper M, Hawksworth J, Tadaki D, Davis TA, Stojadinovic A, Elster E. The majority of US combat casualty soft-tissue wounds are not infected or colonized upon arrival or during treatment at a continental US military medical facility. Am J Surg. 2010;200(4):489–95.
21. Hospenthal DR, Crouch HK, English JF, Leach F, Pool J, Conger NG, Whitman TJ, Wortmann GW, Robertson JL, Murray CK. Multidrug-resistant bacterial colonization of combat-injured personnel at admission to medical centers after evacuation from Afghanistan and Iraq. J Trauma. 2011;71(1):S52–7.
22. Rodriguez C, Weintrob AC, Dunne JR, Weisbrod AB, Lloyd B, Warkentien T, Malone D, Wells J, Murray CK, Bradley W, Shaikh F, Shah J, Carson ML, Aggarwal D, Tribble DR. Clinical relevance of mold culture positivity with and without recurrent wound necrosis following combat-related injuries. J Trauma Acute Care Surg. 2014;77(5):769–73.
23. Vitrat-Hinky V, Lebeau B, Bozonnet E, Falcon D, Pradel P, Faure O, Aubert A, Piolat C, Grillot R, Pelloux H. Severe filamentous fungal infections after widespread tissue damage due to traumatic injury: six cases and review of the literature. Scand J Infect Dis. 2009;41(6–7):491–500.
24. Cannon JW, Hoffman LJ, Glasgow SC, Potter BK, Rodriguez CJ, Cancio LC, Rasmussen TE, Fries CA, Davis MR, Jezior JR, Mullins RJ, Elster EA. Dismounted complex blast injuries: a comprehensive review of the modern combat experience. J Am Coll Surg. 2016;223(4):652–64.
25. Lewandowski L, Purcell R, Fleming M, Gordon WT. The use of dilute Dakin's solution for the treatment of angioinvasive fungal infection in the combat wounded: a case series. Mil Med. 2013;178(4):e503–7.
26. Li J, Topaz M, Li Y, Li W, Xun W, Yuan Y, Chen S, Li X. Treatment of infected soft tissue blast injury in swine by regulated negative pressure wound therapy. Ann Surg. 2013;25(2):335–44.
27. Hospenthal DR, Murray CK, Andersen RC, Blice JP, Calhoun JH, Cancio LC, Chung KK, Conger NG, Crouch HK, D'Avignon LC, Dunne JR, Ficke JR, Hale RG, Hayes DK, Hirsch EF, Hsu JR, Jenkins DH, Keeling JJ, Martin RR, Moore LE, Petersen K, Saffle JR, Solomkin JS, Tasker SA, Valadka AB, Wiessen AR, Wortmann GW, Holcomb JB. Guidelines for the prevention of infection after combat-related injuries. J Trauma. 2008;64(3 Suppl):S211–20.
28. Hamill RJ. Amphotericin B formulations: a comparative review of efficacy and toxicity. Drugs. 2013;73(9):919–34.
29. Caruso J, Weisbrod A, Rodriguez C, Elster E, Jessie E, Dunne J, Burns C, Liston W, Malone D. Vori and Ampho: Not so terrible. Presented at the 33rd Annual Meeting of the Surgical Infection Society, April 12–15, 2013 Las Vegas, NV.
30. Torrance HD, Vivian ME, Brohi K, Prowle JR, Pearse RM, Owen HC, Hinds CJ, O'Dwyer MJ. Changes in gene expression following trauma are related to the age of transfused packed red blood cells. J Trauma Acute Care Surg. 2015;78(3):535–42.
31. Spellberg B, Edwards J Jr, Ibrahim A. Novel perspectives on mucormycosis: pathophysiology, presentation, and management. Clin Microbiol Rev. 2005;18(3):556–69.
32. Trauma-Related Infection Research Program, 8th Annual Investigator's Meeting. Infectious Disease Clinical Research Program. Uniformed Services University of the Health Sciences. March 8–10, 2017 Bethesda, MD.
33. Tribble D. Combat Related Fungal Infection Reports. Curr Fungal Infect Rep. 2014;8:277–86.
34. Heaton SM, Weintrob AC, Downing K, Keenan B, Aggarwal D, Shaikh F, Tribble DR, Wells JM, the IDCRP TIDOS Group. Histopathological techniques for the diagnosis of combat-related invasive fungal wound infections. BMC Clin Pathol. 2016;16:11.

The Rational Care of Burns

15

Gary Vercruysse

Introduction

Currently, most patients suffering complex blast injuries have minimal to no thermal component to their injury complex, but this may change with newer generations of weapons. Burns are a challenge for the deployed physician on many levels. The patients can be very sick and are often subject to penetrating or blunt injury in addition to their thermal injury [1]. Many patients may show up at the same time. The hospital may be full. Resources will be limited, time may be limited, and direction with respect to priorities of care may be challenging [2]. Finally, the comfort level of the average deployed surgeon in caring for patients with burns is wanting. Many if not all of the same things can be said of the civilian physician not intimately familiar with burn care who is faced with multiple burns in a civilian disaster. This chapter is an effort to logically and effectively explain burn care in a way that will make sense to a physician who may at some time in the not-too-distant future indeed find himself or herself deployed or faced with disaster and need to take care of burn patients. It is an effort to go beyond the basics and explain ways of saving resources and the lives of those who might succumb to their burns if these measures are not followed. It is an effort to show the non-burn physician how to adequately care for burn patients with minimal resources in a way that might not be used in ABA-verified burn centers but works well in faraway places and when under duress and faced with a civilian disaster.

Basic Burn Evaluation

When a patient arrives at your facility with a burn, as with any patient, it is important to follow the basic rules of trauma care, that is, the ABCDE.

Airway and Breathing The patient will be breathing, bagged, or intubated. Evaluate their airway. If they are intubated, be sure the tube is in good position and be sure it is an endotracheal tube. King Laryngeal Tube (King Systems) or Combitube (Kendal-Sheridan Corporation) airways have known to be mistaken as endotracheal tubes; if one is present, it should be replaced with an endotracheal tube. The mouth can also be evaluated at this time for carbon or burns (rare). If the patient is intubated on presentation or is obtunded, it can be assumed that the patient has suffered blunt or penetrating trauma in addition to their burn (extremely common in the context of blast injury) and has a head injury or is in hemorrhagic shock or was burned in an enclosed

G. Vercruysse (✉)
University of Michigan School of Medicine,
Ann Arbor, MI, USA
e-mail: vercruys@med.umich.edu

space and has carbon monoxide (more common) or cyanide poisoning (extremely rare). For these reasons burn patients should be transported on 100% oxygen if possible to drive down carboxy-hemoglobin if present. Stat arterial blood gasses should also be sent upon arrival to help confirm this diagnosis.

Intubation

Managing the airway of an acute burn patient is one of the most difficult aspects of the first 24 h of care. Major decisions involve which patients will need intubation and when and where is the best location to intubate [3].

A. Which patients to intubate:
   Very strong indications:
   1. COHb >10% with depressed mental status (note COHb >10% with fairly normal (talking) mental status is in itself not an indicated to intubate).
   2. Burns >50% TBSA – especially in children.
   3. Burns > with full-thickness facial component.
   4. The entire head is burned (both face and scalp) even if it is all just second degree.
   Relative indications:
   (a) Burn occurred indoors with significant smoke inhalation.
   (b) Hoarseness.
   (c) Carbonaceous sputum.
   (d) Partial-thickness burns to the face.
   (e) Very young <1 or very old >75.

Patients with the above findings who have relatively large burns, 40–50% TBSA, often need to be intubated. Patients with the same findings, and smaller burns, can often be successfully observed without intubation.

Findings that are generally not helpful:
(a) Singed nasal hairs (can occur with flash burn, history of burn in a closed space is key to the diagnosis of inhalation injury).
(b) CXR.
(c) Bronchoscopy findings are relatively unhelpful.

B. Thought process – when and where to intubate

In most patients, there is a 4–6-h period of time postburn before edema will occlude the airway. It is important to establish good IV access, check vital signs, and then decide to intubate the patients in a relatively elective fashion.
   (a) Remember to perform a pre-intubation physical exam, especially a neurological exam focusing on other possible injuries beside the burn.
   (b) Oral tracheal intubation is preferred. Try to put in as large an ET tube as possible as these patients may require pulmonary toilet via bronchoscopy at some point in the near future. It is not possible to perform bronchoscopy on an adult with an endotracheal tube smaller than a size 7 in an adult or a 4.5 in a child. As patients swell as a result of their burn, reintubation may be physically impossible.

Tips on intubation:

A. Size of pediatric ET tube: age + 16 = size of ET tube/4. Remember: pediatric ET tubes traditionally were uncuffed. More recently, high volume, low pressure, cuffed and endotracheal tubes have become available. Use a cuffed tube if possible. If an adequate seal does not form between the trachea and ET tube, ventilation will be difficult. Additionally, smaller ET tubes interfere with the removal of secretions and occlude more easily. Try to use a 4.5 ET tube or larger when possible. Cuffed pediatric ET tubes offer better seals when dealing with advanced modes of ventilation.
B. Always listen carefully for breath sounds to avoid a right mainstream intubation. Record the position of the ET tube at the teeth.
C. Carefully secure the ET tube with adhesive tape or umbilical tape. Heavy sedation and/or paralytic drugs and restraints are essential to make certain that the airway is not dislodged. If the patient has a facial burn, tape will not stick to the face; however, it can be used to secure an airway if it is laid on the skin above the upper lip and stapled in place with multi-

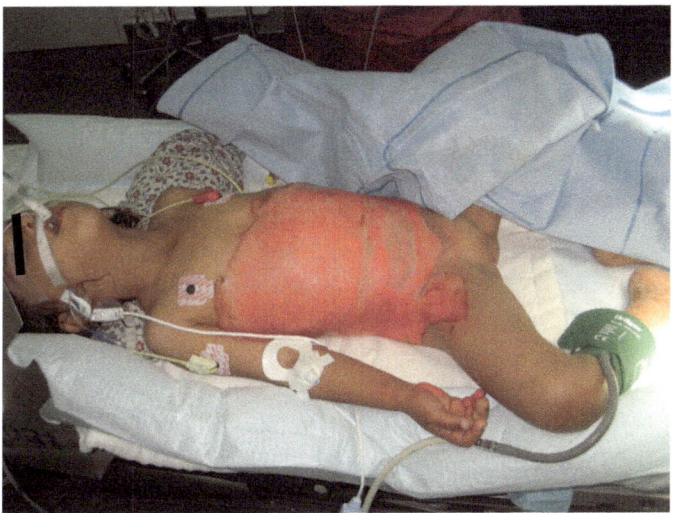

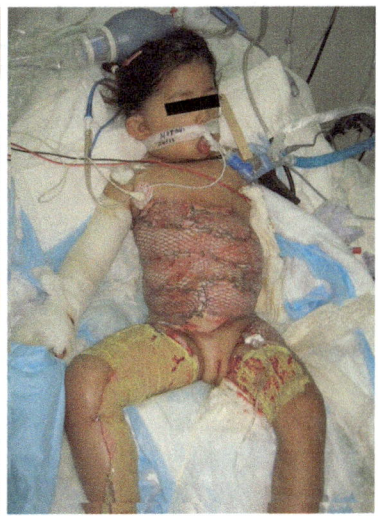

Fig. 15.1 A 4-year-old Iraqi girl presented with a 36% TBSA burn. She was intubated shortly after arrival to facilitate pain control and swelling secondary to resuscitation. The endotracheal tube was secured with silk tape and skin staples to help protect from iatrogenic extubation. The pictures are from postburn day 0 and 7

ple skin staples. This offers a secure airway and allows for facial swelling. A second piece of tape is then often placed over the staples to mitigate family discomfort (Fig. 15.1).

Circulation Most burn patients will have normal or elevated blood pressures in the field and upon arrival. All patients with significant burns should have two large bore intravenous lines placed immediately upon arrival if this is not done in the field. If the burn is large, and an unburned area amenable to IV placement cannot be found, IVs can be placed through the burned skin for initial resuscitation. Once initial resuscitation is started, central access may be advantageous for prolonged access. If an IV cannot be placed, and central lines are not available, a venous cutdown at the ankle or groin or arm (if the legs have been amputated due to blast) should be performed. Pediatric feeding tubes or even a segment of sterile IV tubing is good cannula for a cutdown. Lastly, intraosseous access may be used at the tibial, humeral, or sternal position. This line is less favored due to the fact that these lines are placed in non-sterile conditions, and osteomyelitis, although rare, has resulted after placement.

Disability and Exposure Once the patient has undergone primary survey, and has good IV access, the burn and other injuries can be assessed. These patients should undergo the standard trauma work-up and their skin examined from head to toe to determine the extent of their burns. Head injury, cavitary bleeding, significant long bone and pelvic fractures, pericardial tamponade, hemo- or pneumothorax, and other immediate causes of death should be excluded or ameliorated before caring for the burn. When examining the patient, once pain control has been established, all blisters should be removed to assess the dermis beneath and the % total body surface area calculated to aid in accurate resuscitation. Wash the patients with soap and water or Hibiclens solution if available. Wrap them in a clean sheet. Place a Foley catheter if they have a large (>10% TBSA in children or >20% TBSA in adults or those with burns to the genitalia) burn. Update tetanus status as necessary. This may include tetanus immunoglobulin for unvaccinated civilians or host national forces. Once the need for operative intervention for other causes has been ruled out, the burns can be dressed with antibiotic cream (bacitracin or gentamicin ointments, silver sulfadiazine, or Sulfamylon) and wrapped in Kerlix gauze, ABDs, or other clean dressing materials.

Burn Resuscitation

Basic burn resuscitation is essential for large burns and is complicated by the polytrauma injury patterns associated with dismount complex blast injuries. A large burn is a burn >10% TBSA in those younger than 5 or older than 50 years old and 20% TBSA in the rest of the population. For those with smaller burns, maintenance fluid, and oral intake, or even oral rehydration may suffice [4]. Several formulae are available to guide in resuscitation, but for the purposes of expediency and simplicity, below are two of the easiest and commonest formulas to follow [5].

Rule of Tens (Adults)
- Estimate burn size to the nearest 10% TBSA.
- Multiply % TBSA × 10 = initial fluid rate ml/h for patients 40–80 kg.
- If<40 kg, use Galveston formula.
- For every 10 kg above 80 kg, increase rate by 100 ml/h.
- Use LR (not NS) to avoid hyperchloremic metabolic acidosis.
- Adjust initial fluid rate up or down based on goal Uo 0.5–1 cc/kg/h.

Galveston Formula (Pediatric Burns <40 kg)
- 3–4 mL/kg/%TBSA burn.
- 1/2 volume over first 8 h, second half next 16 h.
- Also infuse maintenance fluid at:
  - 4 ml/kg for first 10 kg body weight
  - 2 ml/kg for the second 10 kg body weight
  - 1 ml/kg for remaining kg body weight
- Use D5LR to avoid hypoglycemia in small children.
- Adjust initial fluid rate up or down based on goal Uo of 1 cc/kg/h.

General Guide to Resuscitation

Resuscitation formulae are guides to resuscitation. The purpose of the formal burn resuscitation is to optimize the amount of oxygen and nutrients that reach the burned skin and avoid loss of other vital functions due to dehydration, such as kidney function. Most burns have a zone of transition that goes from normal skin to partially burned skin (superficial then deep partial-thickness burn) and then full-thickness burn. If the dermis of partial-thickness burns is optimally resuscitated, it may heal and not require grafting. This will often significantly reduce the burn penundrum and allow the patient to heal significantly faster and with less grafting. If the resuscitation is neglected, the patient will become relatively dehydrated and possibly hypotensive. If not hydrated, or if treated with vasopressors instead of fluid, injured dermis will go on to become full-thickness burn as blood is shunted away from the skin and subcutaneous tissues to the central circulation to help maintain blood pressure and heart and brain function. This is referred to as "extension of the burn."

When a patient is being formally resuscitated, fluid rates should be adjusted to match optimal urine output, that is, a goal of 0.5–0.1 cc/kg/h of urine output in an adult and 1 cc/kg/h urine output in a child. Once this goal has been achieved, intravenous fluid rates can gently be adjusted down, and back up as necessary. The JTTS CPG's and JTTS flow sheet can be very helpful as a guide, and way to keep track of vital parameters during resuscitation of the complex blast patient with a burn.

As the vascular endothelium of burn patients is exceedingly leaky, excess intravenous fluid will lead to anasarca and unnecessary pulmonary and even extremity edema. For this reason, formal burn resuscitation mandates avoiding the use of bolus fluids (which will only add to unnecessary edema) and the use of colloid on postburn day 1 after the initial crystalloid resuscitation. A typical dose of colloid would be 5% albumin at the previous crystalloid fluid rate for 24–48 h adjusting for urine output as would be done with crystalloid.

Problems with Resuscitation

The Difficult Resuscitation

The difficult resuscitation is one in which despite optimal fluid delivery, the patient remains oliguric. This may be the result of underestimate of burn size or because of a missed injury leading to early sepsis (hollow viscus injury) or hypotension due to hemorrhagic shock. Once these alternatives have been excluded, an escalation in basic resuscitation strategy should follow.

Difficult Resuscitation Guidelines

- Switch intravenous fluid to 5% albumin.
- Check bladder pressures every 4 h.
- If urine output (UOP) < 30 mL/h in a > 30 kg patient or <1 mL/kg/h in a ≤ 30 kg patient, strongly consider monitoring central venous pressures (CVP) from a subclavian or IJ line along with central venous (ScvO2) saturations (goal CVP 8–10 mmHg, ScvO2 60–65%):
  (a) If CVP is not at goal, then increase fluid rate by 33%.
  (b) If CVP is at goal, then consider dobutamine 5 µg/kg/min (titrate until ScvO2 (if available) at goal). Max dose of dobutamine is 20 µg/kg/min.
  (c) If both CVP and ScvO2 (if available) are at goal, then stop increasing fluids (even if UOP < target). The patient should be considered hemodynamically optimized, and the oliguria is likely a result of established renal insult. Some degree of renal failure should be tolerated and expected. Continued increases in fluid administration despite optimal hemodynamic parameters will only result in "resuscitation morbidity" that is often times more detrimental than renal failure.

Every attempt should be made to minimize fluid administration while maintaining organ perfusion. If UOP >70 mL/h and patient >30 kg, then decrease the fluid rate by 33%. If UOP >2 mL/kg/h and patient is ≤30 kg, then decrease the fluid rate by 33%. Do not decrease below the maintenance IVF rate based on the patient's weight. After 24 h, infusion of lactated Ringer's should be titrated down to maintenance levels and 5% albumin continued until the 48-h mark.

Resuscitation Morbidity

If guidelines for resuscitation are not followed and patients are simply repeatedly bolused large amounts of crystalloid, they will continually extravasate fluid into the interstitial space [6]. If this mode of resuscitation continues unchecked, it may eventually lead to resuscitation morbidity, a consequence of over resuscitation. It is characterized by pulmonary edema, difficult oxygenation despite elevated ventilatory pressures, distended abdomen, and edematous extremities [7]. If not recognized and fluid management optimized, it may lead to abdominal compartment syndrome necessitating laparotomy and an open abdomen and secondary extremity compartment syndrome requiring fasciotomy for limb salvage [8]. It is important to carefully avoid this complication as patients with a 60% TBSA burn and resuscitation morbidity requiring laparotomy and fasciotomy have a very high mortality rate [7]. The use of MTP in the resuscitation of blast injuries would likely not be incongruent with the burn resuscitation. Prior to MTP, trauma resuscitation was historically much like burn resuscitation. It may be that future generations use MTP for burn resuscitation as well. Further research is warranted in this area. It should be noted that if a patient has a known brain injury, and a significant thermal injury, serum sodium should be frequently monitored and corrected to avoid unnecessary cerebral edema.

Escharotomy

In patients with circumferential extremity burns, the arm or leg swells while the burned dermis does not stretch. This can allow pressure to build up under the eschar. When the pressure rises to above tissue perfusion, pressure ischemia will result. First, the nerves will become ischemic, and patients, if conscious, will note tingling. Next, the muscles will become ischemic, and, if nothing is done, rhabdomyolysis and necrosis will result. If left under compression, the patient will develop a compartment syndrome. This is prevented by cutting the eschar and letting the swollen tissue expand. Escharotomies are done for patients with deep 2° and 3° burns that are circumferential around the chest, extremities, abdomen, penis, or neck [9–11].

The most common indication for escharotomies is loss of the palmar arch Doppler signal for upper extremities and loss of the posterior tibial Doppler signal for lower extremities. Other indications are cyanosis of the extremity, paresthesias, and loss of capillary refill/loss of pulse-ox signal from the extremity. In forward locations, if no Doppler or pulse-ox is available, a tight, painful extremity warrants escharotomy.

After giving sedation, cut the eschar with a knife or cautery. This can be relatively painful in an alert patient, so make certain that the alert patient has received sufficient narcotics and perhaps some IV benzodiazepine. Classically, a medial and lateral incision is made on the arms or legs. It is carried down to the subcutaneous fat (but not into the muscular fascia) to allow the extremity to expand. After ensuring hemostasis, apply Silvadene, and wrap the limb with gauze and ace wraps. Avoid cutting through the normal skin during escharotomies if the burned skin is available. Incisions do not need to be strictly medial and lateral but should be adjusted to avoid non-burned skin whenever possible. If a sedated patient has high ventilator pressures and significant full-thickness circumferential chest burns, chest escharotomies may be required.

Always check the patient after an escharotomy has been done to make certain flow has been reestablished. Rarely, a fasciotomy will be needed to reestablish adequate blood flow. Escharotomies are most commonly needed in patients who have circumferential deep 2° or 3° burns on the chest or extremity and who will receive large volumes of fluid for resuscitation. If it is apparent that the patient will eventually need an escharotomy, do not wait until Doppler signals are lost.

Care of the Burn Wound

Once a patient has undergone initial assessment, and %TBSA has been assessed and initial resuscitation accomplished, the wound will need to be cared for until the patient can be evacuated to a burn center. Below are some basic wound care guidelines.

Care of Those That Can Be Evacuated

Civilians in a disaster will be transferred to a burn center as soon as possible. Although they will be transported within a couple days of their injury, they need to be optimized as best as possible prior to a relatively long flight in suboptimal medical conditions [12]. These patients should undergo dressing changes each day prior to and including the day of transport. Dressing changes, accomplished under conscious sedation, consist of removing the old dressing and washing the patient with soap and water to remove all topical antibiotics and remaining dead epidermis (including any blisters that may have formed in the interim) and accompanying bacteria. By performing daily wound care, the burn wound can be reevaluated for progression or healing and bacterial counts reduced to help prevent burn wound infection and eventual burn wound sepsis. The patient should be packaged for flight in clean dry sheets and blankets and Bair Huggers, fluid warmers, and ancillary warming devices utilized to help maintain normothermia during transport. A Foley catheter should be placed in anyone who has a burn requiring formal fluid resuscitation. Other than escharotomy and early tracheostomy (when necessary), operative burn care should not be undertaken until after they are evacuated.

Care of Host Nationals and Coalition Forces

The care of these individuals is challenging. Many host nationals are malnourished, they are not necessarily vaccinated for tetanus and other diseases, parasitic infections are common, there is a large communication barrier, and they may have large burns. In addition, there will be limited resources to care for burn wounds; deployed surgeons may or may not have any experience with burn surgery and will have limited bed space and time given operational constraints [13]. Despite all of these obstacles, good care can be rendered if done in a stepwise, rational fashion. Additionally, the deployed surgeon may be facing one or more burn casualties who are not eligible for evacuation.

Unlike civilian surgeons, the deployed surgeon must balance many competing priorities while providing care to US forces; coalition forces; national, regional, and local police; US and foreign contractors; host nationals; and prisoners of war (aka enemies of peace). Additionally, deployed surgeons must take into account that battle conditions may change abruptly necessitating "clearing" of the beds to accommodate newly wounded soldiers. In an effort to open bed space and provided needed subspecialty care in an expedient fashion, wounded American and coalition forces and civilian contractors are continually evacuated to Europe, and local forces are transferred to local (non-American) military hospitals, and local nationals are given as much care as possible and transferred to local hospitals or home. When more capacity is needed to care for injured soldiers, every effort is made to find a local hospital to care for host nationals, (predictably without burn expertise or the necessary supplies) who will almost universally result in mortality in non-American burn patients with critical needs at the time of transfer. The key to avoiding this situation is to treat thermal injuries in a piecemeal fashion. Allow what will heal to heal with dressing changes. Try to avoid large operations that will require large amounts of fluid resuscitation and ICU recovery, and wean patients from mechanical ventilation between required skin grafts, and follow the following recommendations.

When providing definitive burn care in the deployed environment, one must remember that providing the same standard of care that one would in an American burn center will result in mortality as one cannot provide the same level of critical care, available blood is limited, dressing supplies are precious, infection control is rudimentary, supplemental nutrition may or may not be available, and deployed nurses and physical therapists may have variable to no burn experience. Despite these limitations, with determination, and adaptive care, very acceptable burn care can be rendered and lives saved. The key to acceptable care is not doing so much that the patient requires ICU care for prolonged periods of time. If you can resuscitate the patient and do wound care and grafting in small doses, often ICU level care is not necessary, even for large burns. Opportunities for innovation can be rewarding in and of themselves with the end result being a healed patient who will return to their community and speak well of their experience under American care.

When the surgeon – with the support of the medical unit leadership – decides to undertake the definitive treatment of a burned casualty, the following guidelines and recommendations are offered to assist in providing the best care possible in what can be best described as suboptimal circumstances. What follows is a general philosophy with regard to the definitive treatment of major burns in the deployed setting.

1. When a newly burned patient arrives, take them to the operating room ASAP. This will allow for maintenance of normothermia, adequate analgesia, and evaluation of the burn in a clean environment.
2. Change field lines as soon as possible to ensure the patient has clean lines placed in a relatively sterile environment.
3. Wash all wounds with soap and water or if available Hibiclens solution.
4. Note the size of the burn and try to determine which parts of the burn are superficial partial-thickness (pink and wet dermis), deep partial-

thickness (less pink dermis that may be somewhat dry), and full-thickness (white dermis, leathery texture) burns.
5. Coat with some form of antibiotic salve (silver sulfadiazine, Sulfamylon, bacitracin, or gentamicin ointment all work well), and wrap with gauze.
6. Resuscitate the patient orally if a small burn and according to a prescribed formula if a large burn [14].
7. Rewash the patient with soap and water, or Hibiclens, and change the dressings every 24 h and note the evolution of the burn wounds.
8. Wait 2–3 days before making a decision as to grafting. (Partial-thickness wounds can heal on their own, and sometimes wounds that initially look good will look worse on postburn day 3, and need grafting.)

The Conservative Approach Skin Grafting

Skin grafting is a surgical procedure essential to the survival of the burn patient who has full-thickness burns generally exceeding 20% TBSA. Many surgical specialties include the basic techniques of skin grafting as part of their training programs, but few surgeons perform these as part of their routine practice. Smaller size burns may be amenable to primary excision and closure of the wound, particularly when the wound allows for an elliptical excision. Larger burns and those which involve full-thickness dermal injury generally require tangential excision of the burn and coverage with a split thickness graft harvested from uninjured donor sites. Occasionally, a full-thickness skin graft may be required for smaller burns in cosmetically sensitive areas (i.e., face). Once the burns have "declared" themselves, excise and graft small portions of full-thickness burn approximately every 3 days until:

A. All partial-thickness wounds are healing and all full-thickness sites are covered with graft. In this situation, the patient will not require critical care, will have full coverage, and can return to their community with clinic visits as needed.

B. The patient no longer requires critical care (ventilator, IVF, abx), and wound care can be accomplished daily in an outpatient setting. In this circumstance, some full-thickness eschar will be allowed to separate from the patient. Under this separated eschar, either new skin will be present or a granulation bed. If a granulation bed appears after burn wound separation, this can be grafted in a 3 or 4:1 fashion and will heal without further debridement. If no further grafting can be offered, this wound will eventually heal by secondary intention (contraction), which is not optimal and will lead to scaring and wound contracture, but the patient will live to undergo revisionary surgery at a later date.

In both of these situations, it is assumed that all partial-thickness burns will heal without grafting (Figs. 15.2 and 15.3).

Suggestions for Successful Skin Grafting in the Deployed Environment

1. When the decision has been made to debride and graft a burn, debride only full-thickness wounds. Leave all partial-thickness wounds to heal with dressing changes.
2. Blood is a precious resource. Wrap extremities tightly with an ace wrap to exsanguinate the extremity, and then use a tourniquet whenever possible prior to debridement. Preparation of the wound prior to excision includes cleansing with an antimicrobial cleanser such as Hibiclens. Excision of full-thickness burns may be accomplished by serial tangential passes of a knife or bladed instrument known by several names, to include Blair, Braithwaite, Humby, or Watson. A power dermatome may also be used to excise burns; however, this process will require an ample supply of disposable dermatome blades or experience with a wet or dry sharpening stone, and the efficiency of the

15 The Rational Care of Burns

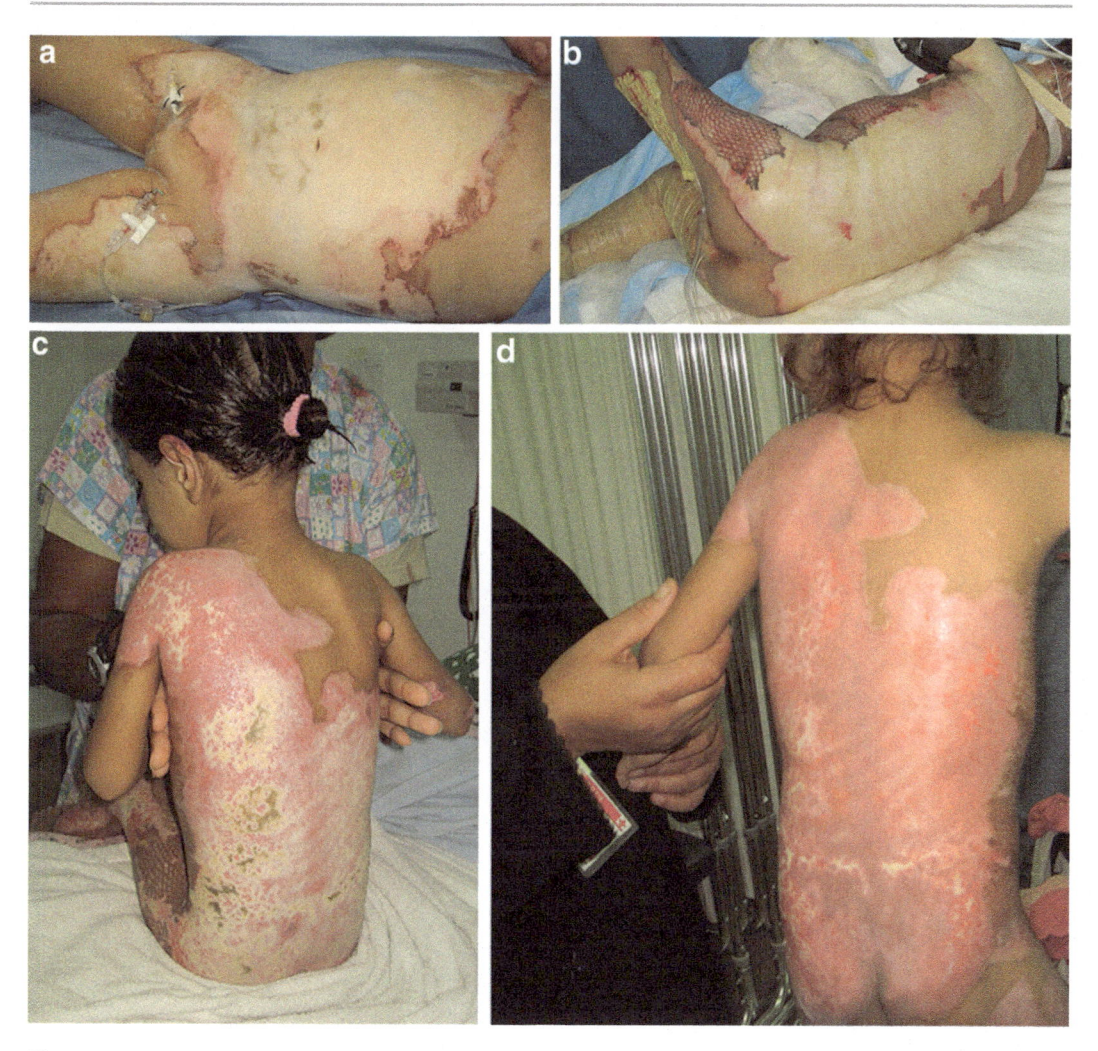

Fig. 15.2 This Iraqi girl came to us after a large (40% TBSA) scald burn. She was intubated and resuscitated and taken to the OR on PBD 3 for excision and grafting of her anterior abdomen and chest as necessary. She was then rapidly diuresed and extubated. She underwent conservative treatment of her back and buttocks as an outpatient and healed without further grafting

process will be related to the power of the dermatome. Alternatively, cautery may be used. This will often result in excision to the level of the fascia but is very useful in minimizing blood loss when debriding wounds that are not located in areas amenable to tourniquet use.

3. If the fat under the dermis is orange, or there is evidence of thrombosed blood vessels, excision will need to be taken to the level of the fascia. If graft is placed on questionable or dead fat, it will not survive.

4. If grafting to granulation tissue, wash with Hibiclens, rinse with NS, and then *lightly* rub with a 4x4 prior to grafting. You don't need to remove all granulation tissue prior to grafting. It has a great blood supply and will take grafts.

5. After extremity wounds have been debrided, spray with bovine thrombin, place Telfa Clear, then dilute epinephrine-soaked gauze, then ace wrap, and then release tourniquet. Wait 10 min, and then take down gauze and stop any bleeding (there shouldn't be much).

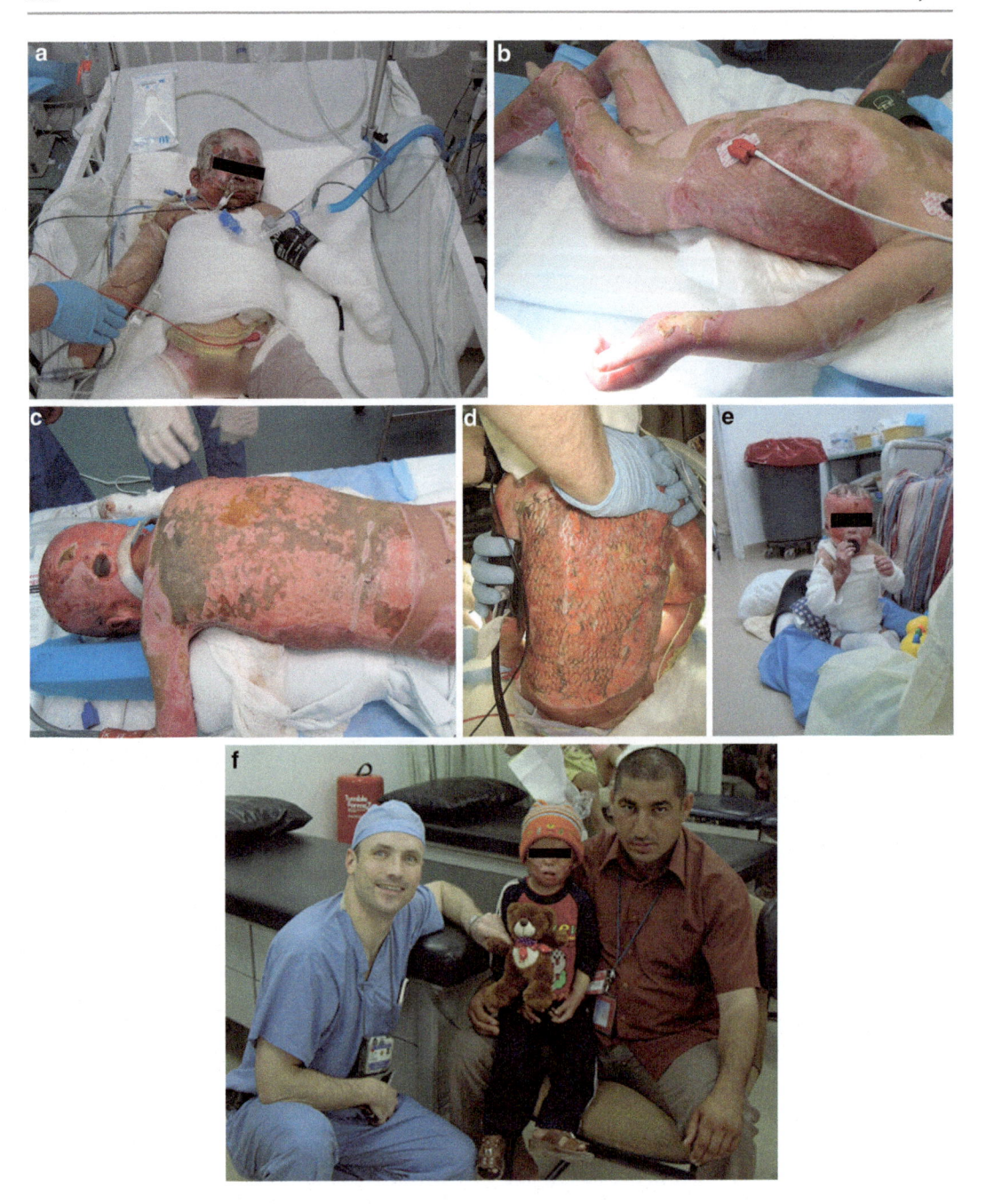

Fig. 15.3 This 2-year-old Iraqi boy was admitted shortly after falling into a bread oven which he could not get out of without help. He was intubated for pain control and expected swelling. He was resuscitated and on postburn day 3 taken to the OR for grafting of his chest and abdomen (legs were donor sites.) As he diuresed, he was extubated, and his back and face wounds were allowed to "separate." With aggressive feeding and daily dressing changes, his wounds separated, but some did require further grafting. This strategy avoided another ventilator course, which saved valuable resources and freed up valuable hospital space

Try not to rub the wound bed as this will result in unnecessary bleeding. For burns not located on extremities, the procedure is similar except that manual pressure is applied to the epinephrine-soaked gauze and no ace wraps are used. Occasionally suture ligatures and electrocautery may be required after the wounds are unwrapped to help achieve hemostasis prior to placing the autografts.

6. Selection of donor sites is important when planning an operation. I generally harvest skin from lateral thighs, anterior thighs, posterior thighs, lower abdomen, back, medial thighs, below knees (calf then shin), chest, and then anywhere else, in that order. Tumescent fluid (NS without epi) can be injected under the skin to be harvested to make harvesting easier. Set dermatome to 10/1000 of an inch. Use mineral oil liberally. Use epinephrine solution (1 amp in 1 L NS) on a lap pad, and apply to harvested area immediately after harvesting to stop bleeding. Xeroform gauze is inexpensive, has antimicrobial properties, is generally readily available even in remote locations, is easy to apply, and serves as an effective donor site dressing. If it is not available, op-site-type dressing can be applied or a thin coat of bacitracin or gentamicin ointment. With good nutrition, donor sites can generally be reharvested in 10–14 days provided that healing is progressive.

7. Securing of split thickness autograft to the wound bed can be accomplished with the use of surgical staples placed intermittently around the periphery of the graft as well as between the seams of adjacent grafts. Absorbable suture can be used in the same manner. The autograft must be protected during the early phases of engraftment. Telfa Clear coated with bacitracin or Dermanet® wound contact layer is a lightweight "veil" material which serves to protect the fresh graft yet allows for coverage with outer gauze or even negative pressure wound dressing. Dressings should typically be left in place for at least 72 h prior to "revealing" and inspecting the wounds.

Special Circumstances

In cases of patients with superficial or deep burns of the dorsum of the hands, palms, or fingers or dorsum of the feet, soles, and/or toes, once initial debridement is done, these wounds can be managed with a plastic bag dressing. This simple dressing is created by placing the hand or foot in a plastic bag containing Silvadene cream. The bag is then taped around the forearm or shank and can remain for up to a week. With time, the Silvadene will admix with perspiration and form a thick liquid that will bathe the hand or foot continuously. The advantage of this dressing is that it is less resource intensive than a daily dressing change and allows visualization of the healing burn as well as allows the patient to do range of motion exercises as tolerated (Fig. 15.4).

1. If grafting of the face is required, sheet grafts have better cosmetic outcome and tend to have less contracture formation in the long term (Fig. 15.5).
2. In extreme cases of extensive full-thickness burns, amputation of the affected body part may be a necessary form of excision, especially if the injury appears to have destroyed the underlying tissue down to and including the bone. This situation is most commonly seen with high-voltage electrical burns but not with DCBI.

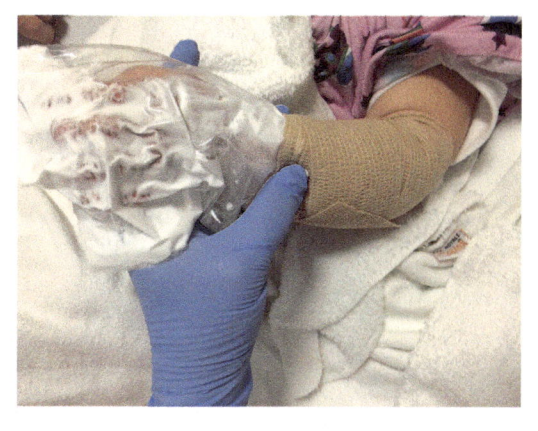

Fig. 15.4 The use of this "plastic bag dressing" allowed for range of motion exercises and daily inspection of the wound while using minimal supplies

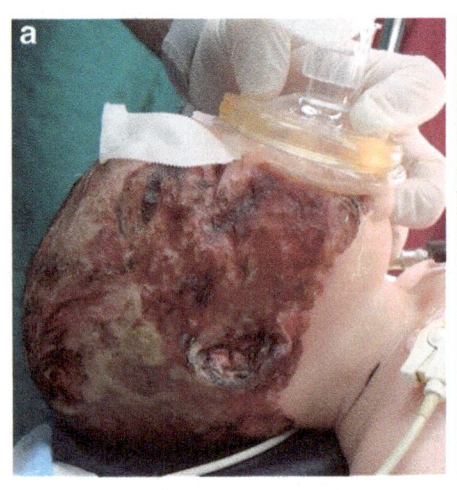

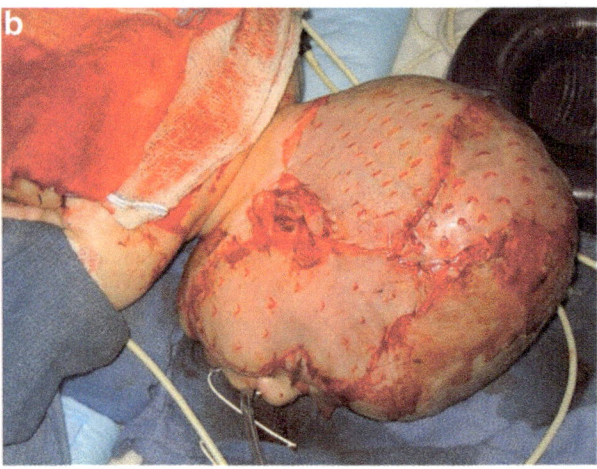

Fig. 15.5 This 15-month-old Iraqi girl required extensive sheet grafting of her face after her parents used gasoline in a kerosene heater resulting in a large explosion and resulting fire. Initially cared for in an Iraqi facility, she came to us on postburn day 7. She was debrided to granulation tissue, and the skin from her back was harvested and used for sheet grafting. Her ear was debrided to viable cartilage and closed primarily

References

1. Ramasamy A, Hill AM, Clasper JC. Improvised explosive devices: patho-physiology, injury profiles and current medical management. J R Army Med Corps. 2009;155:265–72.
2. Jeevaratnam JA, Pandya AN. One year of burns at a role 3 medical treatment facility in Afghanistan. J R Army Med Corps. 2014;160:22–6.
3. Smith DL, et al. Effect of inhalation injury, burn size, and age on mortality—a study of 1447 consecutive burn patients. J Trauma. 1994;37:655–9.
4. Kramer GC, Michell MW, Oliveira H, et al. Oral and enteral resuscitation of burn shock. The historical record and implications for mass casualty care. J Burn Wound Care. 2003;2:1458–74.
5. Chung KK, Salinas J, Renz EM, et al. Simple derivation of the initial fluid rate for the resuscitation of severely burned adult combat casualties: in silico validation of the rule of 10. J Trauma. 2010;69(suppl 1):S49–54.
6. Saffle JR. The phenomenon of "fluid creep" in acute burn resuscitation. J Burn Care Res. 2007;28:382–95.
7. Ivy ME, Atweh NA, Palmer J, et al. Intra-abdominal hypertension and abdominal compartment syndrome in burn patients. J Trauma. 2000;49:387–91.
8. Brownson EG, Pham TN, Chung KK. How to recognize a failed burn resuscitation. Crit Care Clin. 2016;32:567–75.
9. Bennett JE, Lewis E. Operative decompression of constricting burns. Surgery. 1958;43:949–55.
10. Kaplan I, White W. Incisional decompression of circumferential burns. Plast Reconstr Surg. 1961;28:609–18.
11. Pruitt BA, Dowling JA, Moncrief JA. Escharotomy in early burn care. Arch Surg. 1968;96:502–7.
12. Renz EM, Cancio LC, Barillo DJ, et al. Long range transport of war-related burn casualties. J Trauma. 2008;64:S136–45.
13. Venticinque SG, Grathwohl KW. Critical care in the austere environment: providing exceptional care in unusual places. Crit Care Med. 2008;36:S284–92.
14. Dufour D, Kroman Jensen S, Owen-Smith M, et al. Surgery for Victims of War. Geneva, Switzerland: International Committee of the Red Cross, 1998:225. Ref. 0446. Available at: http//www.icrc.org/web/eng/siteeng0.nsf/html/p0446. Accessed 30 Jan 2017.

Soft Tissue Reconstruction of Complex Blast Injuries in Military and Civilian Settings: Guidelines and Principles

16

Corinne E. Wee, Jason M. Souza, Terri A. Zomerlei, and Ian L. Valerio

Background

The recent military operations in the Middle East, Operation Iraqi Freedom (OIF) and Operation Enduring Freedom (OEF), have introduced unparalleled mechanisms and levels of injury, bringing new challenges to military technology, strategy, and medicine. While fairly recent American conflicts such as Vietnam recorded explosions as the cause of less than 50% of casualties, Iraq and Afghanistan have recorded increased rates of explosive and blast casualties, estimated at >70% explosions as the leading cause of modern battlefield injury [1, 2]. The trend toward blast and improvised explosive device (IED) attacks has been evidenced over the course of the most recent conflicts, with explosion-related casualties increasing by 20% from 2003 to 2006. Improvements in personal protective equipment that safeguards the vulnerable thorax and its vital organs, forward surgical teams, greater efficiencies gained in rapid patient transport to definitive care centers, hemorrhage control measures, and massive transfusion protocols have increased the overall battlefield survival rates to the highest levels seen in military medial engagements, with current battlefield survival rates exceeding 97%. These survival gains have resulted in more complex injury patterns, as casualties who survive their initial injuries often suffer from severe blast injuries and have greater injury severity scores (ISS), increased composite type defects (i.e., combined orthopedic and soft tissue injuries such as skin, nerve, and muscle), high numbers of traumatic amputations, and elevated mortality threats given their susceptibility to sepsis and multisystem organ failure [2, 3] (Figs. 16.1 and 16.2).

Furthermore, exposure to dismounted explosives has also been reported to suffer an unprecedented number of perineal, genital, and urinary tract injuries, which not only affect reproduction and genitourinary function, but they also have higher associated risks of suicide secondary to their psychological consequences [4]. The effect of these high-energy blast exposures is further illustrated by the devastating impact of traumatic

C. E. Wee · T. A. Zomerlei
Department of Plastic & Reconstructive Surgery, The Ohio State University Wexner Medical Center, Columbus, OH, USA

J. M. Souza
Department of Plastic & Reconstructive Surgery, Walter Reed National Military Medical Center, Bethesda, MD, USA

I. L. Valerio (✉)
Department of Plastic & Reconstructive Surgery, The Ohio State University Wexner Medical Center, Columbus, OH, USA

Department of Plastic & Reconstructive Surgery, Walter Reed National Military Medical Center, Bethesda, MD, USA
e-mail: Ian.Valerio@osumc.edu

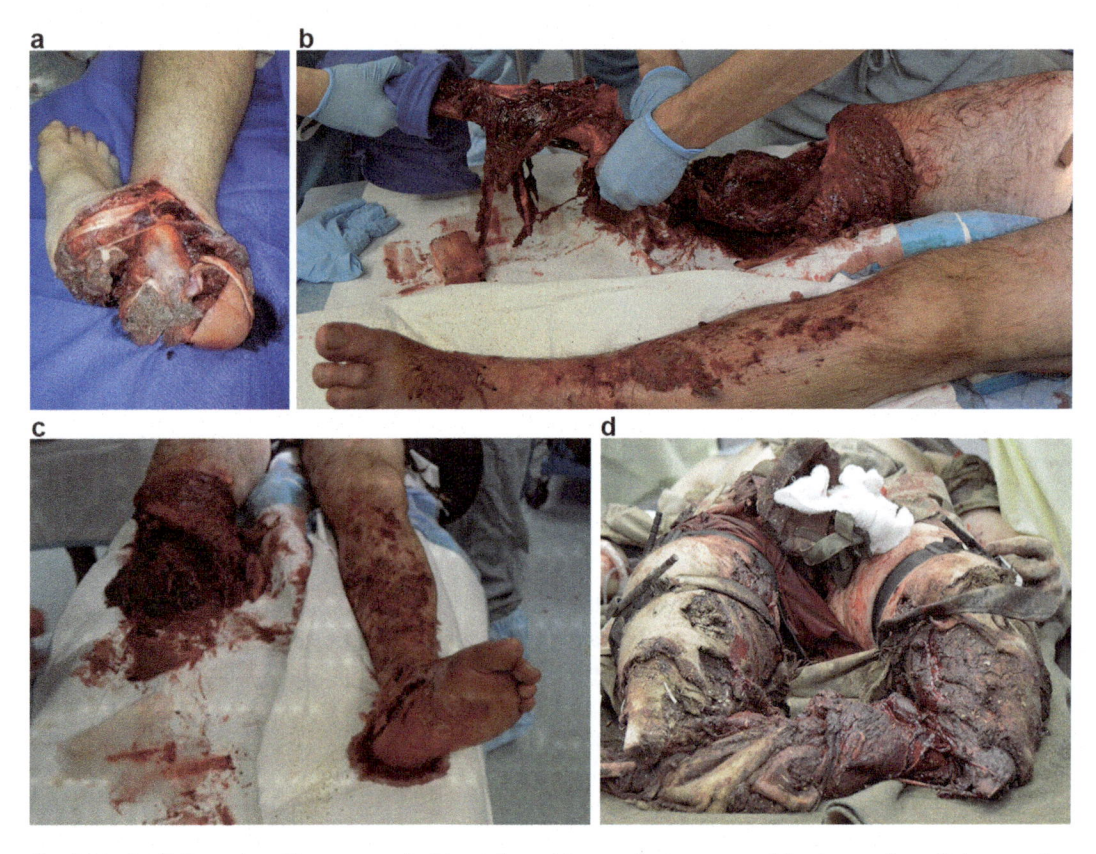

Fig. 16.1 (**a**–**d**) Examples of lower extremity blast injury with extensive trauma resulting in complex soft tissue, orthopedic, and neurovascular injuries

amputation, which beyond its obvious physical impact is also associated with a significant rate of depression and PTSD [5]. During the height of the war, an amputation occurred once every 36 h, which led to the Pentagon in investing over $75 million in the fight against IEDs [6]. In the face of advancing military technology and weapons, reconstructive surgeons are faced with new challenges as well, including a high volume of extensive soft tissue trauma requiring updated techniques and approaches.

Unfortunately, recent events have identified the need for a comprehensive approach to blast trauma management outside of the military setting, with increasing numbers of civilians falling victim to explosive acts of terror. Events such as the 2005 London bus bombings, the 2006 train bombings in Mumbai, the 2013 Boston Marathon bombing, and various global terrorist- and insurgent-backed attacks have seen IEDs targeted toward civilians. Like those servicemembers who have experienced blast injury on the battlefield, survivors of these aforementioned attacks have experienced similarly devastating and complex injuries, ranging from burns and lacerations to craniofacial and extremity trauma to even limb loss and/or permanent blindness [7]. As a result, there is newfound importance for dissemination of surgical techniques and regenerative medicine technologies that were once primarily the domain of the military surgeon. Using knowledge gained from the recent wartime experiences, this chapter will review approaches to soft tissue reconstruction following blast-related injuries, including initial evaluation and planning, timing to definitive reconstruction, operative techniques, and useful emerging regenerative technologies and adjuncts.

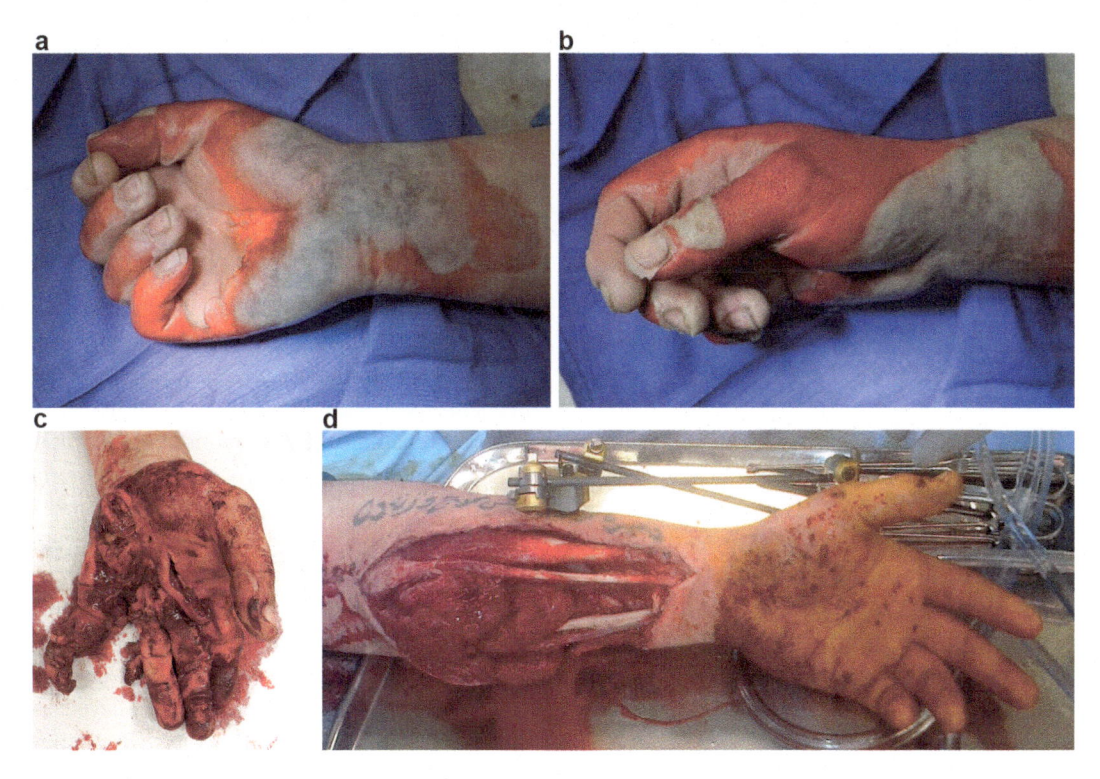

Fig. 16.2 (**a**–**d**) Upper extremity blast injuries; (**a**–**b**) severe upper extremity burns as a result of blast injury

Approach to Reconstruction

The reconstructive approach to blast injuries must be as unique as the injury itself; traditional reconstructive planning may not be sufficient for the patient suffering from extensive polytrauma with systemic complications. Lessons learned from wartime reconstruction regarding surgical timing, management of complex comorbidities, and limb length preservation are helpful in optimizing reconstructive approaches to blast injuries.

Initial Management of Blast Injuries with Severe Soft Tissue Injury and/or Loss

Initial management of blast-related soft tissue injuries still requires a focus on casualty survival efforts including medical stabilization, hemorrhage control, resuscitation, and limb-saving efforts. From the initial point of injury, throughout the casualty transport process and until definitive care of soft tissue and extremity injuries, tourniquets to prevent exsanguination and uncontrolled hemorrhage are critical to prevent additional patient distress and instability. Once triaged to the next level of care, damage control surgery, adequate debridement of devitalized and/or contaminated tissues, transition of previously applied tourniquets to temporary vascular shunts followed by conversion to vascular reconstruction and/or bypass grafting, placement of external fixation devices for orthopedic stabilization, and appropriate soft tissue dressing applications prior to patient transport to higher echelons of care remain important tenants prior to definitive soft tissue reconstruction measures. Soft tissue wound care often consists of serial surgical debridements, local wound care via traditional dressings such as wet-to-dry or wet-to-wet sponges, or Kerlix containing saline or Dakin's solution versus more advanced techniques such as negative pressure therapy with or without instillation. Broad spectrum antibiotics coverage may also require fungal coverage considerations based on certain patterns of injury (e.g., perineal or pelvic disruption injuries) and local environmental flora and contaminants. Once final speciation with susceptibilities of microorganisms is identified, the antibiotic regimen can be modified from broad to more specific antibiotic coverage. However, longer duration of treatment for soft tissue wounds at high risk of fungal contamination is warranted given that fungal culture growth and identification may be delayed (Fig. 16.3).

Goals of Reconstruction

The ultimate treatment goal is to restore or retain limb function though fracture union and soft tissue healing [8]. If the patient is able to participate in surgical planning, reconstructive options and alternatives must be discussed in detail. Often, traditional reconstructive modalities can be augmented with regenerative reconstructive approaches to provide ideal definitive soft tissue coverage. Once medically stable, the first priority of care becomes obtaining a clean wound and limiting secondary infection, through adequate removal of foreign bodies and devitalized tissue.

As previously discussed, this starts with comprehensive debridement in theater. Blast injuries create a unique challenge with regard to infection prevention and control, as the explosives themselves are often highly contaminated and foreign bodies can be buried deep within the soft tissues due to the shockwave mechanism associated with these blasts. This is evidenced by the fact that 63% of blast patients experience bacterial or fungal infection following explosive injury [9, 10]. Thus, unlike in traumatic injuries caused by other mechanisms, it is important to send soft tissue for culture and pathology. Post-debridement cultures should include fungi and acid-fast bacteria (which may be acquired contaminants from the environment) and should be obtained at every operative visit to assist in the administration of appropriate culture-driven antibiotics. While surveillance cultures may not be necessary for many traumatic mechanisms of civilian soft tissue injuries, blast-related soft tissue injuries do have certain characteristics and infection risk profiles which warrant special consideration and care. It is routine for wounds to require serial irrigation and debridement, usually performed every 1–3 days, before the wound is clinically clean enough to proceed with definitive soft tissue

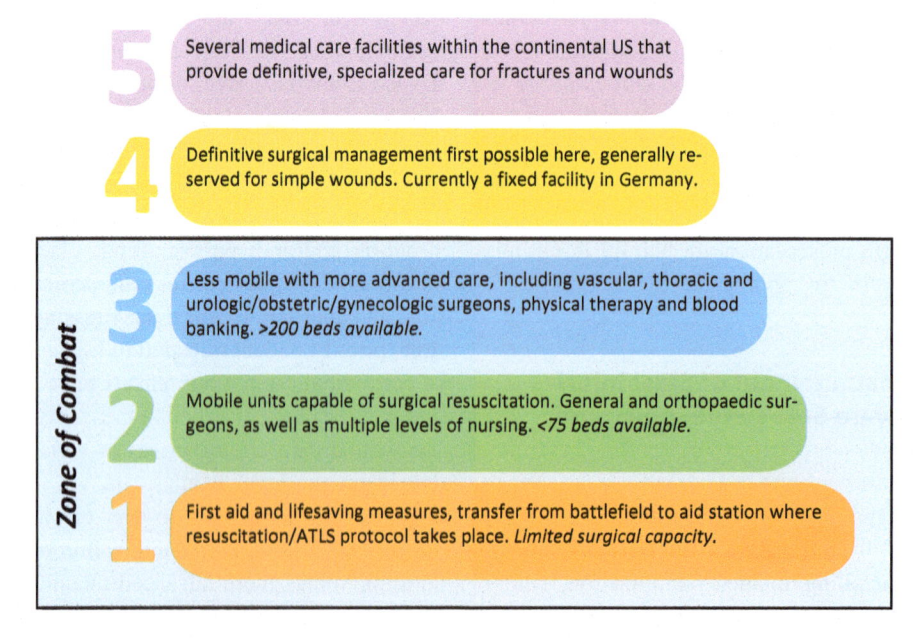

5 Several medical care facilities within the continental US that provide definitive, specialized care for fractures and wounds

4 Definitive surgical management first possible here, generally reserved for simple wounds. Currently a fixed facility in Germany.

Zone of Combat

3 Less mobile with more advanced care, including vascular, thoracic and urologic/obstetric/gynecologic surgeons, physical therapy and blood banking. *>200 beds available.*

2 Mobile units capable of surgical resuscitation. General and orthopaedic surgeons, as well as multiple levels of nursing. *<75 beds available.*

1 First aid and lifesaving measures, transfer from battlefield to aid station where resuscitation/ATLS protocol takes place. *Limited surgical capacity.*

Fig. 16.3 Military echelons of care

reconstruction or coverage. These serial wound debridements are commonly coordinated with orthopedic interventions, as a similarly staged approach to bony fixation is frequently employed, based on the cleanliness of the wound and the quality of the available soft tissue coverage.

Beyond minimizing the discomfort and time associated with conventional dressing changes, the utilization of negative pressure wound therapy (NPWT) between operative visits can aid to decrease bacterial burden by optimizing blood flow, facilitating edema control, and aiding in the evacuation of proteases that may encourage chronic wound formation [11, 12]. The sponge interface of NPWT can be tailored to the wound by using "white" foam, which is hydrophilic and has a small, dense pore allocation, on structures such as exposed bone or tendon that are sensitive to desiccation. The use of silver-impregnated sponges is particularly suited for a wound that has significant contamination, as the oxidative properties of the silver ions impair bacterial growth and have demonstrated effectiveness even against antibiotic-resistant organisms [13, 14]. Negative pressure therapy can also be combined with a system for fluid instillation, which allows clinicians to periodically introduce a solution such as sodium hypochlorite (Dakin's solution), hypochlorous acid (HOCL), or saline into the wound without requiring the need for operative irrigation or a dressing change. This technique has shown promise in decreasing bacterial burden in infected wounds [15] [WG4].

Noted disadvantages associated with NPWT include inability to accurately control applied pressure in geometrically challenging wounds or wounds near or at anatomically sensitive areas where adhesive seals are hard to obtain, bleeding which may be difficult to easily assess secondary to obstruction from the dressing, skin irritation, infection, pain or discomfort, ingrowth of granulation tissue within the dressing materials, machine- or device-related technical problems (e.g., battery failure, inadvertent clamping or compression of suction tubing, leakage of instillation solutions from adhesive dressing, etc.), fibrotic and "woody" scar formation, obscuring tissue planes as granulation tissue sets in, and inability to assess or view the wound until the dressing is completely removed [16]. However, the various advantages of NPWT including decreased dressing changes that can reduce patient discomfort, improved blood flow within the wound bed, edema control and reduction of tissue bed fluid, bacteria load reduction, more ease in large or complex wound management, soft tissue stabilization through transport, better wound healing, favorable tissue and cell deformation properties that trigger favorable intracellular signals for cell turnover, granulation formation, and revascularization of wound bed aid to largely outweigh the disadvantages of NPWT even in the setting of complex war injuries [17]. Complications such as bleeding and infection seen with NPWT in these settings have been attributed to the nature of the injury itself.

While reconstructive planning should commence at the time of the initial surgical evaluation, evolution in the wound appearance, status of concomitant injuries, and fixation requirements necessitate a flexible approach to reconstruction. Once these variables have been delineated and the wound is stable and adequately decontaminated, progress toward definitive reconstruction can be initiated. Though tools for wound assessment continue to be developed, the decision to proceed rests largely on clinical judgment, as there is little objective evidence available to guide this determination. It is rare for injuries to be sufficiently optimized for reconstruction within the acute period of 5 days post injury. Usually, the delay in the definitive reconstruction is a natural consequence of the patient's progression through the military echelons of care and is necessary to allow time for sufficient debridement and demarcation of the injured tissues, conversion of temporary measures to more definitive measures (e.g., vascular shunt conversion to formal vascular bypass), and confirmation versus placement of external fixation for orthopedic fractures. This level of care has more extensive surgical capabilities which also aids in direct transport of severely injured personnel requiring more advanced surgical options, lifesaving measures, and massive transfusion requirements and often triage mass casualty events. After successfully navigating the above echelons of care, recent wartime experience suggests that definitive reconstruction of blast-related trauma is best accomplished in the subacute period, which runs counter to established teaching espousing the benefits of early coverage. In a series of 35 pedicled flap reconstructions, Mathieu et al. performed the reconstruction at an average of 17.8 days, with some patients waiting up to 40 days from injury without evidence of increased complication rates associated with subacute reconstruction [18]. Other case series dealing with blast injuries reported similar delays, approximately 18–22 days, until wounds were clinically clean [19].

The Reconstructive Ladder for Blast Injury

The traditional approach to traumatic reconstruction follows a sequential progression through the rungs of the reconstructive ladder, which provides reconstructive options in order from simplest to most complex [20]. According to this approach, more complex reconstructive options such as composite adjacent tissue transfer and free tissue transfer are pursued only if more basic techniques fail or are unavailable. Blast victims, especially those in the military, are unique in that they are frequently young, active, and healthy prior to injury. In these cases, the patient's optimal premorbid status and heightened expectations for post-morbid function serve to influence the reconstructive approach. Depending on the pattern and extent of injury, the reconstructive tools available to maximize limb function can sometimes be restricted (muscle-sparing is sometimes preferred for rehabilitation purposes) or expanded beyond standard reconstructive approaches. This is exemplified by cases involving sequential free tissue transfer for reconstruction of blast victims [21]. Reconstruction is not limited to skin and soft tissue alone and may also include definitive orthopedic stabilization measures and repair of affected peripheral nerves. While autologous nerve grafting is considered to be the gold standard, processed nerve allografts have shown promising results when applied in the post-traumatic setting and have become more critical in those bilateral amputees where autologous nerve sources are severely lacking or deficient [22, 23].

One of the unique attributes of a high-energy blast injury is the extensive nature of the tissue damage sustained. The extent and distribution of injury in blast patients are often larger than initially anticipated, as percussive waves from the blast may cause significant shearing and avulsion to surrounding muscles, tendons, vessels, and nerves. Consequently, microanatomic structures in tissue that clinically appears to be "spared" may actually be compromised, resulting in an expanded zone of injury [9]. This large zone of injury often precludes stepwise progression through the traditional reconstructive ladder. Local options such as adjacent tissue transfer (ATT) are frequently limited by the dearth of available uninjured donor tissue. In certain cases where the extent of injury renders the use of local tissue reconstruction impossible, free tissue techniques are applied to wound locations that are usually otherwise amenable to coverage via ATT in the setting of conventional trauma mechanisms [WG5].

In those cases where free tissue transfer is often indicated, difficulty with microvascular anastomoses is common due to local vessel damage, risking complications in the postoperative period. However, given the extensive zones of injury associated with blast trauma, in-zone microsurgical anastomoses are often necessary, and thus, careful assessment of the arterial and venous vascular systems for adequate inflow and outflow is critical for in-zone microsurgical success. Careful preoperative vascular assessment with CT or MR angiography or traditional angiography measures can aid in target vessel identification. Intraoperatively, meticulous dissection in the zone of injury is critical to identify and protect intact large vascular source vessels with visualization of pulsatile flow and sufficient arterial flow (spurt testing), and ease in heparinized saline flush within target veins is crucial for improving flap anastomoses, flow restoration to the flap, and ultimately survival of the flap. Additional considerations in these cases include the incorporation of larger parent source pedicles, saphenous vein grafting to extend outside of the zones of injury, and arteriovenous loops to improve blood flow in the setting of a potentially damaged blood supply, further complicating the surgery (Figs. 16.4, 16.5 and 16.6).

Redesigning the Reconstructive Ladder

The challenges presented by blast injuries require an evolved approach to the reconstructive ladder. Recently, the concept of the reconstructive ladder has largely been replaced by the "reconstructive elevator." The reconstructive elevator prioritizes functional and aesthetic outcome over the minimization of resources and complexity. According to this approach, the reconstructive surgeon is justified in bypassing simpler reconstructive options when the combination of defect complexity and patient goals and characteristics is better served by advanced reconstructive techniques. Conversely, the development of advanced technologies and techniques for local wound care have also allowed for modifications to the traditional reconstructive algorithm. Here, we suggest the use of a "hybrid reconstructive ladder," which incorporates the use of these advanced wound care and regenerative medicine modalities to be used alongside traditional reconstructive options to achieve soft tissue coverage [24] (Fig. 16.7).

The application of newer modalities such as dermal regenerative templates (DRT) and extracellular matrices (ECM) at our institution has allowed us to employ simpler reconstructive options for wounds that would typically require more complex coverage. A greater understanding of the modalities described in this chapter may allow reconstructive surgeons to better avoid or minimize the postoperative morbidity associated with traditional techniques or allow surgical coverage options to be used for salvage in the event of a complication.

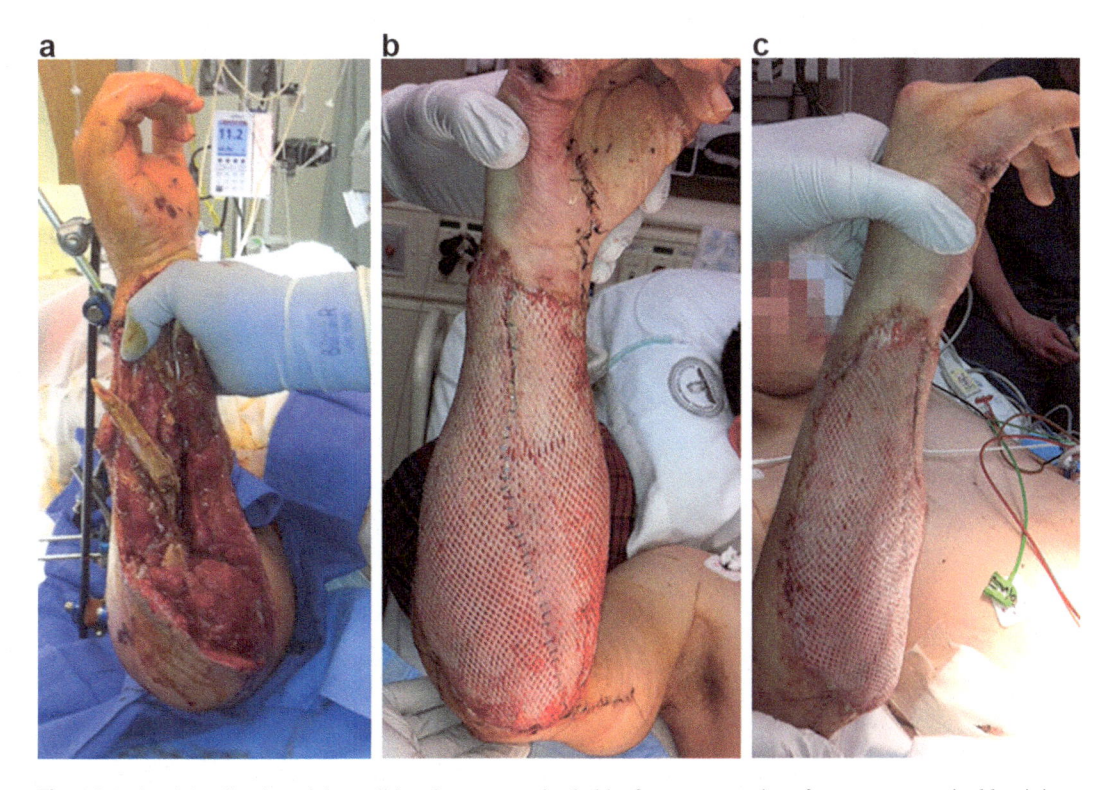

Fig. 16.4 (a–c) Application of the traditional reconstructive ladder for reconstruction after upper extremity blast injury. Patient underwent definitive coverage following ORIF with free tissue transfer and split-thickness skin graft

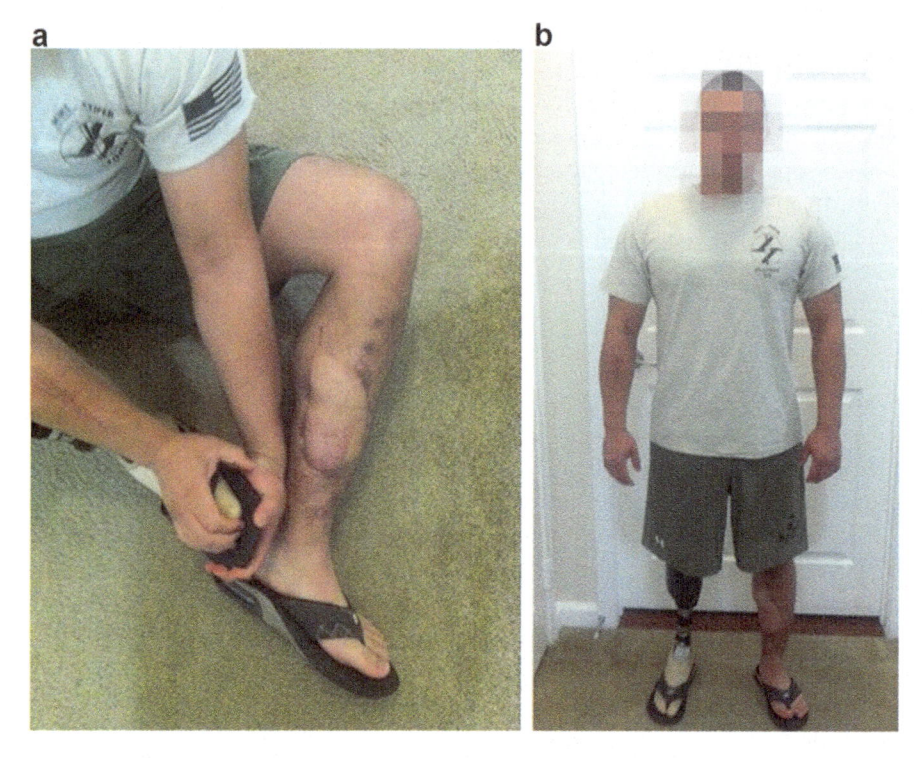

Fig. 16.5 (a–b) Left lower extremity reconstruction for limb salvage with free ALT flap; right lower extremity amputation with adequate soft tissue coverage to allow for comfortable prosthesis wear

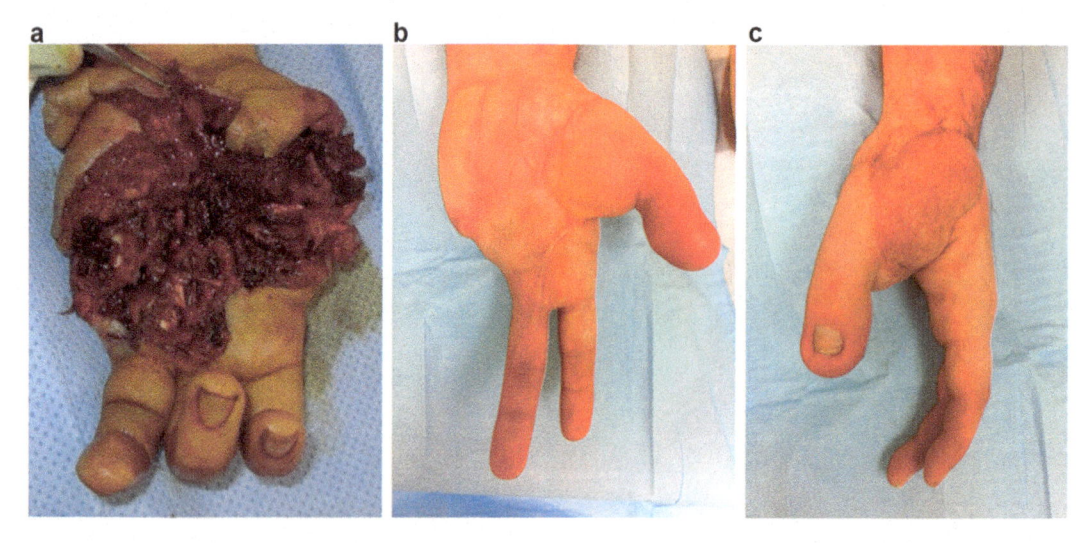

Fig. 16.6 (a–c) Reconstruction of the left hand after blast injury combining free tissue transfer with great toe transplant after ectopic banking for thumb reconstruction

In the case of civilian blast injuries, this concept of the hybrid reconstructive ladder can aid in the design of viable coverage in the face of polytrauma. Unlike more localized wounds which may permit the use of the traditional reconstructive ladder, blast injuries present as large, complex wounds with limited donor tissue in the setting of significant comorbidities such as

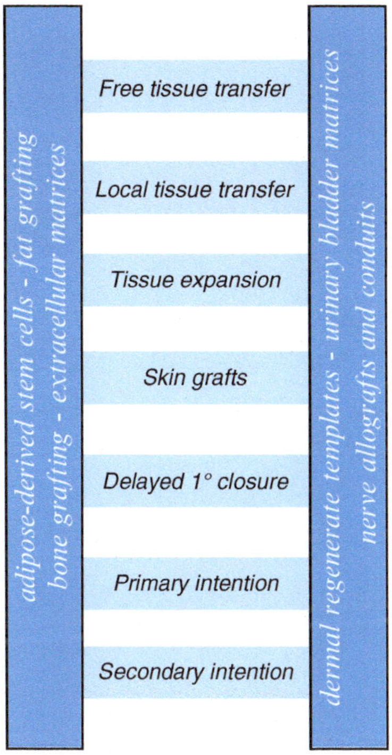

Fig. 16.7 Hybrid reconstructive ladder, showing the incorporation of regenerative modalities which can be inserted into the various rungs of the traditional reconstructive ladder

sepsis, soft tissue, and bone infections. In addition to other comorbidities such as uncontrolled diabetes and vascular disease, these circumstances greatly increase the risk of graft failure. Based on our experience, we present some of the many useful modalities to aid in soft tissue coverage in the setting of complex traumatic wounds.

Regenerative Technologies for Soft Tissue and Skin Replacement

The recent innovation of numerous biologic and synthetic dermal and epidermal regenerative modalities can aid in the treatment of extensive soft tissue defects as the result of blast injury.

Dermal Regenerative Templates

Dermal regenerative templates have been approved for wound care for approximately 20 years and have proven to be advantageous in large blast injuries requiring immediate coverage. At our institution, Integra (Integra LifeSciences, Plainsboro, NJ) is the most commonly used DRT and is composed of two layers. The deeper layer acts as a neodermis and consists of a porous matrix of cross-linked bovine tendon collagen and glycosaminoglycans. The superficial permeable silicone layer acts as a temporary epidermis, limiting water loss and providing strength against tear; this layer is removed in a second stage following integration of the deeper layer. The neodermal layer encourages neovascularization and angiogenesis which facilitates the migration of fibroblasts and keratinocytes into the matrix. During this process, the bovine collagen is absorbed and replaced by the patient's own collagen, signifying integration of the deep layer. Following removal of the silicone layer, the newly integrated dermal layer is covered with an autologous, meshed split-thickness skin graft (Fig. 16.8).

The major advantage of DRTs in civilian blast injuries is the ability to provide immediate coverage in a high-risk patient with a large, heterogeneous, complex wound. Not only is autologous coverage difficult in these settings due to the size of the defect, metabolic disturbances and critical illness due to such injury greatly increase the risk of failure. Early attempts at autologous coverage without optimization of the wound bed can ultimately result in limited coverage options following initial failure of graft take. DRTs are incredibly versatile and have shown to be effective in a variety of wound environments, including burn injuries, necrotizing fasciitis, and degloving injuries with exposed bone and tendon. Burns, concomitant infection, and exposed vital structures may all be present

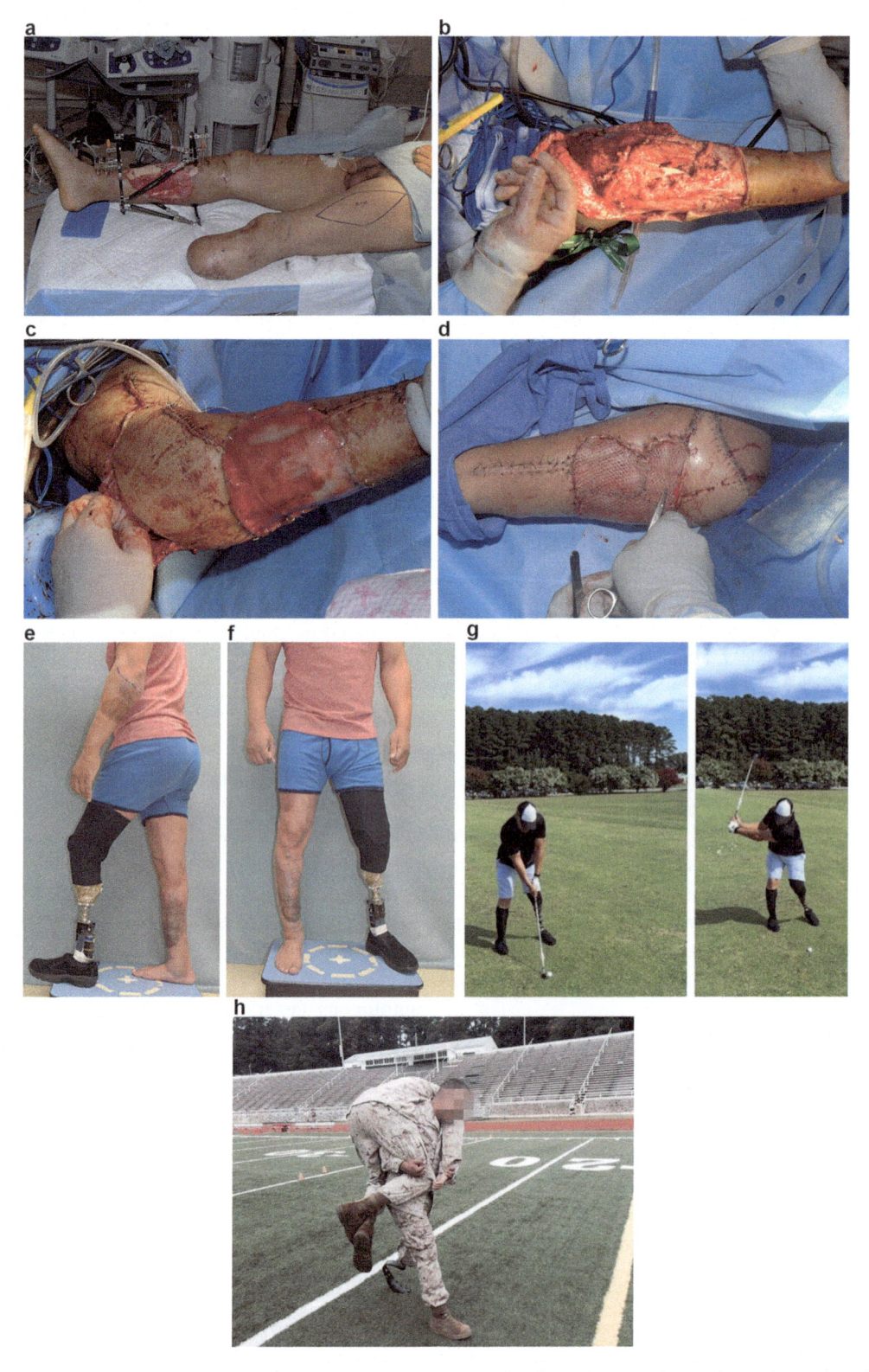

Fig. 16.8 (**a–h**) Complicated blast injury demonstrating principles of the hybrid reconstructive ladder. This patient required unilateral amputation and complex orthopedic and soft tissue reconstruction on both upper and lower

in blast injuries, and the effectiveness of DRTs in each of these settings makes DRT a good candidate for initial coverage. Furthermore, DRTs have shown to improve functional outcomes in patients, reducing contractures and postoperative pain [25].

Biologic-Based Extracellular Matrices

Extracellular matrices can also optimize soft tissue coverage in complex blast wounds, especially those with significant volume deficiency, concern for infection due to particulate matter, or lacking vascular supply. ECMs are derived from various tissue and animal sources and are arranged in a scaffold consisting of collagen, laminin, fibronectin, glycosaminoglycan, and growth factor. Examples include ovine forestomach matrix, urinary bladder matrix (UBM), and small intestinal submucosa (SIS). They can be applied as a powder or as a sheet onto the wound bed. While the exact mechanism remains unknown, ECM leads to the release of VEGF as it is degraded by host cells and has also been shown to modulate the innate immune system. In this way, ECM helps to promote angiogenesis, establish healthy granulation tissue in complex blast wounds, and decrease bacterial loads. In a case series of combat wounds treated at Walter Reed, Valerio et al. reported that incorporating urinary bladder matrix (UBM) into the reconstructive process stimulated production of granulation tissue leading to successful definitive soft tissue coverage [24]. This case series illustrated the benefit of UBM in the case of localized tissues having microvascular compromise, such as with exposed tendons, bone, and/or joint capsules devoid of paratenon, periosteum, or adequate soft tissue coverage over certain exposed vital structures.

Materials derived from pig small intestinal submucosa (SIS) contain additional ECM components important to wound closure such as glycosaminoglycans, proteoglycans, fibronectin, and growth factors [26–28]. These components simulate organization of collagen fibers, angiogenesis, tissue proliferation, and differentiation. SIS has been shown to induce tissue remodeling in a variety of settings, including animal models of urinary bladders, tendon and ligaments, vessels, body wall defects, and skin wounds [29–35].

Advances in Skin Replacement

Following optimization of the wound bed, spray skin technology can be used in conjunction with autologous coverage to provide definitive coverage to a large wound. Currently, these technologies are used in compassionate care cases as they are currently not FDA approved in the United States. Spray skin involves processing a small split-thickness skin sample into a suspension of keratinocytes, Langerhans cells, melanocytes, and fibroblasts which is delivered onto the wound bed by a spray applicator. In addition to reducing skin graft donor site burden by permitting larger meshing ratios, spray skin has also been shown to decrease healing time and hospital stays, improve postoperative pain, improve pigmentation match, and possibly prevent contracture [36–38]. Animal studies performed in both pigs and mice have shown that spray skin is effective in improving epidermal and superficial dermal wound healing, with immunohistologic examination of pig skin showing proper distribution of alpha 6 within the epithelium and basement membrane, as opposed to inappropriate distribution of alpha 6 in untreated pig skin [39]. Furthermore, spray skin technology can be combined with Integra in a one-stage procedure and has been shown to promote more rapid organization and epithelialization both grossly and histologically while still

Fig. 16.8 (continued) extremities. (**a**) Latissimus flap to the right lower extremity; (**b–d**) Integra use to assist in dermal regeneration and improve skin graft take – left to right: upper extremity soft tissue trauma after sufficient I&D in preparation for Integra; placement of Integra; definitive coverage with STSG and ALT flap; (**e–f**) long-term follow-up of RLE latissimus flap and RUE ALT flap/STSG, LLE amputation with stable coverage allowing for functional prosthetic use; (**g–h**) adequate soft tissue envelope and peripheral nerve management after amputation allows for maximum functionality. Long-term follow-up for LLE amputee demonstrating successful recovery following amputation

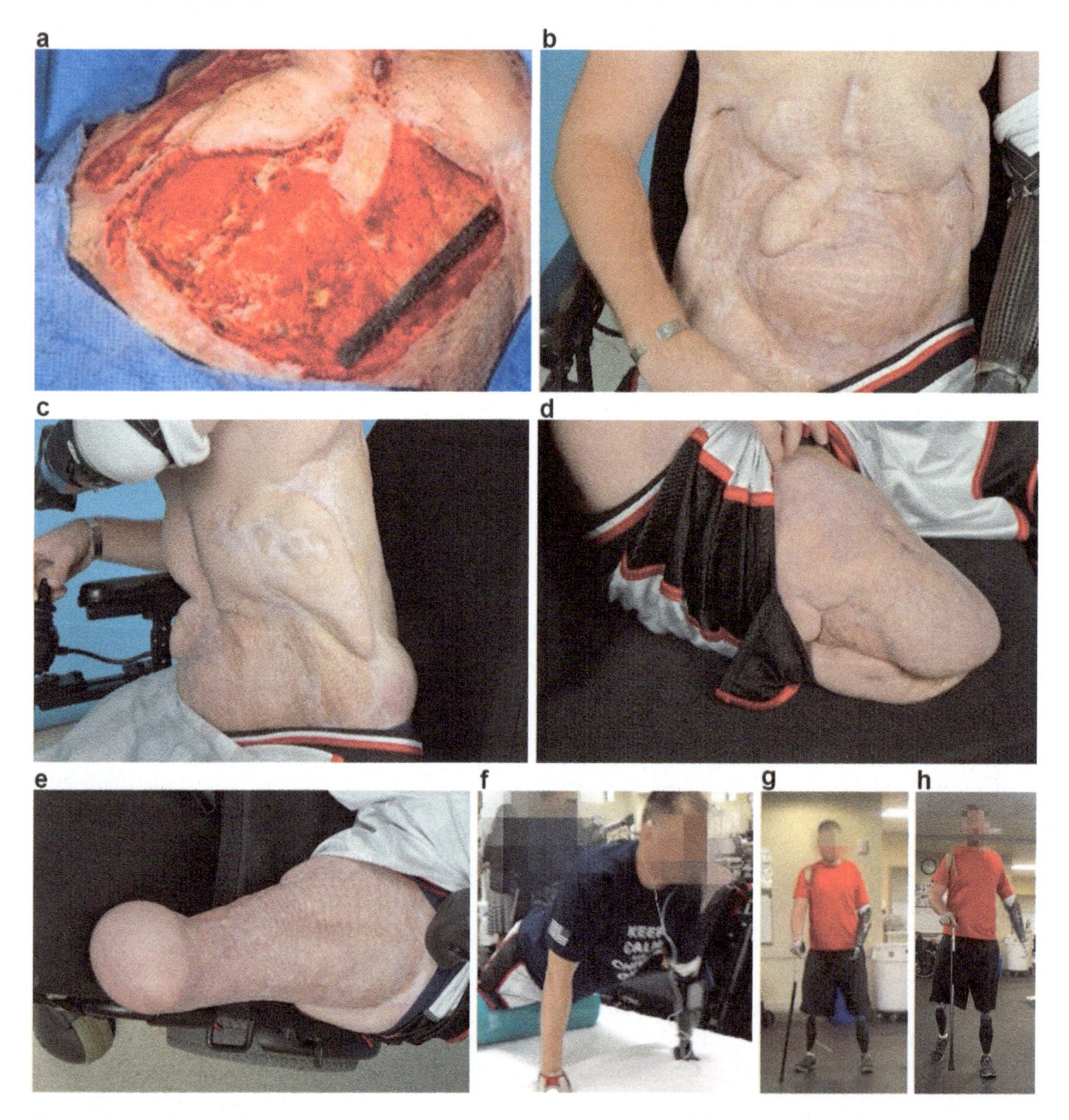

Fig. 16.9 (**a–h**) Application of hybrid reconstructive ladder for abdominal wall and lower extremity defects. (**a**) Significant abdominal defect before reconstruction; (**b–c**) abdominal wall reconstruction utilizing adjacent tissue transfers and spray skin for coverage; excellent pigmentation match was achieved; (**d–e**) lower extremity defects requiring spray skin; amputation with parascapular flap for creation of a sufficient soft tissue envelope to improve pain symptoms and optimize future prosthetic use; (**f–h**) successful definitive coverage allowing for functional prosthetic use and return to an active life

allowing for regeneration of the dermal layer by a dermal regenerative template [37] (Fig. 16.9).

Hammer et al. used spray skin in conjunction with split-thickness skin grafting following first-stage treatment with DRT. Once the DRT was absorbed and replaced with the patient's own collagen, the silicone layer was removed (about 3–5 weeks after DRT placement). Spray skin technology was then utilized by taking a small split-thickness skin sample and preparing it into a suspension containing keratinocytes, melanocytes, Langerhans cells, and fibroblasts. It is estimated that 1cm^2 of donor tissue can be used to cover an 80 cm2 defect. In this study, spray skin allowed surgeons to mesh STSG at a ratio of 6:1 vs. 1.5:1 and 3:1 with STSG alone. Furthermore, the use of spray skin reduced healing time and led to better pigmentation match when compared to STSG alone.

Peripheral Nerve Management

Any consideration of soft tissue coverage or reconstruction following a blast injury should consider the possibility of associated peripheral nerve injuries. It is critical that associated peripheral nerve injuries are appropriately diagnosed and the need for immediate or secondary nerve reconstruction or repair is incorporated into the reconstructive plan. The painful sequelae of neuroma formation have been identified as a major barrier to successful rehabilitation and improved quality of life in those with major limb amputations due to blast injury [40, 41]. Clinically, we have found chronic pain or lack of function secondary to peripheral nerve injury to be the principal driver for elective amputation following successful limb salvage, though there is a paucity of literature on this topic. On occasion, a qualified limb salvage candidate has been averse to the multiple operations and lengthy rehabilitation that is commonly required by limb salvage techniques and has desired early amputation in order to shorten his/her period of convalescence. In this circumstance, peripheral nerve transfers and advanced reconstructive techniques can be combined with amputation to deliver maximal functionality. Peripheral nerve techniques such as targeted muscle reinnervation (TMR) can be performed to provide intuitive and simultaneous control of the prosthesis and have recently been demonstrated to decrease the development of adverse sequelae such as neuromas [42]. TMR involves the transfer of residual, transected peripheral nerves to redundant target muscle motor nerves, with the goal of restoring physiologic continuity and encouraging more organized nerve regeneration. While originally developed to optimize prosthetic control by using target muscles as a bioamplifier for nerve signals, this procedure has been shown to be an effective treatment for neuroma and phantom limb pain [41].

Implantable myoelectric electrode systems (IMES) and advanced detection algorithms and techniques have further enhanced control of advanced prosthetics by improving the quality and consistency of the EMG control signals delivered to the device. Finally, the use of nerve and free tissue transfers in combination with elective amputation was first introduced by Aszmann et al. for management of severe injuries from high-energy trauma [43]. This approach has been embraced by our institution and, by combining complex reconstructive techniques with the most advanced prosthetic capabilities, represents the most recent evolution of the reconstructive elevator.

Future Endeavors

Current projects in regenerative medicine have yielded various options for soft tissue coverage in the recent years, all of which provide promising solutions to patients suffering from extensive soft tissue injuries. Further research in the field should focus not only on tissue substitutes but also on materials aimed to improve take of coverage by mimicking the role of the extracellular matrix. Recent studies have focused on the role of stem cells in creating a favorable wound-healing environment. Both mesenchymal (MSCs) and adipose stem cells (ASCs) are involved in wound healing throughout the body and have been shown to promote angiogenesis, improve epithelial migration, reduce inflammation, and promote formation of the ECM [44].

Currently, dermal substitutes such as Integra have been used in combination with MSCs for full-thickness defects with promising results; future exploration into the use of stem cells is necessary to advance our practice of soft tissue coverage.

Vascularized composite allotransplantation (VCA) has also gained the attention of many reconstructive surgeons and may be a future consideration for those with disfiguring trauma to the face or trunk or extremities. More than 100 VCAs have been performed worldwide, with a major restriction on advancement being the risk of lifelong immunosuppression [45]. Promising results have been achieved by combining decellularized allotransplantation with autologous stem cell transplant to achieve transplantation while avoiding the need for immunosuppression [46, 47].

Conclusion

Explosive attacks due to IEDs often result in devastating trauma with severe physical and psychological consequences. In recent years, blast injuries resulting in extensive soft tissue injury have begun to affect civilians following horrific acts of violence. While principles regarding soft tissue coverage in the setting of significant medical instability have been useful to military physicians in the past, these principles are now applicable to civilian reconstructive surgeons as well. This chapter, based on military management of blast reconstruction, sought to review principles of timing, reconstructive planning, and available technologies as a guide for extensive soft tissue reconstruction. Future studies focusing on stem cell technology, nerve regeneration, and composite allotransplantation will continue to advance our practices.

References

1. Schoenfeld AJ, Dunn JC, Bader JO, Belmont PJ Jr. The nature and extent of war injuries sustained by combat specialty personnel killed and wounded in Afghanistan and Iraq, 2003-2011. J Trauma Acute Care Surg. 2013;75:287–91.
2. Cannon JW, et al. Dismounted complex blast injuries: a comprehensive review of the modern combat experience. J Am Coll Surg. 2016;223:652–664.e8.
3. Kelly JF, et al. Injury severity and causes of death from Operation Iraqi Freedom and Operation Enduring Freedom: 2003–2004 versus 2006. J Trauma. 2008;64:S21–6; discussion S26–7.
4. Grady D. Study Maps 'Uniquely Devastating' Genital Injuries Among Troops. The New York Times. 2017.
5. Doukas WC, et al. The military extremity trauma amputation/limb salvage (METALS) study: outcomes of amputation versus limb salvage following major lower-extremity trauma. J Bone Joint Surg Am. 2013;95:138–45.
6. Zoroya G. How the IED changed the U.S. military. USA TODAY. 2013.
7. Lucy Rodgers Salim Qurashi. July London bombings: What happened that day? BBC News. 2015.
8. Burns TC, et al. Does the zone of injury in combat-related type III open tibia fractures preclude the use of local soft tissue coverage? J Orthop Trauma. 2010;24:697–703.
9. Shin EH, Sabino JM, Nanos GP 3rd, Valerio IL. Ballistic trauma: lessons learned from Iraq and Afghanistan. Semin Plast Surg. 2015;29:10–9.
10. Mossadegh S, Tai N, Midwinter M, Parker P. Improvised explosive device related pelvi-perineal trauma: anatomic injuries and surgical management. J Trauma Acute Care Surg. 2012;73:S24–31.
11. Han G, Ceilley R. Chronic wound healing: a review of current management and treatments. Adv Ther. 2017. https://doi.org/10.1007/s12325-017-0478-y.
12. Venturi ML, Attinger CE, Mesbahi AN, Hess CL, Graw KS. Mechanisms and clinical applications of the vacuum-assisted closure (VAC) device: a review. Am J Clin Dermatol. 2005;6:185–94.
13. Bowler PG, Jones SA, Walker M, Parsons D. Microbicidal properties of a silver-containing hydrofiber?? Dressing against a variety of burn wound pathogens. J Burn Care Rehabil. 2004;25:192–6.
14. Wright JB, Lam K, Burrell RE. Wound management in an era of increasing bacterial antibiotic resistance: a role for topical silver treatment. Am J Infect Control. 1998;26:572–7.
15. Wolvos T. Wound instillation – the next step in negative pressure wound therapy. Lessons learned from initial experiences. Ostomy Wound Manage. 2004;50:56–66.
16. Ollat D, Tramond B, Nuzacci F, Barbier O, Marchalan JP, Versier G. Vacuum-assisted closure: an alternative low cost method without specific components. About 32 cases reports and a review of the literature. Bull Acad Natl Chir Dent. 2008;7:10–5.
17. Maurya S, Bhandari PS. Negative pressure wound therapy in the management of combat wounds: a critical review. Adv Wound Care. 2016;5:379–89.
18. Mathieu L, et al. Soft tissue coverage of war extremity injuries: the use of pedicle flap transfers in a combat support hospital. Int Orthop. 2014;38:2175–81.
19. Tintle SM, Wilson K, McKay PL, Andersen RC, Kumar AR. Simultaneous pedicled flaps for coverage of complex blast injuries to the forearm and hand (with supplemental external fixation to the iliac crest for immobilization). J Hand Surg Eur Vol. 2010;35:9–15.
20. Webster D. Clinical applications for muscle and musculocutaneous flaps. S. J. Mathes and F. Nahai. 285 × 215 mm. Pp. 733 xvi with 1052 illustrations. 1982. London: Year Book. £102.00. Br J Surg. 1983;70:451–2.
21. Valerio IL, et al. Sequential free tissue transfers for simultaneous upper and lower limb salvage. Microsurgery. 2013;33:447–53.

22. Cho MS, et al. Functional outcome following nerve repair in the upper extremity using processed nerve allograft. J Hand Surg Am. 2012;37:2340–9.
23. Ray WZ, Mackinnon SE. Management of nerve gaps: autografts, allografts, nerve transfers, and end-to-side neurorrhaphy. Exp Neurol. 2010;223:77–85.
24. Valerio IL, Campbell P, Sabino J, Dearth CL, Fleming M. The use of urinary bladder matrix in the treatment of trauma and combat casualty wound care. Regen Med. 2015;10:611–22.
25. Cuadra A, et al. Functional results of burned hands treated with Integra®. J Plast Reconstr Aesthet Surg. 2012;65:228–34.
26. Hodde JP, Badylak SF, Brightman AO, Voytik-Harbin SL. Glycosaminoglycan content of small intestinal submucosa: a bioscaffold for tissue replacement. Tissue Eng. 1996;2:209–17.
27. McPherson TB, Badylak SF. Characterization of fibronectin derived from porcine small intestinal submucosa. Tissue Eng. 1998;4:75–83.
28. Mostow EN, Davin Haraway G, Dalsing M, Hodde JP, King D. Effectiveness of an extracellular matrix graft (OASIS Wound Matrix) in the treatment of chronic leg ulcers: a randomized clinical trial. J Vasc Surg. 2005;41:837–43.
29. Badylak SF. In: Tissue Engineering. 1993. p. 179–89.
30. Badylak SF, Lantz GC, Coffey A, Geddes LA. Small intestinal submucosa as a large diameter vascular graft in the dog. J Surg Res. 1989;47:74–80.
31. Badylak SF, et al. The use of xenogeneic small intestinal submucosa as a biomaterial for Achilles tendon repair in a dog model. J Biomed Mater Res. 1995;29:977–85.
32. Aiken SW, Badylak SF, Janas W, Boop FA. Small intestinal submucosa as an intra-articular ligamentous graft material: a pilot study in dogs. Vet Comp Orthop Traumatol. 1994;7.
33. Cobb MA, Badylak SF, Janas W, Boop FA. Histology after dural grafting with small intestinal submucosa. Surg Neurol. 1996;46(4):389–93; discussion 393.
34. Prevel CD, et al. Small intestinal submucosa: utilization as a wound dressing in full-thickness rodent wounds. Ann Plast Surg. 1995;35:381–8.
35. Prevel CD, et al. Small intestinal submucosa: utilization for repair of rodent abdominal wall defects. Ann Plast Surg. 1995;35:374–80.
36. Gravante G, et al. A randomized trial comparing ReCell system of epidermal cells delivery versus classic skin grafts for the treatment of deep partial thickness burns. Burns. 2007;33:966–72.
37. Wood FM, Stoner ML, Fowler BV, Fear MW. The use of a non-cultured autologous cell suspension and Integra® dermal regeneration template to repair full-thickness skin wounds in a porcine model: a one-step process. Burns. 2007;33:693–700.
38. Sood R, et al. A comparative study of spray keratinocytes and autologous meshed split-thickness skin graft in the treatment of acute burn injuries. Wounds. 2015;27:31–40.
39. Graham JS, et al. Medical management of cutaneous sulfur mustard injuries. Toxicology. 2009;263:47–58.
40. Bowen B, et al. Targeted Reinnervation for the amputee: a multi-cohort analysis. J Am Coll Surg. 2016;223:S102–3.
41. Souza JM, et al. Targeted muscle reinnervation: a novel approach to postamputation neuroma pain. Clin Orthop Relat Res. 2014;472:2984–90.
42. Tintle LTSM, Keeling CJJ, Shawen LSB, Forsberg LJA, Potter MBK. Traumatic and trauma-related amputations. J Bone Joint Surg Am Vol. 2010;92:2852–68.
43. Aszmann OC, et al. Bionic reconstruction to restore hand function after brachial plexus injury: a case series of three patients. Lancet. 2015;385:2183–9.
44. Tartarini D, Mele E. Adult stem cell therapies for wound healing: biomaterials and computational models. Front Bioeng Biotechnol. 2015;3:206.
45. Bueno EM, et al. Vascularized composite allotransplantation and tissue engineering. J Craniofac Surg. 2013;24:256–63.
46. Gonfiotti A, et al. The first tissue-engineered airway transplantation: 5-year follow-up results. Lancet. 2014;383:238–44.
47. Siemionow M. Vascularized composite allotransplantation: a new concept in musculoskeletal regeneration. J Mater Sci Mater Med. 2015;26:266.

Rehabilitation of the Blast Injury Casualty with Amputation

Keith P. Myers, Tirzah VanDamme, and Paul F. Pasquina

Introduction

In recent conflicts blast injuries have become very common, resulting in the recognition of an injury pattern now known as "dismounted complex blast injury" or "DCBI." According to the Report of the Army Dismounted Complex Blast Injury Task Force issued in 2011, a DCBI is defined as trauma inflicted upon a person on foot that produces a specific pattern of injury. It involves traumatic amputation of at least one lower limb with severe injury to at least one other extremity as well as pelvic, abdominal, or urogenital wounding [1]. A traumatic brain injury (TBI) is also often sustained, though this is not an explicit part of the Task Force's definition. Rates of such injuries have been high during the conflicts in Iraq and Afghanistan, increasing steadily after 2006 [2]. This reflects the tactical requirement and emphasis on dismounted patrols and engagements in an environment where improvised explosive devices (IEDs) and land mines have become more and more common. Improvements in emergency medical care and medical evacuation (MEDEVAC) procedures have resulted in fewer deaths from such injuries, which increased the number of very severely injured service members requiring extensive treatment interventions [3]. As of February 2018, greater than 1700 service members with amputations had been treated at one of three major military treatment facilities (MTFs). Of these, approximately 30% had multiple limb loss, and 18% had upper limb loss [4].

In the general population, trauma accounts for approximately 30,000 new amputations per year and is the leading cause of upper limb amputation in the United States. Vascular disease is eight times more common than trauma and so remains the leading cause of overall limb loss. This is due to the disproportionately higher number of individuals with vascular disease requiring lower limb amputation compared to upper limb. Most victims of a traumatic amputation are male between the ages of 15 and 30 [5]. Blast injuries that result in limb amputation are of considerable concern to the military. Such injuries are especially complex to care for because of the extent of associated soft tissue damage, high incidence of complications (e.g., infection and heterotopic ossification), as well as the high frequency of other comorbid injuries. These comorbid injuries can take the form of other musculoskeletal traumas, traumatic brain injury (TBI), paralysis, psychological trauma, and other sensory impairments, including vision and hearing dysfunction [6].

K. P. Myers · T. VanDamme · P. F. Pasquina (✉)
Department of Rehabilitation, Walter Reed National Military Medical Center, Bethesda, MD, USA

Department of Physical Medicine & Rehabilitation, Uniformed Services University of the Health Sciences, Bethesda, MD, USA
e-mail: paul.pasquina@usuhs.edu

Comprehensive care of individuals with traumatic amputation is challenging and requires an interdisciplinary team effort. Rehabilitative interventions should start as early during the acute phase of treatment as possible. This should include helping surgeons decide on the optimal level of amputation to maximize function with or without a prosthesis. Other early interventions include patient and family education, mitigation of secondary complications (e.g., contractures, deconditioning, decubitus ulcers), and initiation of therapy to maximize functional independence. While a discussion of all aspects of rehabilitation care for blast trauma casualties is beyond the scope of this chapter, the following sections will highlight many of the unique needs of those with amputation.

Immediate Post-op Rehabilitation

Rehabilitation professionals should be consulted in the immediate postoperative period of care for blast trauma casualties with amputation. Rehabilitative interventions should not be delayed until the patient is ready to be fit with a prosthetic device, as a significant delay will lead to reduced function and poorer outcomes [7]. A physician specialist in physical medicine and rehabilitation (PM&R) is a key component in this process. The PM&R specialist can assist the trauma team in assessing the patient's medical, surgical, behavioral health, pain, and rehabilitative needs. Further a PM&R specialist is skilled in initiating and enhancing patient and family education, coordinating interdisciplinary care, and helping with disposition planning. During the acute postoperative period, the patient can begin immediate physical and occupational therapy. Physical therapy services provided can include basic range of motion and strengthening exercises, bed mobility, transfer training, wheelchair training, core strengthening, as well as balance assessment and crutch mobility for those that can stand without a prosthetic device. In addition occupational therapists will work with the patient, family, and other caregivers on achieving independence with activities of daily living (ADLs), such as feeding, bathing, dressing, toileting, etc. For individuals with upper limb amputation, especially individuals who lose their dominant hand, this can be especially challenging. Occupational therapists will begin assessing upper residual limb function and patient goals, including potential myoelectric sites of control. They will initiate discussion with the PM&R specialist and prosthetist in regard to which type of prosthesis would likely be most advantageous for the patient.

Evidence suggests that the sooner the patient is introduced to the therapy suite where other individuals with amputation are being rehabilitated, the better [8]. This allows the patient to immediately see their potential and can help improve their outlook while setting new goals. The patient should be given "shrinker socks" or "shrinkers" as soon as possible after bulky dressings are removed [9]. A shrinker sock is similar to an elastic compression stocking but designed to fit over the residual limb. This assists in reducing swelling and can help relieve pain. Shrinker socks come in different sizes to accommodate upper and lower residual limbs. Immediately following surgery, significant swelling is typically present, which will persist or worsen if a shrinker sock is not worn consistently [10] (Fig. 17.1).

Prosthetic device fitting and training begins when the surgical team gives clearance for weight-bearing on the affected limb. While weight-bearing is typically not a consideration for upper limb amputees, the patient may require use of their upper limbs for transferring in and out of a bed or commode, propelling a wheelchair, or ambulating with crutches. Therefore, consideration should be given to the amount of forces that will likely be placed on the residual limbs after both upper and lower limb amputations. This is especially true for individuals with multiple limb loss. In general once the sutures are removed from the surgical site and healing has progressed as expected with no wound breakdown, the patient can be safely fit with a prosthetic socket [11].

Initial socket fitting is typically achieved by placing a sock over the residual limb and taking a mold of the limb with plaster, although some

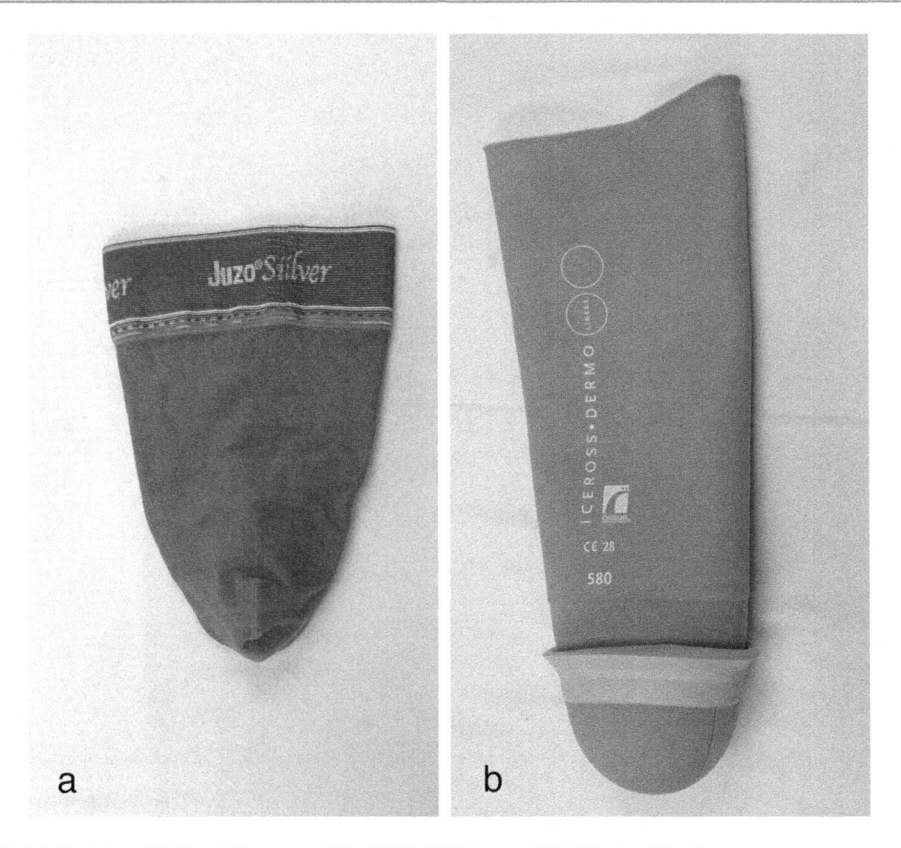

Fig. 17.1 (**a**) Shrinker, (**b**) liner (Courtesy of Dr. Keith P. Myers and Dr. Yinting Chen)

prosthetists may prefer to use a 3-D scanning technique. Once a positive mold of the residual limb is achieved, a custom socket can be built out of a moldable clear plastic ThermoLyn material that hardens after cooling. This serves as the initial "check socket" for the patient and is readily adjustable by using a heat gun and/or filing to increase comfort for the patient (Fig. 17.2a). As the size of the residual limb shrinks over time, further layers of socks can be worn by the patient to maintain a good socket fit. When a patient is nearing a 15-ply thickness of sock, a new socket is needed [12].

Depending on the extent of injuries, level of amputation(s), and functional capacity of the patient, ambulation with or without a prosthetic device may be significantly delayed, if achieved at all. Therefore, an appropriate wheelchair should always be considered for each patient. While a complete discussion of wheelchair types and features is beyond the scope of this chapter, providers are advised to consult assistive technology (AT) specialists, who are often physical or occupational therapists that have received certification training in AT or bioengineers that may often have a degree in AT. Some basic concepts regarding wheelchair design include whether it should be motorized, manually operated, or have a manual power-assist feature. Manual wheelchairs require choosing between a rigid or collapsible frame. Additionally the optimal seat cushion, seat dimensions, wheel height, and distance from the patient's center of mass must be determined. Finally, patients require training in wheelchair use in order to maximize function and reduce secondary injury from wheelchair propulsion [13, 14]. Most patients with lower limb amputation, particularly those who are expected to walk with a prosthesis, will find that a rental wheelchair is most appropriate for their immediate postoperative and subacute rehabilitative period. Typically their wheelchair needs will

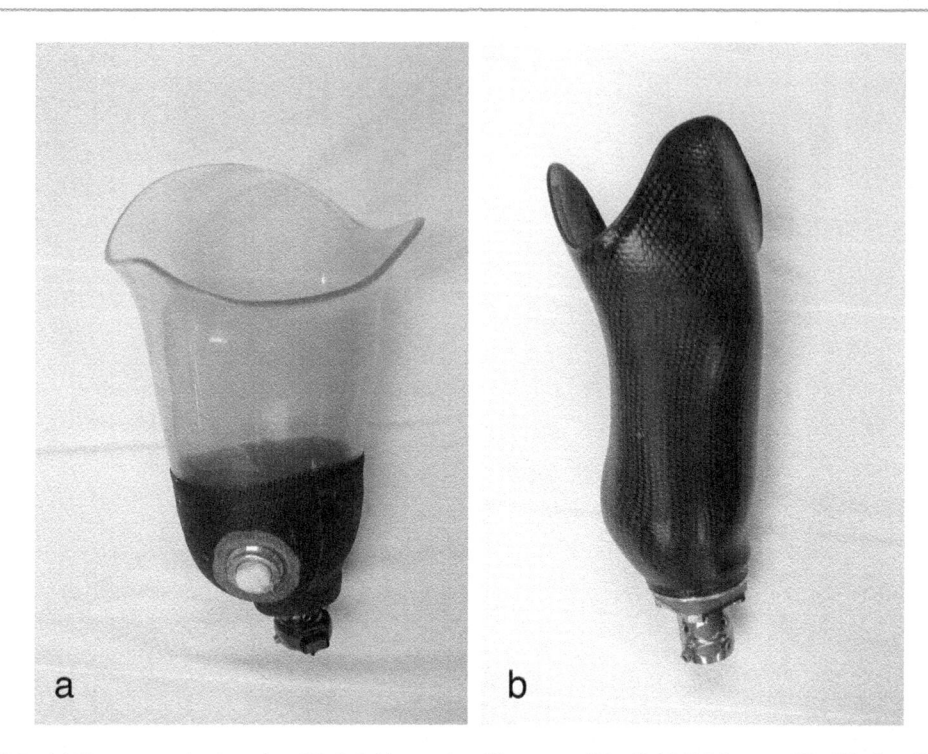

Fig. 17.2 (a) Temporary check socket, (b) definitive socket (Courtesy of Dr. Keith P. Myers and Dr. Yinting Chen)

change significantly as they begin fitting and training with a prosthetic device. Therefore, custom wheelchair fitting should be postponed until a time when the patient's body mass/dimensions are stable and when their ambulation and mobility needs are most apparent. It is important to note that even young trauma casualties who become proficient, lower limb prosthetic device users will often rely on a wheelchair as a backup mobility device [15].

Psychological Support

Trauma casualties require psychological support and counseling during the early stages of injury and recovery. Counseling should also extend to families, especially to the children of trauma casualties. Dealing with a parent's injury may be especially challenging for developing children, who may seek unhealthy coping strategies [16]. The loss of a limb can often be as emotionally challenging as losing a loved one, and the patient may go through a similar grieving process. Changes in body image and functional capabilities require a period of adjustment that may need guidance and specialized counseling [3]. Reestablishing and redefining relationships with friends and family may also be challenging. Likewise learning to use a prosthetic device and function daily without a limb can seem overwhelming. A patient's progress through the rehabilitation process can be impeded by insufficient support from caregivers or family members, feelings of social isolation, low self-esteem and depression, or social anxiety related to body image discomfort. Substance abuse issues may develop if the patient continues to have chronic pain or adjustment problems. Post-traumatic stress disorder (PTSD) may develop months after the actual injury, resulting in nightmares, depression, recurrent thoughts of their accident or injury, avoiding situations that remind them of the event, or feelings of being "keyed up" (hyperarousal) [17]. The patient may also experience "survivor's guilt" if others were severely injured or killed in the incident. Depression and anxiety are common after traumatic amputation and may significantly impair socioeconomic status, relationship with others, and overall quality of life [18]. Behavioral health professionals should be involved in the patient's care as soon as possible following their injury and should continue to monitor and assist the patient throughout the course of their rehabilitation [19]. While such symptoms may improve during inpatient rehabilitation, they can rise again upon discharge, requiring continued follow-up [20]. In addition to behavioral health and family support, patients also report significant value in peer support visitation [21].

Prosthetic Fitting

Prosthetists are licensed professionals typically with a master's degree level of education. They can guide the provider and patient in the proper choice of prosthetic components. As soon as the surgical team gives clearance for weight-bearing on the residual limb, the prosthetist can begin fitting of the prosthetic device. The use of shrinker socks aids the patient's residual limb in reducing in size due to swelling as well as encouraging it to assume a shape more appropriate for fitting into a socket [10]. This shrinking and shaping take place over several weeks to months. Therefore, the patient is fitted initially with a temporary thermoplastic socket or "check" socket as noted above. This socket allows for adjustments to accommodate painful areas and will likely need to be replaced multiple times as the patient's residual limb continues to shrink and change shape. A patient typically will go through anywhere between three and six thermoplastic sockets. When the patient's residual limb has finally stabilized to a consistent size and shape that is maintained over a consecutive period of 8–12 weeks, they are then fitted with a "definitive" socket. Definitive sockets are usually made of carbon fiber, which is much lighter and more durable than a thermoplastic socket (Fig. 17.2b). Definitive socket fitting usually occurs at around 6–18 months following the amputation surgery or last revision surgery, depending upon the extent of any comorbid injuries [3].

Lower Limb Prosthetics

Achieving a well-fitting and comfortable socket is fundamental to the success of using a lower limb prosthetic device. The socket is the interface between the patient's residual limb and his or her prosthetic device. It encloses the residual limb and attaches the prosthetic device to the patient. Many patients benefit from a gel liner (typically made of silicone) that the patient wears like a sock prior to donning the prosthetic socket (Fig. 17.1b). Suspension of the prosthetic limb can be achieved through suction between the liner and socket or by a metal pin that is embedded at the end of the gel liner and locks into the bottom of the socket upon inserting. Sockets for individuals with a very proximal transfemoral amputation, hip disarticulation, or hemipelvectomy are extremely challenging to fit and fabricate and require an experienced and highly skilled prosthetist [22].

For patients with a transfemoral amputation, appropriate prosthetic knee selection is very important. The knee can be of a simple mechanical design or feature varying resistance controlled by an integrated computer chip, referred to as a microprocessor knee. Mechanical knees may provide basic locking when standing and unlocking when sitting or more sophisticated hydraulic fluid resistance depending on advanced activities (Fig. 17.3). Over the last decade, significant advances have been made in microprocessor-controlled knees, which allow for more efficient and safer variable cadence ambulation [23]. Microprocessor-controlled knees have "onboard" computer devices that sense the speed and ground reactive forces of the prosthesis to adjust the resistance of the knee to better accommodate different walking speeds and create a smoother gait (Fig. 17.4). These devices can also prevent the knee from suddenly flexing while standing, creating a safer and more stable device. Microprocessor knees can also be programmed to work in various "modes" to accommodate various sports or recreational activities. In addition to microprocessor knees, powered lower limb prosthetic devices have recently emerged in clinical use. These have actuator motors strong

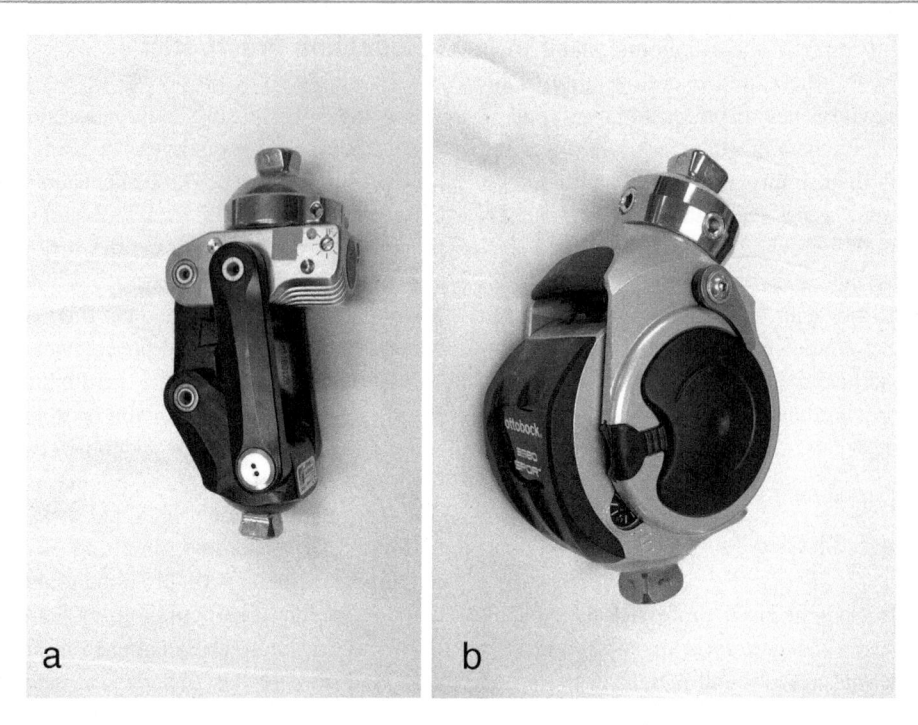

Fig. 17.3 Mechanical knees (Courtesy of Dr. Keith P. Myers and Dr. Yinting Chen)

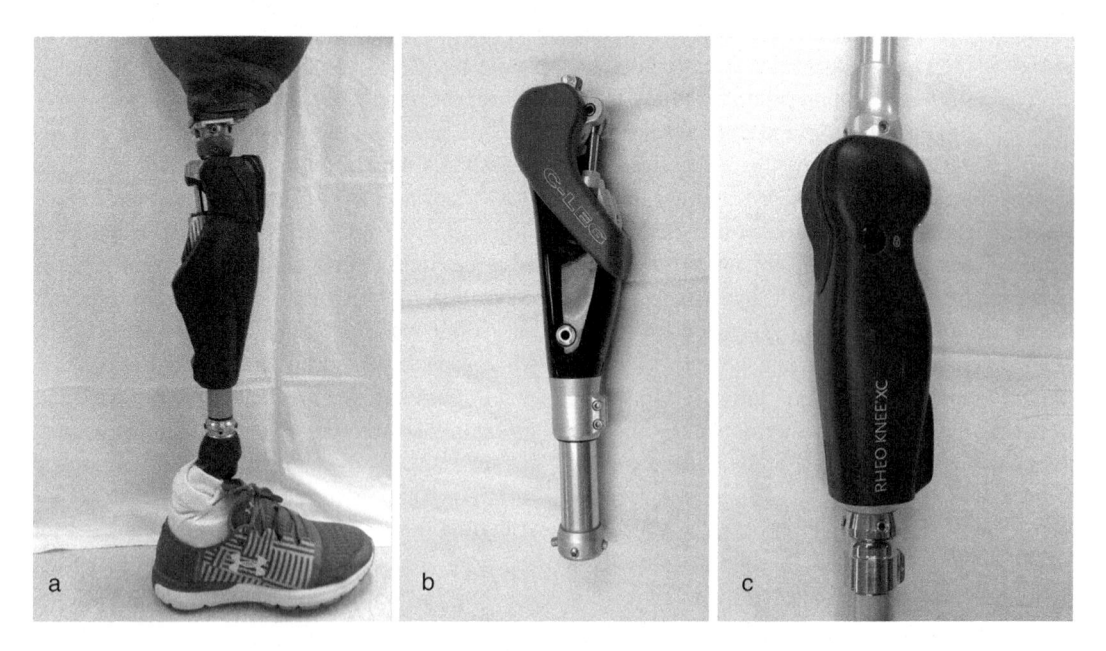

Fig. 17.4 Microprocessor knees (Courtesy of Dr. Keith P. Myers and Dr. Yinting Chen)

enough to propel a patient up ramps or steps [24]. This motor actively extends the knee of the device and moves the lower leg forward during the swing phase of gait, greatly decreasing the amount of energy expended by the patient. It can also actively assist the patient in standing from a seated position or in climbing stairs.

A pylon is used to connect the prosthetic knee to the foot for individuals with transfemoral amputation or the socket to the foot for individuals with transtibial amputation. Some pylons include shock-absorbing capabilities to make the patient's gait smoother and more comfortable or a small pump that creates a negative pressure within the socket to improve fit [25].

Prosthetic feet vary widely, depending on desired functional activities and patient preference. Most are made of carbon fiber and designed to give various levels of energy return when the patient loads them with their weight while walking or running. As the patient transfers their weight forward toward the "toe" of the prosthetic foot, the carbon fiber strut bends and absorbs energy like a spring and then releases this energy as the person continues their stride, simulating push-off into the next step. Some designs also accommodate side-to-side motion within the foot through a split keel that mimics pronation and supination to improve ambulation over uneven terrain [26] (Fig. 17.5a, b). Specialized prosthetic feet without heels are made specifically for running. These feet are often referred to as running "blades" and are useful for individuals who desire to return to long-distance running or sprinting [27]. Powered ankle devices are also now available and provide motor actuation to simulate active plantarflexion. This supports a more efficient gait and provides greater ease with long-distance walking or walking at faster speeds, especially on stairs or slopes [28] (Fig. 17.5c).

Upper Limb Prosthetics

Similar to lower limb prosthetics, successful upper limb prosthetic device use requires a well-fitting and comfortable socket. While self-suspending sockets exist for upper limb amputees, often axillary straps and harnesses are used for both suspension and control. These harnesses typically go across the shoulder and axilla of the contralateral side and have embedded cables that provide elbow and terminal device control for "body-powered" prosthetics. Through motions such as scapular protraction and shoulder flexion, patients are able to transmit tension through the cable system to open or close a terminal hand or hook (Fig. 17.6a). In addition to these "body-powered" upper limb prosthetic devices, externally powered myoelectric devices are also available for individuals with upper limb amputation. These devices are usually self-suspended through a suction socket and have embedded sensors that pick up surface EMG signals of the remaining flexors and extensors of the residual limb (Fig. 17.6b).

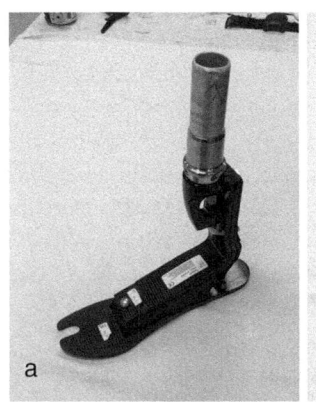

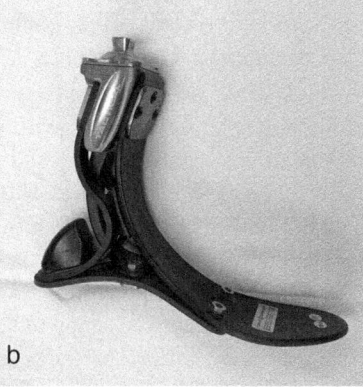

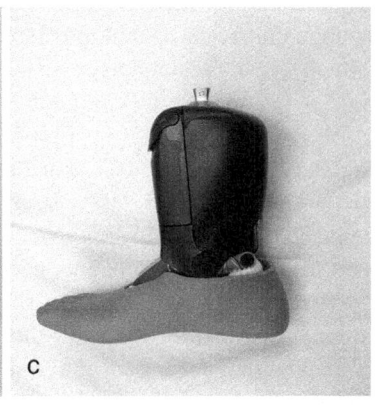

Fig. 17.5 (a–b) Energy return feet, c. powered ankle (Courtesy of Dr. Keith P. Myers and Dr. Yinting Chen)

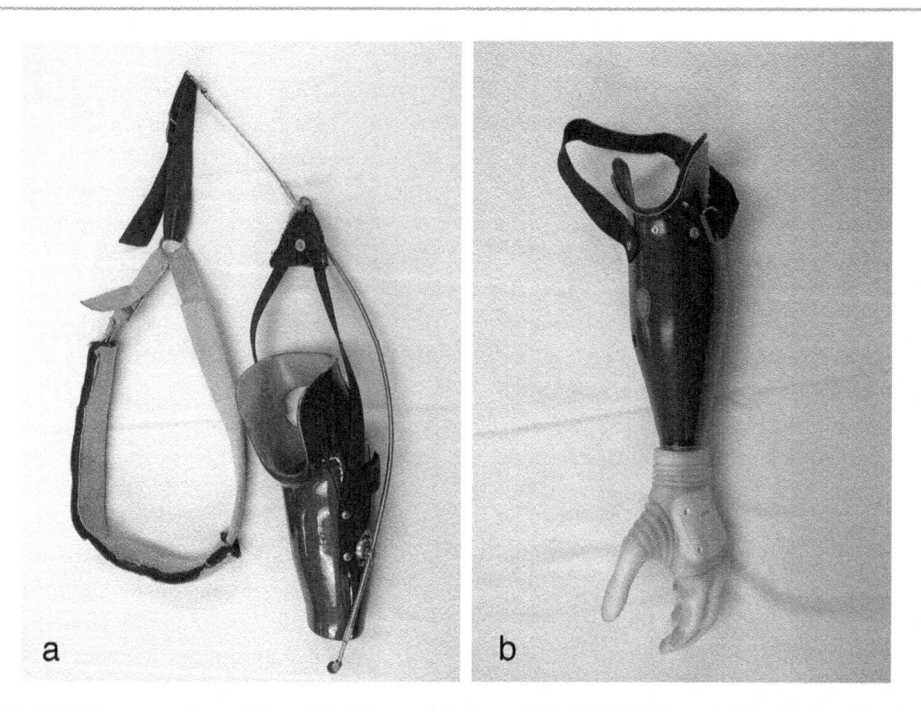

Fig. 17.6 (**a**) Body-powered arm, (**b**) myoelectric arm (Courtesy of Dr. Keith P. Myers and Dr. Yinting Chen)

Contraction of the residual limb muscles are recorded by these EMG sensors, which then trigger prosthetic elbow or terminal device motion. They can also be used to control motorized elbow flexion/extension, wrist pronation/supination, or terminal device opening/closing. Terminal devices range from simple hooks to full biomimetic hands with fingers and a thumb that can actually grasp like a human hand [29]. Specialized terminal devices also exist to support various activities including fishing, racket sports, weight lifting, archery, etc. (Fig. 17.7). It is common for individuals with upper limb amputation to have multiple terminal devices which they can interchange as needed depending on the specific task or sport in which they wish to participate [30]. High-definition cosmetic covers can also be created that match the patient's intact hand very closely (Fig. 17.8). Advances continue to be made in upper limb prosthetic devices including advanced strategies for human control [31] and the integration of robotic technology to allow the simultaneous manipulation of elbow, wrist, hand, and finger functioning [32, 33].

Phases of Rehabilitation

Comprehensive rehabilitative care of blast trauma casualties with amputation should be aimed at restoring the highest possible level of independent function. The elements of rehabilitation are often divided into four phases: (1) initial management, (2) preprosthetic, (3) prosthetic/ambulation, and (4) progressive activities/return to daily life.

As noted earlier, physical therapy can begin immediately during the postoperative period. As soon as the patient is able, he or she can begin working on functional activities such as bed mobility, transfers, dressing, hygiene and grooming, and contracture prevention/positioning measures. This will quickly progress to bedside strengthening and range of motion exercises, as well as wheelchair training and crutch mobility as needed. When the patient is able to go to the therapy suite, they can begin more extensive strengthening and stretching activities. Such exercises may include core strengthening/stabilization, balance, cardiovascular endurance, and ambulation with assistive devices. Once the

17 Rehabilitation of the Blast Injury Casualty with Amputation

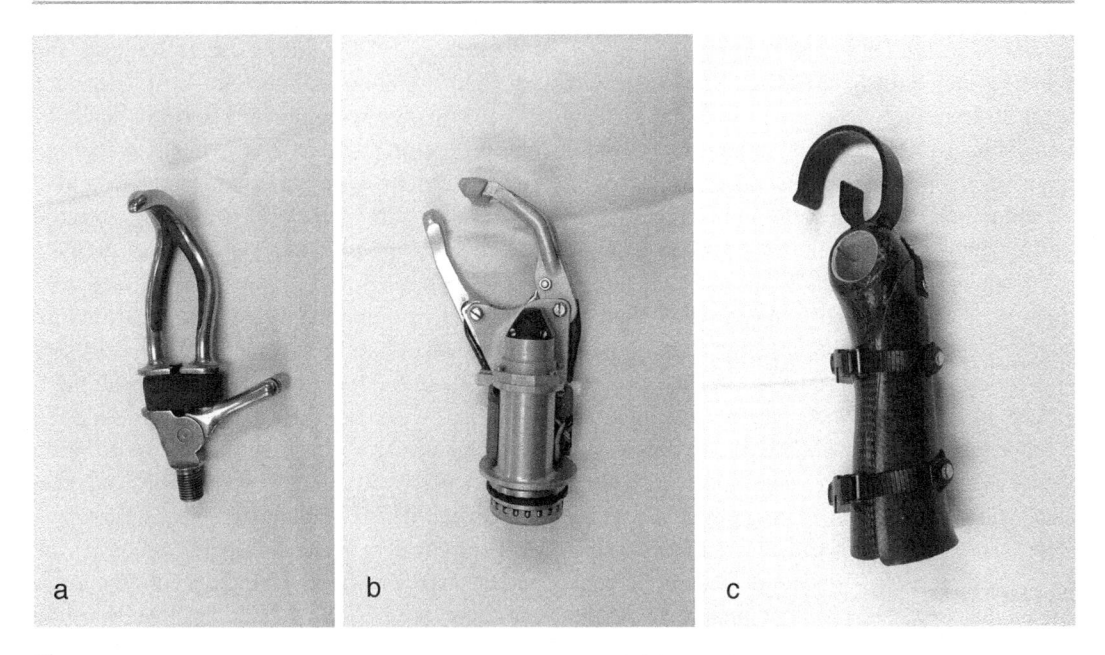

Fig. 17.7 Terminal devices (Courtesy of Dr. Keith P. Myers and Dr. Yinting Chen)

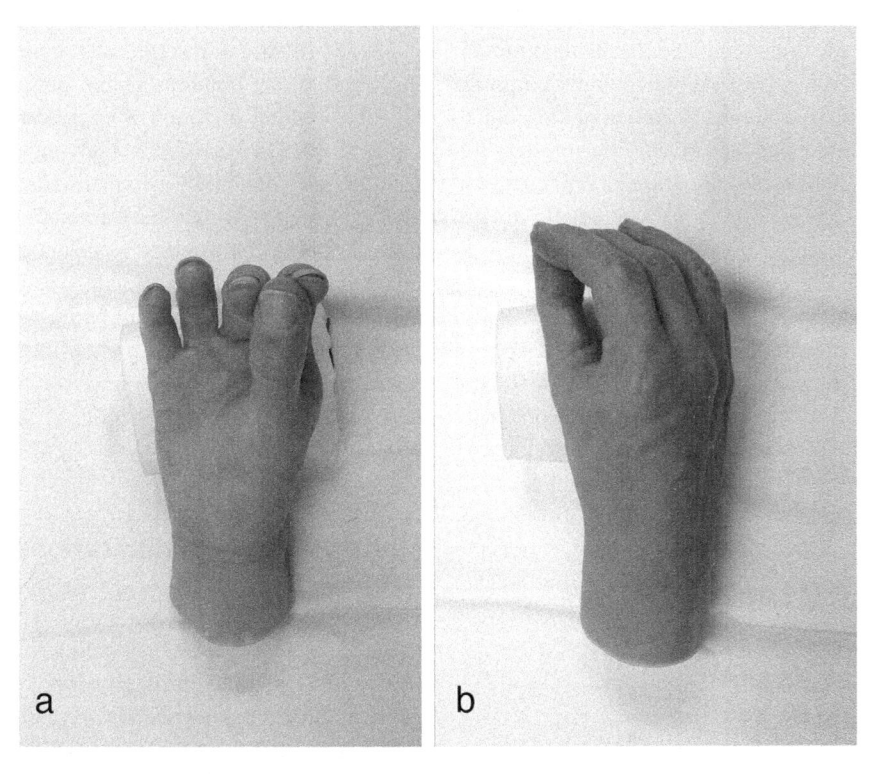

Fig. 17.8 Cosmetic cover (Courtesy of Dr. Keith P. Myers and Dr. Yinting Chen)

patient is cleared for weight-bearing, they can be fitted for their prosthetic device. They then will begin to learn how to don and doff the device, transition from sitting to standing positions, improve their standing tolerance, and begin weight transferring and early ambulation. Much of this begins at the parallel bars, with or without overhead harness weight support. Initial close monitoring is conducted to the residual limb to ensure tolerance of the prosthetic device, to appropriate socket fit, and to prevent skin or wound breakdown. Once patients are able to walk on level ground with or without an assistive device (e.g., single point cane or walker), they can begin training on navigating obstacles, stairs, slopes, and uneven or irregular surfaces using their prosthetic leg. When the patient demonstrates that they can use their prosthetic device safely and effectively, they are then allowed to take the device home with them and begin using it in their daily life.

In addition to their physical therapy, occupational therapy is also initiated during the immediate postoperative phase of care. Initial emphasis is made on assessing and initiating training to maximize independence in activities of daily living (ADLs). Patients are trained on functional tasks both with and without a prosthetic device. Patients are taught proper residual limb care as well as donning and doffing techniques for upper limb prosthetics. Patients receiving "body-powered" prosthetics begin training on control strategies. For those who receive myoelectric prosthetics, occupational therapists work with the physician, prosthetist, and patient to identify and isolate strong muscle contractions that can be used as myoelectric sites of control. Virtual reality training devices now exist to allow patients to practice myoelectric control even before socket fitting [34].

Sports and Recreation

Involving patients in sports and recreational therapy and/or music/art therapy may also be very helpful in supporting proficiency in prosthetic use, improving psychological well-being, improving fitness, avoiding social isolation, and enhancing quality of life. Not only does this allow a patient to return to activities that they enjoyed prior to their injury, it has also been shown to help with pain management, depression, and self-image [35]. Activity-specific prosthetic components and wheelchairs are now available that allow an individual with amputation or other impairments from trauma to return to high-level sports and recreational activities [36, 37]. Individuals with lower limb amputation that wish to resume running should be involved in a "return to run" therapy program that focuses specifically on strength, balance, and technique for running.

Throughout the rehabilitation process, the patient may also be receiving specific therapies for other injuries [38]. Injuries other than the amputation itself may complicate the rehabilitation process. For example, patients with coexisting hand injuries may have significant problems donning prosthetic devices or developing independence in ADLs. Patients with comorbid pelvic fractures or fractures in the non-amputated leg may remain in a non-weight-bearing status for a protracted period, not allowing prosthetic standing or ambulation. Patients with significant abdominal injuries may have impaired core stability, limiting their ability to balance and walk on a prosthetic device. Finally, patients with moderate to severe traumatic brain injuries may have problems understanding or implementing instructions from their therapists or have problems with balance, coordination, or sequencing of motor routines.

Management of Complications

Pain is a very common complaint after an amputation. This may be pain originating from trauma to the residual limb itself (somatic pain), pain generated from the nerves that were damaged or severed (neuropathic pain), or pain that the brain perceives as coming from the missing limb (phantom pain). Non-painful sensations from the phantom limb are referred to as "phantom sensations" and occur in the majority of patients with traumatic amputation. Even sensations that are not perceived as painful can be very annoying and somewhat alarming to a patient [39]. Phantom pain has been reported in approximately 80% of individuals with traumatic limb amputation and may manifest in a variety of uncomfortable sensations (e.g., cramping, sharp lancinating, burning, contorted positioning) [40]. Regardless of the source of pain that the patient might experience after a blast trauma, a multimodal management approach is typically most effective.

Somatic pain related to the injury and subsequent surgery often requires management with opioid medications. Opioid use should be carefully monitored because of common side effects such as impaired cognition, constipation, addiction, and misuse. Opioids should be tapered off and discontinued as soon as possible. Supplementation with NSAIDs and/or acetaminophen may help decrease opioid requirements. For patients that require opioids to achieve adequate pain relief, long-term preparations are often used to avoid peaks and troughs of opioid levels. These are given on a scheduled basis and titrated to adequately control the patient's pain while minimizing side effects. A short-acting opioid or opioid combination medication should be provided on an as-needed basis for "breakthrough" pain. These would be taken if the effect of the patient's long-acting opioid is wearing off and pain is returning prior to the next scheduled dose. The use of one or two doses of a short-acting medication between scheduled doses of the long-acting medication should be considered typical. If the patient is requiring increasing doses of a short-acting medication, this is an indication that the dosage of long-acting medication needs to be increased. Conversely, if the patient is not requiring any short-acting medication for breakthrough pain, then decreasing the dosage of the long-acting medication should be considered. The patient can also be transitioned off of the long-acting opioid and use only the short-acting medication as needed. Short-acting opioids can also be helpful as a means of pretreatment prior to therapy sessions in order to allow the patient to fully participate in rehabilitation, provided excessive drowsiness is not experienced [41].

Phantom limb pain and phantom sensations typically diminish over time after the patient begins wearing their prosthetic device [42]. The patient can be taught simple "desensitization" measures by their physical therapist such as tapping the end of their residual limb with their fingers, applying alternating warm and cold contrast water baths, or rubbing their residual limb with varying textures of fabric such as silk, faux fur, and burlap. "Mirror therapy" can also be performed. This is typically done during physical or occupational therapy sessions by having the patient look into a mirror that reflects their intact limb and makes it appear to take the place of their missing limb. They then think of moving both limbs through various motions while watching in the mirror. Medications such as gabapentin, pregabalin, and duloxetine can also be helpful in managing persistent phantom pain. Finally, other non-pharmacological therapies such as transcutaneous electrical nerve stimulation (TENS) and acupuncture may also be helpful in pain management [43].

A small number of patients may develop chronic and recalcitrant pain of either a somatic or neuropathic nature. An interventional pain management specialist should then be consulted, and procedures such as sympathetic nerve blocks, regional nerve blocks, a trial of IV ketamine, or the placement of a spinal cord stimulator may be considered.

A frequent source of residual limb pain after surgical amputation is a neuroma. A neuroma occurs in all transected nerves and is generally considered the equivalent of scaring of the distal nerve ending. Neuromas can range in size from slightly wider than the original nerve to several times the normal diameter of the nerve. While a full discussion of the surgical management of peripheral nerves during amputation surgery is beyond the scope of this chapter, most surgeons try to embed the distal end of the nerve deep within muscle and soft tissue to provide protection. This is thought to reduce the likelihood of developing a large neuroma as well as provide it with "cushioning" so that it is less sensitive. Current surgical practice often also includes consideration for reconnecting the distal nerve to remaining residual limb muscle, referred to as "targeted muscle reinnervation" (TMR) [44]. Neuromas can cause significant pain when they are compressed while using a prosthetic device. A prosthetist can make adjustments to the patient's socket to reduce the amount of pressure over a neuroma and improve comfort. The neuropathic pain generated by a neuroma can be treated with medications such as gabapentin, pregabalin, or duloxetine. If the neuroma can be visualized via the use of musculoskeletal ultrasound, the area immediately around it can be injected with a mixture of triamcinolone and lidocaine. This may provide relief from pain for several months or more. If the effect is only temporary, then using ultrasound guidance to ablate the neuroma with pulsed radiofrequency stimulation may provide longer relief. If the neuroma is recurrent or persistent and limiting the patient's ability to wear their prosthetic device, it will likely require surgical excision [45].

Low back pain (LBP) is a common complication following lower extremity amputation. Up to 50–70% of lower limb amputees will have back pain at some point, and it is more common in individuals with more proximal lower limb amputations [46]. Leg length discrepancy, excessive lumbar lordosis, excessive trunk motion, and altered gait symmetry are all factors that may contribute to LBP. Patients that have been the victim of a blast injury may have experienced a direct injury to their lower back that further complicates the presentation. The presence of LBP can have a strong impact on the patient's disability, function, and rehabilitation and so should be monitored closely [47]. The patient's prosthetist may need to make adjustments to the fit and alignment of the patient's prosthetic device to relieve stresses on the lower back. Patients with persistent or chronic lower back pain should be referred to a spine specialist for further assessment and appropriate treatment.

Heterotopic ossification (HO) is another common complication associated with traumatic amputation, especially blast-related trauma. HO is thought to be the formation of the bone from pluripotent mesenchymal cells within the muscles of the residual limb. While the exact mechanism for this bone formation is unclear, it is relatively common and may manifest within weeks to months of the injury. Depending on the location and extent of bone formation, HO may lead to restricted range of motion or pain, particularly with prosthetic socket wear. The patient's prosthetist can make adjustments to the patient's socket such as "blowouts," "cutouts," or adding padding to relieve pressure over an affected area. When accommodations cannot be made to the socket, surgical removal might be necessary. Surgical resection is typically delayed until the heterotopic bone is thought to be "mature" and has stopped growing, which may take between 6 and 12 months. Nonsteroidal anti-inflammatory drugs and bisphosphonates may be used to help prevent the formation of HO or to slow its growth [48].

Lastly, individuals with traumatic amputation frequently develop skin problems on their residual limbs. Having patients establish a routine of daily skin inspection and care is fundamental in preventing complications. A skin problem that is ignored has the potential of leading to secondary complications such as infection or the need for possible revision surgery. Most skin problems are related to the wearing of the prosthetic socket. Simple mechanical shear forces, friction, and stretching within a socket can stress vulnerable areas of the skin and lead to irritation and breakdown. While covering the residual limb with a silicon liner may offer some protection, it may also lead to significant sweating and potential skin maceration. Folliculitis is common and if not properly treated may become infected and lead to abscess formation. Excessive movement within the socket or underlying heterotopic ossification may also contribute to areas of friction within the socket. Patients who have had complicated wounds, including skin or soft tissue flaps are particularly susceptible to poor wound healing and future skin problems. In addition to frequent inspections, patients should be advised to wash their residual limb and their liners daily with a mild soap and water. Excessive hair growth on the residual limb can be associated with recurrent folliculitis. Shaving the hair often just increases the likelihood of developing folliculitis, so referral to a dermatologist for laser hair removal at the areas of the limb covered by the liner and socket should be considered if folliculitis becomes a recurrent problem. A patient may also develop a contact dermatitis when exposed to some shrinker sock or liner materials requiring a switch to a different material, manufacturer, or suspension system. In situations where the prosthetic socket has more pressure proximally than distally, this may create a "choke syndrome" and lead to "verrucous hyperplasia," a condition that develops over time leading to the skin at the distal residual limb becoming thickened and discolored giving a "warty" or "verrucous" appearance. This can usually be corrected by replacing the socket.

Lifelong Care

Despite the advances in prosthetic technology, ambulating on a prosthetic device requires greater energy and effort as compared to the patient's premorbid status. For individuals with traumatic transtibial amputation, the metabolic cost for ambulation increases by 25%, and for those with transfemoral amputation, energy demand increases by 63% [49]. Therefore, it is very important to encourage patients to maintain a healthy lifestyle in order to mitigate risks of cardiovascular disease, obesity, diabetes, and deconditioning that may lead to increased morbidity and mortality. Patients should be encouraged to avoid smoking, maintain a healthy diet, and exercise regularly to maintain their strength, endurance, and healthy body weight. Evidence suggests that after traumatic amputation, patients are at greater risk of developing hypertension, cardiovascular disease, obesity, diabetes, and depression than age-matched controls without amputation [5]. In addition, alterations in gait and body biomechanics increase their risk of developing degenerative joint disease in the lumbar spine and remaining intact joints of the lower extremities [50]. For those who frequently use crutches or a wheelchair for mobility, there is an increased risk for developing shoulder problems, entrapment neuropathies, or other upper limb overuse injuries, and these should be monitored over time. Finally, psychological issues such as PTSD, depression, and anxiety may persist in the long term in survivors of blast trauma and therefore should be followed closely.

Summary

Rehabilitation of blast trauma casualties with amputation is a complex process that requires a holistic interdisciplinary team approach. Support from friends, family, and peers is very important for the patient's recovery. Rehabilitative interventions should commence as early as possible to mitigate secondary complications, improve functional independence, and begin preparation for successful prosthetic fitting and training. Medical comorbidities and associated injuries should receive close attention and integrated care so as not to impair recovery and participation in rehabilitation. Providers, patients, and family members should be alerted to the common complications following traumatic amputation and employ strategies to prevent or treat them as quickly as possible. Individuals with limb amputation will require lifelong care and monitoring to help prevent or manage long-term health risks such as hypertension, cardiovascular disease, and diabetes. Furthermore, programs to promote independence, community participation, and resumption of sports and recreational activities can greatly enhance recovery and quality of life.

References

1. Ficke JR, Eastridge BJ, Butler FK, Alvarez J, Brown T, Pasquina PF, Stoneman P, Caravalho J. Dismounted complex blast injury report of the army dismounted complex blast injury task force. Journal of Trauma and Acute Care Surgery. 2012;73(6):S520–S534.
2. Cannon JW, Hofmann LJ, Glasgow SC, Potter BK, Rodriguez CJ, Cancio LC, Rasmussen TE, Fries CA, Davis MR, Jezior JR, Mullins RJ, Elster EA. Dismounted Complex Blast Injuries: A Comprehensive Review of the Modern Combat Experience. J Am Coll Surg. 2016;223(4):652–664.
3. Pasquina P, Cooper R. Care of the Combat Amputee. In: Lenhart M, editor. Textbooks of military medicine.

1st ed. Fort Sam Houston: Office of the Surgeon General, Department of the Army, United States Army and US Army Medical Department Center and School; 2009.
4. Extremity Trauma and Amputation Center of Excellence (EACE), 2017. Conflict Related Amputee Monthly Statistics Report, March 2017.
5. Meier RH 3rd, Heckman JT. Principles of contemporary amputation rehabilitation in the United States, 2013. Phys Med Rehabil Clin N Am. 2014;25(1):29–33.
6. Pasquina PF, Shero JC. Rehabilitation of the combat casualty: lessons learned from past and current conflicts. US Army Med Dep J. 2016;(2–16):77–86.
7. Pasquina PF. Twenty years forward. J Rehabil Res Dev. 2013;50(10).
8. Dillingham TR, Pezzin LE, Mackenzie EJ. Limb amputation and limb deficiency: epidemiology and recent trends in the United States. South Med J. 2002;95:875–83.
9. Gajewski D, Granville R. The United States armed forces amputee patient care program. J Am Acad Orthop Surg. 2006;14(10):S183–7.
10. Levy W, MF A, Barnes G. Skin problems of the leg amputee. JAMA. 1962:85–121.
11. Pasquina P, et al. Advances in amputee care. Arch Phys Med Rehabil. 2006;87(3):34–43.
12. Kuiken T, Huang M, Harden N. Perioperative rehabilitation of the transtibial and transfemoral amputee. Phys Med Rehabil. 2002;16(3).
13. Flemmer CL, Flemmer RC, et al. Disabil Rehabil Assist Technol. 2016;11(3):177–87.
14. Morgan KA, Engsberg JR, Gray DB. Important wheelchair skills for new manual wheelchair users: health care professional and wheelchair user perspectives. Disabil Rehabil Assist Technol. 2017;12(1):28–38.
15. Laferrier JZ, McFarland LV, Boninger ML, Cooper RA, Reiber GE. Wheeled mobility: factors influencing mobility and assistive technology in veterans and servicemembers with major traumatic limb loss from Vietnam war and OIF/OEF conflicts. J Rehabil Res Dev. 2010;47(4):349–60.
16. Cozza SJ, Cohen JA, Dougherty JG. Disaster and trauma. Child Adolesc Psychiatr Clin N Am. 2014;23(2):xiii–xvi. https://doi.org/10.1016/j.chc.2014.01.005.
17. Cavanagh S, Shin L, Karamouz N, Rauch S. Psychiatric and emotional sequelae of surgical amputation. Psychosomatics. 2006;47(6):459–64.
18. Mckechnie PS, John A. Anxiety and depression following traumatic limb amputation: a systematic review. Injury. 2014;45(12):1859–66.
19. Mohta M, Sethi A, Tyagi A, Mohta A. Psychological care in trauma patients. Injury. 2003;34(1):17–25.
20. Singh R, Ripley D, Pentland B, Todd I, Hunter J, Hutton L, Philip A. Depression and anxiety symptoms after lower limb amputation: the rise and fall. Clin Rehabil. 2009;23(3):281–6.
21. PasquinaPF TJW, Collins DM, Chan BL, Charrow A, Karmarkar AM, Cooper RA. Quality of medical care provided to service members with combat-related limb amputations: report of patient satisfaction. J Rehabil Res Dev. 2008;45(7):953–60.
22. Kralovec ME, Houdek MT, Andrews KL, Shives TC, Rose PS, Sim FH. Prosthetic rehabilitation after hip disarticulation or hemipelvectomy. Am J Phys Med Rehabil. 2015;94(12):1035–40.
23. Hafner B, et al. Evaluation of function, performance, and preference as Transfemoral amputees transition from mechanical to microprocessor control of the prosthetic knee. Arch Phys Med Rehabil. 2007;88(2):207–17.
24. Windrich M, Grimmer M, Christ O, Rinderknecht S, Beckerle P. Active lower limb prosthetics: a systematic review of design issues and solutions. Biomed Eng Online. 2016;15(Suppl 3):140. https://doi.org/10.1186/s12938-016-0284-9.
25. Klute G, Kallfelz C, Czerniecki J. Mechanical properties of prosthetic limbs: adapting to the patient. J Rehabil Res Dev. 2001;38(3):299–307.
26. Ko C-Y, et al. Comparison of ankle angle adaptations of prosthetic feet with and without adaptive ankle angle during level ground, ramp, and stair ambulations of a transtibial amputee: a pilot study. Int J Precis Eng Manuf. 2014;15(12):2689–93.
27. Rahman M, et al. Finite element analysis of prosthetic running blades using different composite materials to optimize performance. Am Soc Mech Eng Proc. 2014;10.
28. Yu T, et al. Testing an electrohydrostatic powered ankle prosthesis with transtibial and transfemoral amputees. IFAC-Papers Online. 2016;49(21):185–91.
29. Carey S, Lura D, Highsmith MJ. Differences in myoelectric and body-powered upper-limb prostheses: systematic literature review. J Rehabil Res Dev; Washington. 2015;52(3):247–62.
30. Behrend C, Reizner W, Marchessault J, Hammert W. Update on advances in upper extremity prosthetics. J Hand Surg. 2011;36(10):1711–7.
31. Pasquina PF, Evangelista M, Carvalho AJ, Lockhart J, Griffin S, Nanos G, McKay P, Hansen M, Ipsen D, Vandersea J, Butkus J, Miller M, Murphy I, Hankin D. First-in-man demonstration of a fully implanted myoelectric sensors system to control an advanced electromechanical prosthetic hand. J Neurosci Methods. 2015;244:85–93.
32. Resnik L, Klinger S, Etter K. The DEKA arm: its features, functionality, and evolution during the veterans affairs study to optimize the DEKA arm. Prosthetics Orthot Int. 2014;38(6):492–504.
33. Modular Prosthetic Limb, Johns Hopkins Applied Physics Lab. http://www.jhuapl.edu/prosthetics/scientists/mpl.asp.
34. Lambrecht JM, Pulliam CL, Kirsch RF. Virtual reality environment for simulating tasks with a myoelectric prosthesis: an assessment and training tool. J Prosthet Orthot. 2011;23(2):89–94.
35. Laferrier JZ, Teodorski E, Cooper RA. Investigation of the impact of sports, exercise, and recreation participation on psychosocial outcomes in a population of veterans with disabilities: a cross-sectional study. Am J Phys Med Rehabil. 2015;94(12):1026–34.

36. De Luigi AJ, Cooper RA. Adaptive sports technology and biomechanics: prosthetics. PM R. 2014;6(8 Suppl):S40–57.
37. Cooper RA, De Luigi AJ. Adaptive sports technology and biomechanics: wheelchairs. PM R. 2014;6(8 Suppl):S31–9.
38. Goldgerg K, et al. Integrated musculoskeletal rehabilitation care at a comprehensive combat and complex casualty care program. J Manip Physiol Ther. 2009;32(9):781–91.
39. Flor H. Phantom-limb pain: characteristics, causes, and treatment. Lancet Neurol. 2002;1(3):182–9.
40. Luo Y, Anderson TA. Phantom limb pain: a review. Int Anesthesiol Clin. 2016;54(2):121–39.
41. Chan MH, Pasquina PF, Tsao JW. Chapter 55: chronic pain after amputation in atlas of amputations and limb deficiencies. 4th ed. AAOS; 2016.
42. Weiss T, et al. Decrease in phantom limb pain associated with prosthesis-induced increased use of an amputation stump in humans. Neurosci Lett. 1999;272(2):131–4.
43. Alviar MJ, Hale T, Dungca M. Pharmacologic interventions for treating phantom limb pain. Cochrane Database Syst Rev. 2016;(10):CD006380.
44. Morgan EN, Kyle Potter B, Souza JM, Tintle SM, Nanos GP 3rd. Targeted muscle reinnervation for transradial amputation: description of operative technique. Tech Hand Up Extrem Surg. 2016;20(4):166–71.
45. Schnell M, Bunch W. Management of pain in the amputee. In: *Atlas of limb prosthetics: surgical, prosthetic, and rehabilitation principles*. Rosemont, IL: American Academy of Orthopedic Surgeons; 2002.
46. Kulkarni J, et al. Chronic low back pain in traumatic lower limb amputees. Clin Rehabil. 2005;19(1):81–6.
47. Ehde D, et al. Back pain as a secondary disability in persons with lower limb amputations. Arch Phys Med Rehabil. 2001;82:731–4.
48. Nauth A, et al. Heterotopic ossification in orthopaedic trauma. J Orthap Trauma. 2012;26(12):684–8.
49. Schmalz T, Blumentritt S, Jarasch R. Energy expenditure and biomechanical characteristics of lower limb amputee gait: the influence of prosthetic alignment and different prosthetic components. Gait Posture. 2002;16(3):255–63.
50. Gailey R, et al. Review of secondary physical conditions associated with lower-limb amputation and long-term prosthesis use. J Rehabil Res Dev. 2008;45(1):15–29.

Mild Traumatic Brain Injury Rehabilitation

18

Bruno S. Subbarao, Rebecca N. Tapia, and Blessen C. Eapen

Definition of Mild Traumatic Brain Injury

Mild traumatic brain injury (mTBI) and concussion are monikers that can be used interchangeably, although there lacks a consensus on a single definition. Several professional entities including the Department of Veterans Affairs/Department of Defense (VA/DoD), American College of Rehabilitation (ACRM), Centers for Disease Control and Prevention (CDC), and World Health Organization workgroups have offered attempts at a medical definition [1–3]. The VA/DoD Clinical Practice Guideline for the Management of Concussion/Mild Traumatic Brain Injury definition parallels these entities and defines traumatic brain injury (TBI) as a "traumatically induced structural injury and/or physiological disruption of brain function as a result of an external force and is indicated by new onset or worsening of at least one of the following clinical signs immediately following the event: any period of loss of or a decreased level of consciousness; any loss of memory for events immediately before or after the injury (posttraumatic amnesia); any alteration in mental state at the time of the injury (e.g., confusion, disorientation, slowed thinking, alteration of consciousness/mental state); neurological deficits (e.g., weakness, loss of balance, change in vision, praxis, paresis/plegia, sensory loss, aphasia) that may or may not be transient; intracranial lesion [1]." In this context, external forces not only encompass a direct blow from blunt objects but also acceleration/deceleration movements, penetrating trauma, and blast exposure mechanisms (Fig. 18.1).

B. S. Subbarao, D.O.
Polytrauma / Transition and Care Management Programs, Phoenix VA Health Care System, Phoenix, AZ, USA

R. N. Tapia, M.D.
Polytrauma Network Site, South Texas Veterans Health Care System, San Antonio, TX, USA

Department of Rehabilitation Medicine, University of Texas Health Science Center San Antonio, San Antonio, TX, USA

B. C. Eapen, M.D. (✉)
Polytrauma Rehabilitation Center, South Texas Veterans Health Care System, San Antonio, TX, USA

Department of Rehabilitation Medicine, University of Texas Health Science Center San Antonio, San Antonio, TX, USA
e-mail: blessen.eapen2@va.gov; eapen@uthscsa.edu

Demographics

According to the CDC, 2.5 million emergency department visits, hospitalizations, or deaths were associated with traumatic brain injuries in 2010 in the United States largely due to falls, blunt trauma, and motor vehicle accidents [5]. The true demographics of mTBI in the civilian population are difficult to accurately assess due to an unknown percentage who do not seek treatment after injury or who sought treatment outside of the emergency department. The CDC estimates that 75% of all

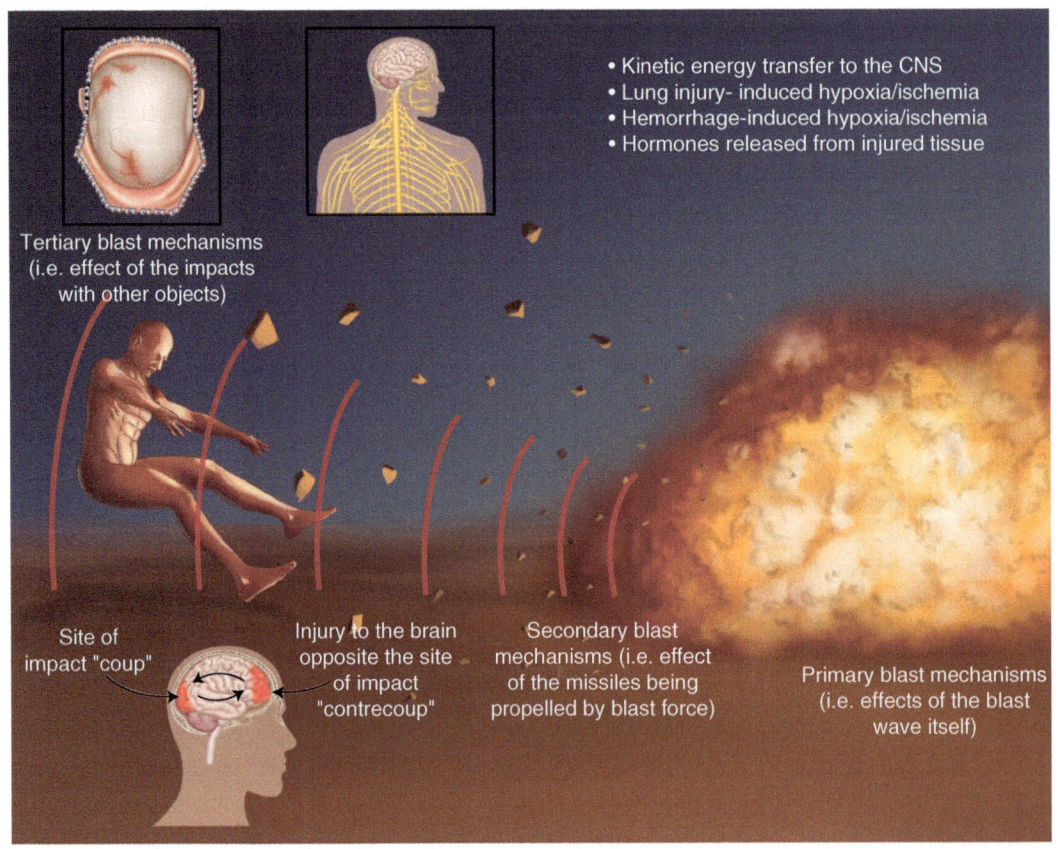

Fig. 18.1 Mechanisms of traumatic brain injury secondary to blast exposure (Adapted from Cernak and Noble-Haeusslein [4]. Sage. Web)

traumatic brain injuries in a given year are mild in severity [6]. From 2000 to 2016, there were 290,214 documented cases of mTBI in military personnel. The mTBI severity category accounted for 82.3% of all brain injury diagnoses (the remainder as moderate or severe) and an estimated 80% of mTBI occurred in garrison [7, 8].

Acute Assessment

Acute mTBI assessments are aimed at determining the appropriate level of care, including the need for possible transfer to emergency care, and minimizing exposure to additional injury (e.g., removing player from game). The history and physical examination should screen for "red flag" symptoms including an extended length of loss of consciousness, focal neurological signs, persistent confusion, or low Glasgow Coma Scale [9]. Physical examination should begin with a structured neurological examination and evaluation of the cervical spine for possible fracture or instability to assess the need for immediate immobilization [10, 11]. Persistent vomiting has also been shown to correlate with intracranial abnormalities after concussion [12]. Serial pupillary examination may be of benefit for determination of serious pathology and for prognostication in the long term [13]. Immediate

CT scan recommendations are based on the Canadian CT Head Rule, which has shown to be highly sensitive for intracranial injuries requiring intervention [14]. Patient risk factors are divided into high-risk and medium-risk categories and include the following:

- Presence of the aforementioned red flags
- Greater than or equal to two episodes of vomiting
- Age greater than 65
- Any sign of basilar, open, or depressed skull fracture
- Retrograde amnesia greater than 30 min
- Any dangerous mechanism, which consists of motor vehicle versus pedestrian, ejection from motor vehicle, or fall from more than 3 feet or more than five stairs [15]

In theater real-time concussion screening is performed by administration of the Military Acute Concussion Evaluation (MACE). It was devised for quick assessment and should be administered within 12 h of the blast or blunt force injury, as delay will diminish sensitivity and specificity below clinical utility [16]. The MACE is comprised of two parts that are essentially a concussion-specific history and focused physical examination. The Service Member will first be asked questions relevant to the event that led to their concussion followed by an assessment of orientation, memory, concentration, and a brief neurological examination [17]. If the MACE identifies concussion symptoms or a cognitive score less than 25, a consultation to a medical provider for higher level of care is recommended.

Other neurocognitive assessment tools may be employed for enhanced detection of symptoms of traumatic brain injury and/or to monitor recovery patterns. In the military setting, the Automated Neuropsychological Assessment Metrics (ANAM) is one such tool. It is a computer-based assessment battery administered at various points in time to assess reaction time, attention, cognitive abilities, and memory [18]. The ANAM is offered in the pre-deployment setting for baseline measures, during deployment for acute assessment within 72 h after sustaining concussion, and in the post-deployment stages to monitor recovery [19].

In the setting of contact sports, the Sport Concussion Assessment Tool (SCAT) is administered and combines brief neurocognitive screens, physical examination, orientation questions, and other objective findings in concussion for efficient sideline assessment [20]. The SCAT version 2 was widely implemented as a sideline concussion tool and even adopted by the National Football League and the National Hockey League [21]. It recently underwent a third revision, bolstering up physical examination findings and creating a pediatric adaptation, the Child-SCAT3 [22]. The utility of SCAT testing has been validated through extensive research in the athletic population, and recent studies demonstrated a high sensitivity for TBI symptoms in the emergency room setting as well [23].

Normal Recovery Patterns

A study on the clinical course of concussion after sport-related mTBI in high school and college demonstrated complete symptom resolution in 80–90% of athletes at the 2-week mark without medical intervention. Approximately 2.5% had no objective findings 45 days post-injury but continued to report symptoms related to their concussion [24]. Outside of athletes, concussion recovery patterns appear similarly predictable, with most individuals being able to expect full recovery without persistent sequelae after concussion in a matter of days, even in the absence of medical interventions. However, those with poor premorbid health conditions or who have suffered significant psychological distress tend to be at higher risk for development of persistent symptoms [25].

Post-concussive Syndrome

Post-concussive syndrome (PCS) is a nebulous diagnosis that encompasses the numerous physical, cognitive, and behavioral symptomatologies that continue to persist beyond the normal timeframe (> 3 months) for resolution. Symptoms can include headaches, insomnia, depression, anxiety, photophobia, phonophobia, irritability, dizziness/

Table 18.1 Post-concussive symptoms by domain

Domains	Common symptoms
Physical	Headache
	Vertigo/dizziness
	Fatigue
	Hearing difficulties
	Visual deficits
Emotional	Insomnia
	Neuropsychiatric illness
	Post-traumatic stress disorder
Cognitive	Poor memory, attention, concentration, processing speeds

Adapted from VA/DoD Clinical Practice Guidelines for Management of Concussion/Mild Traumatic Brain Injury, 2016 [27]

vertigo, poor concentration/attention, poor memory, and fatigue. However, these symptoms are certainly not specific to concussion and can be seen in great frequency in patients with diagnoses such as fibromyalgia, post-traumatic stress disorder, depression, chronic pain, and even those who are otherwise healthy [26]. A comprehensive approach including a thorough history and physical examination is imperative (Table 18.1).

Neuropsychological testing may help clarify contributors to post-concussive complaints. This will assist in future management of the patient, as treatment of PCS is primarily symptom-specific so long as no other disease entities are implicated. Feedback sessions following neuropsychological testing may enhance education and reassurance interventions which continue to be the cornerstone of treatment.

Post-traumatic Headaches

Post-traumatic headaches (PTHA), as defined by the International Classification of Headache Disorders 3rd beta edition, are secondary headache disorders that present within 7 days of trauma to the head. If loss of consciousness is involved, or if medications that impede normal recognition of headaches are started after the trauma, then the 7-day window begins after regaining consciousness or after cessation of the medication, respectively [28]. PTHA is defined as either acute (< 3 months) or chronic (> 3 months), with treatment based on primary headache type (e.g., migraine, tension type, etc.).

In developing a treatment plan, the clinician must consider other confounding factors such as post-traumatic stress disorder, depression, insomnia, anxiety, substance abuse, medication overuse, and any contributing musculoskeletal complaints which may precipitate headache symptoms [29]. Prophylactic medications are recommended in patients with high-frequency (three or more per week) or functionally limiting headaches and in the context of concurrent treatment of comorbid conditions [30]. The most common primary headaches and treatment options are provided in Table 18.2 below.

Cognitive Deficits

A recent systematic review of meta-analyses on the cognitive sequelae of mTBI demonstrated resolution in most individuals within 90 days after the injury. Cognitive sequelae in TBI can encompass issues affecting processing speed, attention, memory, or executive functions, with executive function being the domain most susceptible to multiple concussions [31]. A Cochrane review of multidisciplinary rehabilitation after mTBI suggested that education may be the most appropriate treatment for cognitive complaints after concussion [32]. A recent review of the pharmacologic treatment of the chronic cognitive deficits after TBI concluded that there remains insufficient evidence to recommend any agent at this time [33]. Thus, for the small percent of the patient population with persistent cognitive symptomatology, initial management should focus on behavioral modification interventions including improvement of sleep; reduction of stress; avoidance of alcohol, tobacco, and caffeine; adherence to daily exercise; maintenance of a balanced diet; and prevention of further brain injury [34]. Consideration of therapist-directed cognitive rehabilitation is warranted as a recent randomized controlled trial demonstrated significant improvement of day-to-day functional cognitive abilities of military personnel after concussion with chronic cognitive sequelae [35].

Table 18.2 Common post-traumatic headache types, characteristics, and treatment options

Headache type	Headache characteristics	Pharmacologic treatments

Migraines	Last >4 h
	+/− Aura
	Nausea
	Severe intensity
	Throbbing pain
	Not typically associated with muscle tenderness
		Abortive:
		  NSAIDs
		  Acetaminophen
		  Triptans
		  Ergotamines
		  Tramadol[a]
		  Opioids[a]
		Prophylaxis:
		  Avoidance of triggers
		  Regular exercise
		  Stress reduction
		  Improvement of sleep
		  Cold compress
		  Biofeedback
		  Tricyclic antidepressants
		  SSRI
		  Beta-blockers
		  Anticonvulsants

Tension	Typically associated with muscle tenderness
	Dull / pressure pain
		Abortive:
		  NSAIDs
		  Acetaminophen
		  Aspirin
		Prophylaxis:
		  Relaxation training
		  Biofeedback
		  Daily exercise
		  Physical therapy
		  Topiramate
		  Tricyclic antidepressants
		  Onabotulinum toxin A

Medication overuse headache	Chronic overuse of analgesic headache medication can cause rebound headaches Typically tension-like	Education on limiting abortive medications to no more than three times per week Analgesic holiday

Adapted from VA/DoD Clinical Practice Guidelines for Management of Concussion/Mild Traumatic Brain Injury, 2016 [27]

[a]The use of opioids for the treatment of headaches remains controversial, due to the high abuse potential and the need for regular monitoring and prescreens. Additionally, any analgesic medication has the potential to cause medication overuse headaches with excessive frequency of consumption

Vestibular Dysfunction

Vestibular dysfunction is reported in 20–50% of community patients and 80% of military personnel after suffering a mild to moderate traumatic brain injury [36]. Vestibular dysfunction can present as balance impairments, dizziness, vertigo, blurred vision, or an inability to manage busy environments. Interestingly, examination of sports concussions in a study of 107 high school football players demonstrated dizziness as the only on-field symptom predictive of a protracted recovery pattern [37]. Because of crossover and similarities between oculomotor dysfunction and impairment of the vestibular systems, clinical testing should focus on a thorough vision exam and balance assessment [38]. Despite a high prevalence of vestibular dysfunction after concussion, there is a dearth of quality research into the efficacy of rehabilitative approaches for management and treatment [39]. Treatment options may include a trial of vestibular rehabilitation, canalith repositioning maneuvers, and tai chi. Pharmaceutical management with anticholinergics or antihistamines in this population is limited by risk of worsening cognitive complaints or delaying recovery. For visual disturbances, gaze stability training or graded exposure to stimulus via virtual reality devices can be considered as well [40, 41].

Sleep Disturbances

A 2004 review demonstrated that up to 70% of patients suffered insomnia after traumatic brain injury [42]. Sleep may be disturbed because of an increased prevalence of obstructive sleep apnea (OSA), periodic limb movements, and hypersomnia in the post-traumatic brain injured population [43]. In the military TBI population, post traumatic stress disorder (PTSD) may affect perceived sleep quality, and depression may negatively impact both perceived sleep quality and cause alterations in sleep patterns [44]. Recognition and management of sleep disturbances are mainstays of concussion treatment, as recent studies demonstrated correlations between sleep disturbances and impairment in cognitive processes including executive functioning, memory, attention, and processing speeds [45, 46].

A non-pharmaceutical approach should be considered first and entails sleep hygiene measures which include:

- Routinely establishing times to go to sleep and wake up
- Minimizing stimulation from electronics or lights before bed
- Limiting caffeine intake
- Regulating diet
- Promoting daily exercise routines
- Designating the bedroom for only sleep, not work

A trial of cognitive behavioral therapy may help augment lifestyle modifications to improve sleep [47]. Evaluation for sleep apnea is strongly advised if suspected clinically as addressing this condition can improve multiple domains of outcomes including areas of cognition, pain, and mood. A pharmacological approach must be pursued with caution, as sedating medications in this patient population can interfere with function, slow cognitive processes, or prevent neural plasticity. Agents for consideration include melatonin agonists, melatonin, and trazodone, although an evidence base is still lacking [48]. Therefore, as with most medications, start low, go slow, and monitor closely for side effects.

Second Impact Syndrome

Second impact syndrome (SIS) is the catastrophic and possibly fatal event in which there is diffuse cerebral edema as a result of suffering a second traumatic brain injury before complete resolution of a first [49]. Although SIS is a rare and fairly controversial entity occurring once every 205,000 player seasons, SIS education on prevention is warranted, if for nothing more than protective measures against repeat brain injury [50, 51].

Return to Play (Zurich Guidelines)

In November of 2012, the 4th International Conference on Concussion in Sport was held in Zurich, Switzerland, which aimed to create consensus among a variety of pressing topics within the field, including an updated return to play guideline [20]. The stepwise progression has been outlined in Table 18.3. After a 24 to 48 h period of physical and cognitive rest, and once asymptomatic a gradual introduction of activity begins, and advancement occurs if the individual remains clear of post-concussive symptomatology. Each step warrants a 24-h period of symptom-free activity as described, with full return to play ideally achieved in 1 week [24].

Table 18.3 Comparison of return to play (Zurich) guidelines with return to activity (DVBIC) guidelines

Return to play (Zurich)		Return to activity (DVBIC)	
Activity level	Functional exercise	Activity level	Guidelines
1. None	Physical/cognitive rest	1. Rest	RPE 6-8, HR < 40% of TMHR, basic activities of daily living
2. Light aerobic exercise	Less than 70% of max heart rate	2. Light activity	RPE 7-11, HR < 55% of TMHR, light aerobics
3. Sport-specific exercise	Run drills	3. Light occupational activities	RPE 10-12, HR < 65% of TMHR, increased aerobics
4. Noncontact training	Resistance training	4. Moderate activity	RPE 12-16, HR 70–85% of TMHR, noncontact sports, light resistance training
5. Full-contact training	All training acceptable	5. Intense activity	RPE 16+, HR 85–100% of TMHR, weapon and driving training, increased resistance training
6. Return to play		6. Return to activity	

Adapted from McCrory [20] and McCulloch [52]

Return to Activity (DVBIC Guidelines)

The Defense and Veteran Brain Injury Center (DVBIC) in conjunction with the Office of the Army Surgeon General developed practical guidelines to standardize the management and return to activity protocols implemented in the military setting. Similar to the Zurich guidelines, the DVBIC recommends a stepwise approach beginning with rest and proceeding to increasing activity levels as tolerated. The DVBIC bases progression criteria on Neurobehavioral Symptom Inventory (NSI) scores and symptomatology at exercise tolerances based on Borg's Rate of Perceived Exertion (RPE) scale and theoretical maximum heart rate (TMHR) calculated using 220 minus years of age. If symptoms are graded a 2 or higher on the NSI, another 24 h at the individual's prior level is warranted. Beyond 6 days, referral to a higher level of care is justified [52]. Table 18.3 compares the return to activity guidelines with the Zurich return to play guidelines.

In the combat zone, after a Service Member suffers a potentially concussive event, a 24-h rest period is mandatory, unless their commander determines that their mission objectives override the medical recommendations. If this was a first concussion, the minimum rest time would be 24-h, with additional time as guided by clinical examination and symptom burden. If a second concussion is obtained within a year of the first, the mandatory rest period is extended to 1 week after resolution of symptoms. If a third concussion occurs in under 1 year, return to duty requires completion of a recurrent concussion evaluation, which includes neurological examination, neuroimaging, functional assessment, and neuropsychological assessment [53].

Conclusion

Mild traumatic brain injuries are complex entities, involving intracerebral disruptions that may temporarily affect a patient's physical, cognitive, and behavioral domains. Persistent symptoms are both challenging and multifactorial, often requiring expert clinical skills including a comprehensive, symptom-based and patient-centric approach. Education on the natural course of recovery, prevention of repeat head injury, and reassurance continue to be key components of management. Return to play/activity guidelines can help identify resolution of concussion or the need for higher levels of care.

References

1. Management of Concussion/mTBI Working Group. VA/DoD clinical practice guideline for management of concussion/mild traumatic brain injury. J Rehabil Res Dev. 2009;46:CP1–68.
2. Menon DK, Schwab K, Wright DW, Maas AI. Position statement: definition of traumatic brain injury. Arch Phys Med Rehabil. 2010;91:1637–40.
3. Carroll L, Cassidy JD, Peloso P, Borg J, von Holst H, Holm L, Paniak C, Pépin M. Prognosis for mild traumatic brain injury: results of the who collaborating centre task force on mild traumatic brain injury. J Rehabil Med. 2004;36:84–105.
4. Cernak I, Noble-Haeusslein LJ. Traumatic brain injury: an overview of pathobiology with emphasis on military populations. J Cereb Blood Flow Metab. 2010;30(2):255–66.
5. CDC – Traumatic Brain Injury – Injury Center. http://www.cdc.gov/traumaticbraininjury/. Accessed 5 Feb 2014.
6. TBI: Get the Facts|Concussion|Traumatic Brain Injury|CDC Injury Center. http://www.cdc.gov/traumaticbraininjury/get_the_facts.html. Accessed 26 Nov 2016.
7. DoD Worldwide Numbers for TBI|DVBIC. http://www.dvbic.org/dod-worldwide-numbers-tbi. Accessed 2 Apr 2013.
8. Helmick KM, Spells CA, Malik SZ, Davies CA, Marion DW, Hinds SR. Traumatic brain injury in the US military: epidemiology and key clinical and research programs. Brain Imaging Behav. 2015;9:358–66.
9. Su JK, Ramirez JF. Management of the athlete with concussion. Perm J. 2012;16:54–6.
10. Broglio SP, Cantu RC, Gioia GA, Guskiewicz KM, Kutcher J, Palm M, TC VML, National Athletic Trainer's Association. National Athletic Trainers' association position statement: management of sport concussion. J Athl Train. 2014;49:245–65.
11. Hyden J, Petty B. Sideline management of concussion. Phys Med Rehabil Clin N Am. 2016;27:395–409.
12. Bainbridge J, Khirwadkar H, Hourihan MD. Vomiting – is this a good indication for CT head scans in patients with minor head injury? Br J Radiol. 2012;85:183–6.

13. Hoffmann M, Lefering R, Rueger JM, Kolb JP, Izbicki JR, Ruecker AH, Rupprecht M, Lehmann W, Trauma Registry of the German Society for Trauma Surgery. Pupil evaluation in addition to Glasgow Coma Scale components in prediction of traumatic brain injury and mortality. Br J Surg. 2012;99(Suppl 1):122–30.
14. Papa L, Stiell IG, Clement CM, Pawlowicz A, Wolfram A, Braga C, Draviam S, Wells GA. Performance of the Canadian CT Head Rule and the New Orleans Criteria for predicting any traumatic intracranial injury on computed tomography in a United States Level I trauma center. Acad Emerg Med Off J Soc Acad Emerg Med. 2012;19:2–10.
15. Stiell IG, Clement CM, Grimshaw JM, et al. A prospective cluster-randomized trial to implement the Canadian CT Head Rule in emergency departments. CMAJ Can Med Assoc J J Assoc Medicale Can. 2010;182:1527–32.
16. Coldren RL, Kelly MP, Parish RV, Dretsch M, Russell ML. Evaluation of the military acute concussion evaluation for use in combat operations more than 12 hours after injury. Mil Med. 2010;175:477–81.
17. Stone ME, Safadjou S, Farber B, Velazco N, Man J, Reddy SH, Todor R, Teperman S. Utility of the military acute concussion evaluation as a screening tool for mild traumatic brain injury in a civilian trauma population. J Trauma Acute Care Surg. 2015;79:147–51.
18. Kelly MP, Coldren RL, Parish RV, Dretsch MN, Russell ML. Assessment of acute concussion in the combat environment. Arch Clin Neuropsychol Off J Natl Acad Neuropsychol. 2012;27:375–88.
19. Reeves DL, Winter KP, Bleiberg J, Kane RL. ANAM genogram: historical perspectives, description, and current endeavors. Arch Clin Neuropsychol Off J Natl Acad Neuropsychol. 2007;22(Suppl 1):S15–37.
20. McCrory P, Meeuwisse W, Aubry M, et al. Consensus statement on concussion in sport – the 4th international conference on concussion in sport held in Zurich, November 2012. Clin J Sport Med Off J Can Acad Sport Med. 2013;23:89–117.
21. Okonkwo DO, Tempel ZJ, Maroon J. Sideline assessment tools for the evaluation of concussion in athletes: a review. Neurosurgery. 2014;75(Suppl 4):S82–95.
22. Yengo-Kahn AM, Hale AT, Zalneraitis BH, Zuckerman SL, Sills AK, Solomon GS. The sport concussion assessment tool: a systematic review. Neurosurg Focus. 2016;40:E6, 1–14.
23. Bin Zahid A, Hubbard ME, Dammavalam VM, et al. Assessment of acute head injury in an emergency department population using sport concussion assessment tool – 3rd edition. Appl Neuropsychol Adult. 2016;1–10.
24. McCrea M, Guskiewicz K, Randolph C, Barr WB, Hammeke TA, Marshall SW, Powell MR, Woo Ahn K, Wang Y, Kelly JP. Incidence, clinical course, and predictors of prolonged recovery time following sport-related concussion in high school and college athletes. J Int Neuropsychol Soc JINS. 2013;19:22–33.
25. Cassidy JD, Cancelliere C, Carroll LJ, et al. Systematic review of self-reported prognosis in adults after mild traumatic brain injury: results of the international collaboration on mild traumatic brain injury prognosis. Arch Phys Med Rehabil. 2014;95:S132–51.
26. Wäljas M, Iverson GL, Lange RT, Hakulinen U, Dastidar P, Huhtala H, Liimatainen S, Hartikainen K, Öhman J. A prospective biopsychosocial study of the persistent post-concussion symptoms following mild traumatic brain injury. J Neurotrauma. 2015;32:534–47.
27. Management of Concussion-mild Traumatic Brain Injury (mTBI) (2016) – VA/DoD Clinical Practice Guidelines. http://www.healthquality.va.gov/guidelines/Rehab/mtbi/. Accessed 26 Nov 2016.
28. Headache Classification Committee of the International Headache Society (IHS). The international classification of headache disorders, 3rd edition (beta version). Cephalalgia Int J Headache. 2013;33:629–808.
29. Theeler B, Lucas S, Riechers RG, Ruff RL. Post-traumatic headaches in civilians and military personnel: a comparative, clinical review. Headache. 2013;53:881–900.
30. Lucas S. Headache management in concussion and mild traumatic brain injury. PM R. 2011;3(10 Suppl 2):S406–12. https://doi.org/10.1016/j.pmrj.2011.07.016
31. Karr JE, Areshenkoff CN, Garcia-Barrera MA. The neuropsychological outcomes of concussion: a systematic review of meta-analyses on the cognitive sequelae of mild traumatic brain injury. Neuropsychology © 2013 American Psychological Association. 2014;28:(3)321–36.
32. Turner-Stokes L, Pick A, Nair A, Disler PB, Wade DT. Multi-disciplinary rehabilitation for acquired brain injury in adults of working age. Cochrane Database Syst Rev. 2015;CD004170.
33. Dougall D, Poole N, Agrawal N. Pharmacotherapy for chronic cognitive impairment in traumatic brain injury. Cochrane Database Syst Rev. 2015;CD009221.
34. Flynn FG. Memory impairment after mild traumatic brain injury. Contin Minneap Minn. 2010;16:79–109.
35. Cooper DB, Bowles AO, Kennedy JE, Curtiss G, French LM, Tate DF, Vanderploeg RD. Cognitive rehabilitation for military service members with mild traumatic brain injury: a randomized clinical trial. J Head Trauma Rehabil. 2016. https://doi.org/10.1097/HTR.0000000000000254.
36. Chamelian L, Feinstein A. Outcome after mild to moderate traumatic brain injury: the role of dizziness. Arch Phys Med Rehabil. 2004;85:1662–6.
37. Lau BC, Kontos AP, Collins MW, Mucha A, Lovell MR. Which on-field signs/symptoms predict protracted recovery from sport-related concussion among high school football players? Am J Sports Med. 2011;39:2311–8.
38. Broglio SP, Collins MW, Williams RM, Mucha A, Kontos AP. Current and emerging rehabilitation for concussion: a review of the evidence. Clin Sports Med. 2015;34:213–31.
39. Bland DC, Zampieri C, Damiano DL. Effectiveness of physical therapy for improving gait and balance in

individuals with traumatic brain injury: a systematic review. Brain Inj. 2011;25:664–79.
40. Pavlou M, Davies RA, Bronstein AM. The assessment of increased sensitivity to visual stimuli in patients with chronic dizziness. J Vestib Res Equilib Orientat. 2006;16:223–31.
41. Hoffer ME, Gottshall KR, Moore R, Balough BJ, Wester D. Characterizing and treating dizziness after mild head trauma. Otol Neurotol Off Publ Am Otol Soc Am Neurotol Soc Eur Acad Otol Neurotol. 2004;25:135–8.
42. Ouellet M-C, Savard J, Morin CM. Insomnia following traumatic brain injury: a review. Neurorehabil Neural Repair. 2004;18:187–98.
43. Castriotta RJ, Wilde MC, Lai JM, Atanasov S, Masel BE, Kuna ST. Prevalence and consequences of sleep disorders in traumatic brain injury. J Clin Sleep Med JCSM Off Publ Am Acad Sleep Med. 2007;3:349–56.
44. Babson KA, Blonigen DM, Boden MT, Drescher KD, Bonn-Miller MO. Sleep quality among U.S. military veterans with PTSD: a factor analysis and structural model of symptoms. J Trauma Stress. 2012;25:665–74.
45. Wilde MC, Castriotta RJ, Lai JM, Atanasov S, Masel BE, Kuna ST. Cognitive impairment in patients with traumatic brain injury and obstructive sleep apnea. Arch Phys Med Rehabil. 2007;88:1284–8.
46. Mahmood O, Rapport LJ, Hanks RA, Fichtenberg NL. Neuropsychological performance and sleep disturbance following traumatic brain injury. J Head Trauma Rehabil. 2004;19:378–90.
47. Ponsford JL, Ziino C, Parcell DL, Shekleton JA, Roper M, Redman JR, Phipps-Nelson J, Rajaratnam SMW. Fatigue and sleep disturbance following traumatic brain injury – their nature, causes, and potential treatments. J Head Trauma Rehabil. 2012;27:224–33.
48. Larson EB, Zollman FS. The effect of sleep medications on cognitive recovery from traumatic brain injury. J Head Trauma Rehabil. 2010;25:61–7.
49. Bey T, Ostick B. Second impact syndrome. West J Emerg Med. 2009;10:6–10.
50. Cantu RC. Second-impact syndrome. Clin Sports Med. 1998;17:37–44.
51. McCrory P. Does second impact syndrome exist? Clin J Sport Med Off J Can Acad Sport Med. 2001;11:144–9.
52. McCulloch KL, Goldman S, Lowe L, Radomski MV, Reynolds J, Shapiro R, West TA. Development of clinical recommendations for progressive return to activity after military mild traumatic brain injury: guidance for rehabilitation providers. J Head Trauma Rehabil. 2015;30:56–67.
53. Conaton E. DoD policy guidance for management of mild traumatic brain injury/concussion in the deployed setting. Wash. DC Dep. Def. 2012.

Moderate and Severe Traumatic Brain Injury Rehabilitation

William Robbins and Ajit B. Pai

Introduction

Moderate and severe traumatic brain injury (TBI) results in a vast amount of morbidity and mortality each year. Immediately after TBI, the focus is on preventing secondary injury by stabilizing the individual both medically and surgically. Despite the outstanding care within the robust military, veterans, and civilian healthcare sectors, TBI still results in complex symptoms and sequelae that include physical, cognitive, psychological, and spiritual dysfunction. It is for this reason that care for the individual with TBI spans from the emergency department (or forward operating base) to the rehabilitation center.

Epidemiology

TBI was identified as "the signature injury" of the OEF/OIF conflicts. Blast injuries account for 81% of all OEF/OIF injuries [1, 2]. According to data from the Defense and Veterans Brain Injury Center (DVBIC), 313,816 military personnel sustained a TBI between the years 2000 and 2014. Of these TBIs, 83% were classified as mild, 8% moderate, and 1% severe in initial severity [3]. In the civilian setting, per the Centers for Disease Control and Prevention, TBI results in 2.5 million emergency department visits annually and contributed to the deaths of 50,000 people. However, the leading causes are different from the military setting, as most injuries are from falls in the civilian population [4]. Any system of care for persons injured by a blast mechanism in either the military or civilian setting must include robust and evidence-based practices, algorithms, and protocols for the evaluation, management, and rehabilitation of TBI.

Moderate and Severe Traumatic Brain Injury (TBI) Grading

Severity of injury is based upon several measures: length of coma (LOC), length of posttraumatic amnesia (PTA), and Glasgow Coma Scale (GCS) at time of emergency department evaluation. The severity is graded as the most severe of the measures, if a person exhibits different grading based on the three measures (Table 19.1). It is important to know that prolonged LOC and PTA have been associated with worse outcomes. Additionally, PTA and LOC tend to be better

W. Robbins
Polytrauma Transitional Residential Program, Hunter Holmes McGuire VA Medical Center, Richmond, VA, USA
e-mail: William.robbins@va.gov

A. B. Pai (✉)
Physical Medicine & Rehabilitation, Polytrauma Rehabilitation Center, Hunter Holmes McGuire VA Medical Center, Richmond, VA, USA
e-mail: Ajit.Pai@va.gov

indicators of outcome prognosis in patients with moderate to severe TBI. In comparison, initial GCS scoring may be complicated by intubation, sedation, and/or intoxication; thus, it is not as useful for prognostication.

Description of Injury

Brain injury can be further characterized by the biomechanics of the injury, findings of contusions, intracranial bleeding, and diffuse axonal injury (DAI) on neuroimaging, description and location of skull fractures, and presence of penetrating trauma. An open, or penetrating, head injury occurs when the head is struck by any object that breaks the skull and penetrates the dura mater. Brain contusions typically occur along bony prominences of the basilar skull, most commonly on the undersurface of the frontal and anterior temporal lobe but can also be seen along the occiput and cerebellum. DAI, a result of tensile strain and disruption of the axons due to rapid angular acceleration, is indicative of a more severe injury. Superficial axons and axons at the gray-white matter junction are most vulnerable. Neurons in the corpus callosum and midbrain also are susceptible to DAI. Thus, DAI can also be graded based upon anatomic location of injury. Table 19.2 describes the classification grading scale for DAI.

Neuroimaging, Intracranial Bleeding, and DAI

Computed tomography (CT) scan is the initial imaging of choice for persons with moderate to severe TBI. CT scan provides early detection of bleeds, skull fractures, contusions, and shift of the brain past its midline. CT is also considered standard of care when monitoring progression of injury and complications such as hydrocephalus or rebleed. MRI is recommended in the subacute and chronic setting. MRI is more sensitive in diagnosis and determining the extent of diffuse axonal injury.

Epidural hematomas (Fig. 19.1) result from local impact and injury to dural veins and arteries. Subdural hematomas (Fig. 19.2) result from inertial forces and tearing of bridging veins and are associated with falls. Subarachnoid hemorrhage (Fig. 19.3) results from angular acceleration and shearing of vessels located in the subarachnoid space.

Table 19.1 Severity classification of TBI

	GCS	PTA	LOC
Mild	13–15	<1 day	<30 mins
Moderate	9–12	1–7 days	30 min–24 h
Severe	<8	>7 days	>24 h

Table 19.2 Classification of diffuse axonal injury

Grade	
Grade I	Involves cortical gray-white matter junctions. At times can involve periventricular regions of gray-white matter
Grade II	Involves the corpus callosum in addition to grade I areas
Grade III	Involves the brain stem, usually the midbrain, in addition to areas involved in grade II

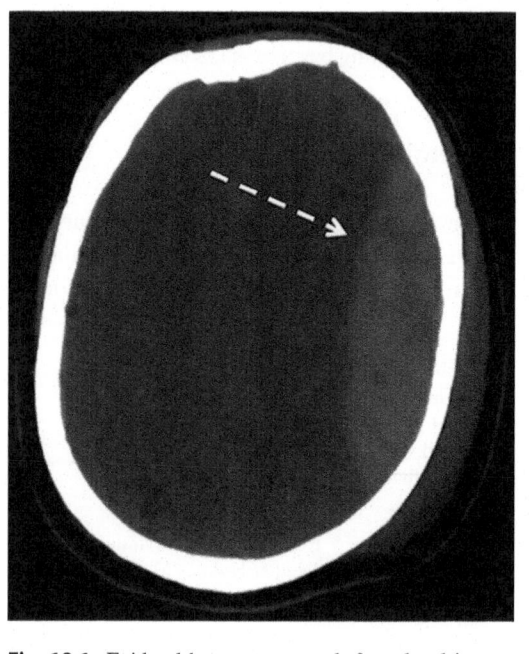

Fig. 19.1 Epidural hematomas result from local impact and injury to dural veins and arteries

19 Moderate and Severe Traumatic Brain Injury Rehabilitation

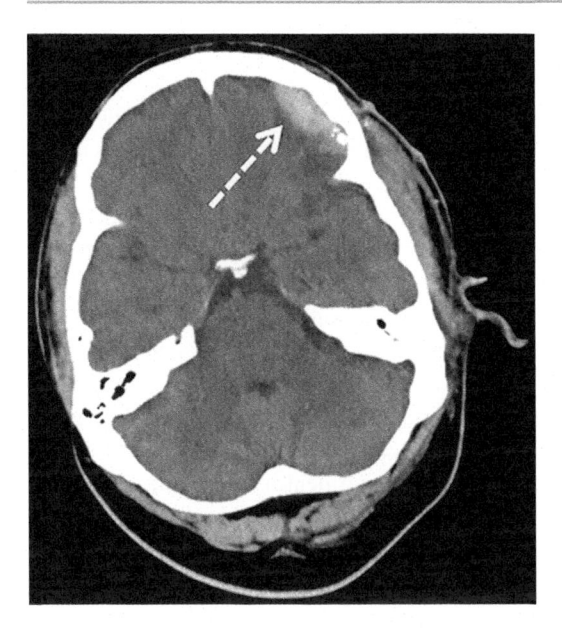

Fig. 19.2 Subdural hematomas result from inertial forces and tearing of bridging veins

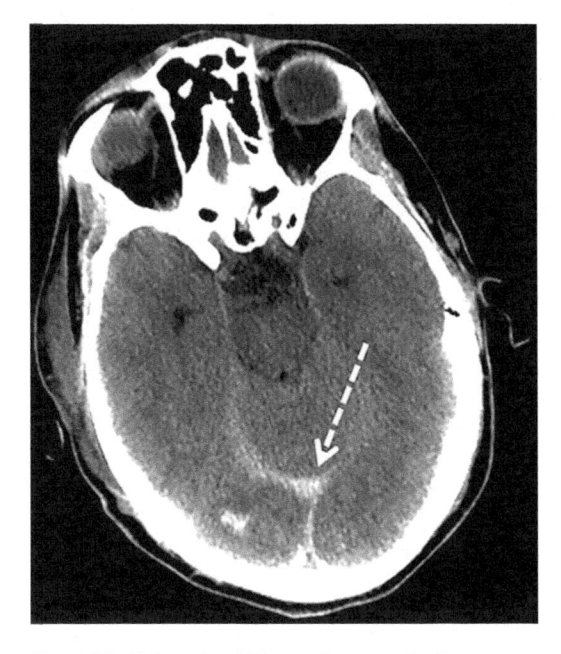

Fig. 19.3 Subarachnoid hemorrhage results from angular acceleration and shearing of vessels located in the subarachnoid space

Pathophysiology

Primary injury occurs at the time of impact and is caused by mechanical forces that lead to direct disruption of the brain tissue. These include focal areas of injury such as contusions and disruption of the vasculature leading to intracranial bleeding as well as more diffuse injury seen in DAI. Depressed skull fractures and penetrating trauma also lead to focal areas of injury by direct contact and/or direct disruption of vasculature.

Secondary injury develops over the hours and days after initial impact and is associated with alterations in normal brain metabolism, cerebral blood flow, cerebral edema, neurochemical and ionic changes, and anoxia leading to cellular injury and eventual cell death. Cerebral edema results in elevated intracranial pressure (ICP) and decreased cerebral perfusion pressure. Moreover, an increase in extracellular glutamate, free radicals, and inflammatory markers coupled with intracellular ionic influx leads to further cell death. The brain is in a hypermetabolic state during this time.

Blast Injuries

Blast-related TBI is comprised of four distinct components termed primary, secondary, tertiary, and quaternary [5, 6]. Primary blast injury is caused by blast wave-induced atmospheric changes. Secondary blast injury is caused by projectiles striking and/or penetrating the skull and brain. Tertiary blast injury is due to acceleration and deceleration of an individual put in motion by a blast and then stopped by a stationary object. Quaternary injury is the result of thermal and toxic detonation products that injure the head, face, scalp, and/or respiratory tract.

Along with the brain, hollow organs such as the lungs, gastrointestinal tract, and middle ear are most susceptible to primary blast injuries, as these organs are more susceptible to barotrauma. Pulmonary barotrauma may include pulmonary contusion, air emboli to the brain or spinal cord, and ARDS. Acoustic barotrauma can lead to tympanic membrane rupture, hemotympanum, as well as ossicle fracture. Mechanisms of secondary and tertiary blasts may lead to direct internal injury, as well as mutilation and amputation of the extremities. Advances in Kevlar® body armor, helmet technology, and other protective equipment, as well as improved acute trauma care, have increased the survival rate of injured personnel that would have likely proven fatal in prior conflicts [7].

Acute Medical Management

Initial assessment should include ABCs, full C-spine immobilization, initial GCS scores, head CT scan, lab work including type and screen and coagulation profiles, and monitoring ICP when indicated. If a patient has a GCS of 8 or less, or initial imaging shows signs of cerebral edema or midline shift, ICP should be monitoring in an ICU setting. Normal ICP is 15 mmHg with sustained elevations greater than 20 mmHg resulting in ischemia and possible herniation. Large depressed skull fractures, open depressed skull fractures, CSF leakage, evacuation of large bleeds, and midline shift of greater than 5 mm are the most common indications for immediate surgical intervention. Early decompression, specifically, the emergence of early craniectomy in order to relieve pressure around the brain has improved survival rates in the OEF/OIF conflicts.

Disorders of Consciousness

States of altered consciousness after severe TBI are referred to as disorders of consciousness (DOC). They are categorized as coma, vegetative state, and minimally conscious state (MCS). Emergence from a MCS is characterized by consistent functional object use and functional interactive communication [8]. Tracking progression is done with assessment tools such as the JFK Coma Recovery Scale-Revised. The goal in this stage of recovery is to prevent secondary medical complications while controlling the external environment to increase cortical stimuli with goal of emergence. Amantadine has been shown to promote recovery for persons with DOC.

Cognitive Disorders After TBI

Cognitive deficits are among the most debilitating and complex aspects of TBI to manage. Arousal is one of the most basic cognitive functions and is commonly affected after moderate to severe brain injury, especially in the acute phase. It is required to engage in all higher levels of cognition; norepinephrine is central to its function. Attention is also commonly impaired after moderate to severe TBI. Attention is a widely distributed cognitive function with impairments of attention affecting many other cognitive domains.

Memory impairment is one of the most common symptoms following brain injury, and it is estimated that time and cost of care would be reduced if effective medical treatments were found to improve memory [9]. Executive functions refer to higher-level cognitive functions that are primarily mediated by the frontal lobes. These functions include insight, awareness, judgment, planning, organization, problem-solving, multitasking, and working memory [10]. The frontal lobes tend to be one of the brain areas most likely to be injured following trauma [11].

In early stages of recovery, treatment can include interaction with family, early patient education, and orientation to medical situation. Later in recover, treatment can include cognitive remediation and retraining in independent living skills. Cognitive therapy may also be used to provide compensatory strategies for impairments across many cognitive domains, mainly in memory and executive functioning.

Pharmacologic treatment of cognitive dysfunction after TBI is largely based upon mechanism of action of the medication and literature for treatment of other disorders that present with cognitive dysfunction. There is evidence that donepezil may improve attention and short-term memory in subacute and chronic periods of recovery after moderate to severe TBI [12]. Methylphenidate may be used to enhance arousal, attention, and speed of cognition. Bromocriptine may be used to enhance aspects of executive functioning [12].

Neurobehavioral Dysfunction and Management

Agitation is commonly seen acutely in patients with moderate to severe TBI. This particular behavior indicates the patient is in the awakening phase of their recovery, but it is one of the more difficult behavioral and/or emotional impairments to manage for both the rehabilitation team and family [13]. It may present as periods of verbal or physical aggression, motor restlessness, and/or sexual disinhibition. Agitation is commonly assessed using the Agitated Behavior Scale, a 40-point scale that can be completed by a trained staff member effectively and reliably. A score of > = 21 indicates agitation.

Reducing environmental stimuli, limiting the number of visitors and staff in the room at a given time, and calm redirection and reorientation to the patient's situation are typical first-line treatment for posttraumatic agitation. One-to-one staff supervision and the use of soft restraints should be considered if the patient is at risk for pulling out lines or tubes, high fall risk, or at risk of self-harm. It is imperative to know that liberal use of restrains may increase agitation as persons with TBI in cognitive suppressed states may feel overly restricted.

First line of pharmacologic treatment is typically beta-blockers and mood-regulating antiepileptics. Neuroleptics, antidepressants, and benzodiazepines may also be used. When treating agitation pharmacologically on an as needed basis, it is often helpful to set parameters for use based on ABS scoring to help guide staff in appropriate administration.

Hypoarousal and sleep disturbances are common in moderate to severe TBI. It is important to rule out any underlying condition or medication that may be contributing. Focus should be placed on restoring sleep-wake cycle and implement proper sleep hygiene. The therapeutic schedule and task intensity should be adjusted to prevent fatigue.

Mental Health Disorders

Depression and anxiety are common residual symptoms regardless of TBI severity. Early treatment can help optimize recovery and improve quality of life. Treatment is similar to treatment in individuals without a traumatic brain injury and usually involves intervention with pharmacologic and non-pharmacologic treatment. It is important to rule out any underlying conditions such as endocrine dysfunction that may mimic depression.

Patients with more severe injuries who are amnestic to their traumatic event are associated with lower incidence of PTSD. However, case studies [14–19] and cohort studies [20] have noted the existence of PTSD developing following severe TBI. PTSD should be screened for if there is clinical suspicion regardless of TBI severity.

Role of Neuropsychological Testing

Neuropsychological testing is commonly used in assessment of multiple cognitive domains after TBI. The purpose of neuropsychological testing varies depending on the stage of recovery. Full neuropsychological tests batteries are usually not administered until several months after a moderate to severe brain injury. These tests may be used to help determine return to work, employability, capacity, ability to manage finances, and to assess ongoing cognitive recovery. However, testing may be used during TBI rehabilitation to assist with diagnosis and treatment planning.

Medical Complications in Moderate to Severe TBI

Autonomic storming is a result of sympathetic imbalance and presents with hypertension, hyperthermia, tachycardia, and diaphoresis. This is mostly seen in the acute stage but can occur any time after TBI. First-line treatment includes propranolol, morphine, and baclofen.

Posttraumatic seizures (PTS) are classified in three categories: immediate, within 1 day of injury; early, within 1 week of injury; and late, occurring after 1 week. Prophylactic treatment with an antiepileptic for 7 days can prevent early seizures but has not been proven to prevent PTS or posttraumatic epilepsy. Patients that have an early or late PTS are at higher risk for seizures in the future and often time require long-term treatment. Risk factors for developing posttraumatic epilepsy have been identified, including biparietal contusion, dural penetration, multiple intracranial surgeries, subdural hematoma with evacuation, focal temporal or frontal lesions, and midline shift >5 mm [21–23].

Heterotopic ossification (HO) usually affects the hips, shoulders, and elbows following severe TBI but can affect any joint or muscle tissue. It is more common after moderate or severe TBI with significant physical impairment. Symptoms include pain, decreased range of motion, redness, and swelling. Untreated HO can lead to permanent loss of range across a joint, pain, and nerve compression. First-line treatment is range of motion exercises. The use of calcium-chelating agents and NSAIDs can halt progression. The use of calcium-chelating agents should be avoided in patients with multiple healing fractures. Surgical intervention is reserved for mature lesions.

Spasticity is commonly managed with range of motion, splinting, oral agents, and local chemodenervation. Intrathecal baclofen pumps can be used for more severe lower extremity spasticity. Common first-line oral agents such as baclofen, tizanidine, and diazepam all cause cognitive slowing. Dantrolene, which acts peripherally, can be used to avoid cognitive slowing.

Hydrocephalus can occur with or without increased intracranial pressure. Signs of hydrocephalus include gait ataxia, urinary incontinence, altered mental status, and headaches. Neuroimaging may show signs of hydrocephalus. A large volume lumbar tap can be diagnostic and therapeutic by temporarily alleviating symptoms. Definitive treatment is placement of an intraventricular shunt, which typically drains into the pleura or the peritoneum.

The pituitary gland can be damaged given its anatomic location either by direct trauma, disruption of its blood supply, or by hypoxia and ischemia. Sodium abnormalities such as SIADH and diabetes insipidus can commonly be seen in the acute and subacute phases of injury, and electrolytes should be closely monitored during this time. Routine screening is not recommended in the acute phase; however, it is recommended at three and six months for patients with moderate to severe TBI [24–26]. However, there is no general consensus on screening at this time. Screening panel includes morning cortisol, thyroid panel, FSH, LH, testosterone in men, and estrogen in women.

Appropriate venous thromboembolism (VTE) prophylaxis, speech therapy, and enteral feeding methods can prevent other common injuries such as blood clots and aspiration [27]. Constipation is also very common in the acute and subacute stages of injury and should be treated with an aggressive bowel regiment to prevent complications. Patients with moderate to severe TBI are at higher risk for obstructive sleep apnea both in the acute and chronic stages and should be screened when clinically indicated.

VA-DoD Continuum of Care

Due to the complex needs of active duty service members (ADSM) injured in combat, VA and DoD created an integrated continuum of care to optimize the health of ADSMs with TBI. The parts of this continuum are known as the Joint Theater Trauma System in DoD and the Polytrauma System of Care (PSC) in VA. Within the DoD, there are five levels of care that are utilized: Level I is in theater care provided by the medic; Level II is stabilization provided by the surgical team in the forward operating base; Level III is the intensive and subspecialty care provided at the combat support hospital; Level IV is the care received at the medical evacuation point, typically Landstuhl Regional Medical Center; and lastly, Level V is the continued care at an military treatment facility in the continental United States, such as Walter Reed National Military Medical Center.

After patients are stabilized and ready for rehabilitation, ADSMs are often transferred to VA's PSC. There are five Level I centers located in Richmond, VA; Minneapolis, MN; San Antonio, TX; Palo Alto, CA; and Tampa, FL. These centers provide acute inpatient rehabilitation with additional services such as vision rehab, kinesiotherapy, driver's rehabilitation, and other specialized treatments. In addition, each site has a residential community reentry program for individuals with TBI. These programs allow a full reintegration into society with some outcomes including return to duty and work.

Conclusion

TBI is one of the "hallmark" injuries suffered by blast-injured patients in both the military and civilian settings. The rehabilitation of persons with TBI requires a number of healthcare providers from the field to the rehabilitation center and beyond. The amount of care these persons require stretches the resources of any system; thus, it is imperative that cross collaboration between DoD, VA, and the civilian sector occurs. Coordinated care is instrumental in allowing individuals with brain injury to fully recover. Additional research and innovation in strategies to treat TBI patients in order to maximize not only survival but also long-term functional and psychological outcomes is sorely needed.

References

1. Brenner LA, Homaifar BY, Adler LE, Wolfman JH, Kemp J. Suicidality and veterans with a history of traumatic brain injury: precipitants events, protective factors, and prevention strategies. Rehabil Psychol. 2009;54(4):390–7.
2. Barnes DE, Kaup A, Kirby KA, Byers AL, Diaz-Arrastia R, Yaffe K. Traumatic brain injury and risk of dementia in older veterans. Neurology. 2014;83(4):312–9.
3. Defense Medical Surveillance System (DMSS), Theater Medical Data Store (TMDS) provided by the Armed Forces Health Surveillance Center (AFHSC), prepared by the Defense and Veterans Brain Injury Center (DVBIC). PDF available for download at: http://dvbic.dcoe.mil/dod-worldwide-numbers-tbi.
4. Centers for Disease Control and Prevention. Traumatic Brain Injury Get the Facts. 2016 [cited 2016 Nov 28]. Available from: http://www.cdc.gov/traumaticbraininjury/get_the_facts.html.
5. Rosenfeld JV, McFarlane AC, Bragge P, Armonda RA, Grimes JB, Ling GS. Blast-related traumatic brain injury. Lancet Neurol. 2013;12(9):882–93.
6. Warden D. Military TBI during the Iraq and Afghanistan wars. J Head Trauma Rehabil. 2006;21(5):398–402.
7. Okie S. Traumatic brain injury in the war zone. N Engl J Med. 2005;352(20):2043–7.
8. Giacino JT, Ashwal S, Childs N, et al. The minimally conscious state: definition and diagnostic criteria. Neurology. 2002;58(3):349–53.
9. McLean A Jr, Stanton KM, Cardenas DD, Bergerud DB. Memory training combined with the use of oral physostigmine. Brain Inj. 1987;1:145–59.
10. Lezak MD. Neuropsychological assessment. 2nd ed. New York: Oxford University Press; 1983.
11. Greenwald BD, Burnett DM, Miller MA. Congenital and acquired brain injury. 1. Brain injury: epidemiology and pathophysiology. Arch Phys Med Rehabil. 2003;84:S3–7.
12. Bayley M, Teasell R, Kua A, Marshall S, Cullen N, Colantonio A. ABIKUS evidence based recommendations for rehabilitation of moderate to sever acquired brain injury. 1st ed. Ontario Neurotrauma Foundation; Toronto, 2007.
13. Luauté J, Plantier D, Wiart L, Tell L, SOFMER group. Care management of the agitation or aggressiveness crisis in patients with TBI. Systematic review of the literature and practice recommendations. Ann Phys Rehabil Med. 2016;59(1):58–67.
14. Bryant RA. Posttraumatic stress disorder, flashbacks, and pseudomemories in closed head injury. J Trauma Stress. 1996;9:621–9.
15. Bryant RA, Harvey AG. Traumatic memories and pseudomemories in posttraumatic stress disorder. Appl Cogn Psychol. 1998;12:81–8.
16. Koch WJ, Taylor S. Assessment and treatment of motor vehicle accident victims. Cogn Behav Pract. 1995;2:327–42.
17. Layton BS, Wardi Zonna K. Posttraumatic stress disorder with neurogenic amnesia for the traumatic event. Clin Neuropsychol. 1995;9:2–10.
18. McMillan TM. Post-traumatic stress disorder and severe head injury. Br J Psychiatry. 1991;159:431–3.
19. McMillan TM. Posttraumatic stress disorder following minor and severe closed head injury: 10 single cases. Brain Inj. 1996;10(10):749–58.
20. Bryant RA, Marosszeky JE, Crooks J, Gurka JA. Posttraumatic stress disorder after severe traumatic brain injury. Am J Psychiatry. 2000;157:629–31.
21. Temkin NR. Risk factors for posttraumatic seizures in adults. Epilepsia. 2003;44(Suppl 10):18–0.
22. Englander J, Bushnik T, Duong TT, et al. Analyzing risk factors for late posttraumatic seizures: a prospective, multicenter investigation. Arch Phys Med Rehabil. 2003;84(3):365–73.

23. Yablon SA. Posttraumatic seizures. Arch Phys Med Rehabil. 1993;74(9):983–1001.
24. Powner DJ, Boccalandro C, Alp MS, Vollmer DG. Endocrine failure after traumatic brain injury in adults. Neurocrit Care. 2006;5:61–70.
25. Powner DJ, Boccalandro C. Adrenal insufficiency following traumatic brain injury in adults. Curr Opin Crit Care. 2008;14:163–6.
26. Schneider HJ, Schneider M, Saller B, et al. Prevalence of anterior pituitary insufficiency 3 and 12 months after traumatic brain injury. Eur J Endocrinol. 2006;154:259–65.
27. Pai AB, Robbins WA. Darko. Moderate to severe TBI. In: Batmangelich I, Cristian S, editors. Physical medicine and rehabilitation patient centered care: mastering the competencies. New York: Demos; 2014.

Management of Dismounted Complex Blast Injury Patients at a Role V Military Treatment Facility: Special Considerations

20

John S. Oh and Ashley E. Humphries

Introduction: WRNMMC – Brief History as an OIF/OEF Role V

From 2001 to 2011, the Walter Reed Army Medical Center in Washington, DC, and the National Naval Medical Center in Bethesda, Maryland, were just 5 miles apart but functioned as independent military Role V hospitals in the National Capital Area. Together, they cared for over **3500** combat wounded evacuated from Iraq and Afghanistan with over **1200** having sustained traumatic extremity amputation.

Since the 2009 surge into Afghanistan, a significant number of these patients presented with a very distinct injury pattern caused by improvised explosive devices encountered while on foot patrol – the dismounted complex blast injury (DCBI). DCBI consists of blast-related traumatic amputation of at least one lower extremity and significant injury to a second extremity (upper or lower) combined with concomitant injuries to the perineum, external genital, pelvis, or abdomen. This pattern was first described by the Army DCBI Task Force in 2011, and as can be anticipated, DCBI patients present with complex, multi-system injuries requiring comprehensive, multidisciplinary, and coordinated plans of care [1].

To address the complexity of these injuries and the intricacies of care, both WRAMC and NNMC had formal trauma programs in place with fellowship-trained medical directors, trauma program managers, and process improvement programs. In addition to establishing their local programs, both trauma directors provided timely performance improvement data and were able to address quality assurance concerns to all levels throughout the continuum of care through participation in the weekly Joint Trauma System teleconferences. While only WRAMC provided inpatient rehabilitation, both institutions functioned as military Role V medical centers by providing access to definitive surgical reconstruction and advanced critical care.

In early autumn 2011, Walter Reed Army Medical Center closed its doors in Washington, DC, and combined with the National Naval Medical Center in Bethesda, Maryland. The newly formed institution, physically located at the NNMC campus, was renamed the Walter Reed National Military Medical Center (WRNMMC). At WRNMMC, the concept of a multidisciplinary trauma team led by a fellowship-trained trauma director continued where combat-wounded patients were cared for

J. S. Oh (✉)
Department of Surgery, Division of Trauma, Milton S. Hershey Medical Center, Hershey, PA, USA
e-mail: johnoh1@hmc.psu.edu

A. E. Humphries
Department of General Surgery, Walter Reed National Military Medical Center, Bethesda, MD, USA

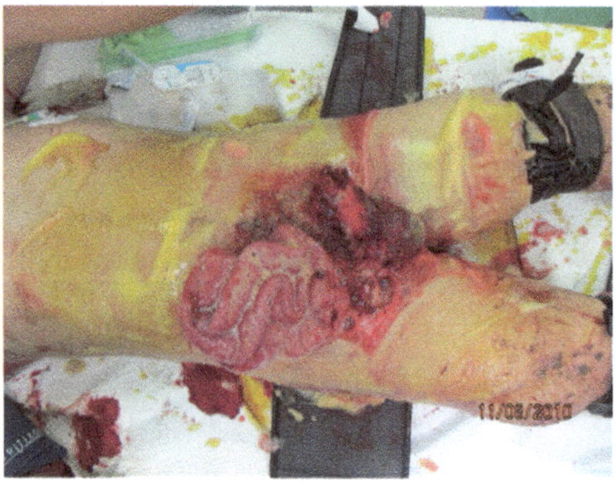

Fig. 20.1 Through a combination of blunt and penetrating mechanisms, blast injuries represent the pan-ultimate in polytrauma. The patient seen here required general, orthopedic, vascular, and plastic surgery for wound stabilization and reconstruction

Table 20.1 Multidisciplinary trauma team

Trauma surgeons	Federal recovery coordinators
Orthopedic surgeons	Warrior Transition Unit (Army)
Anesthesia (pain management)	Marine Corps Liaison
Behavior health	Navy Liaison
Neuropsychologists/TBI	Surgical intensive care unit
Physical medicine and rehabilitation	VA Liaisons
Plastic surgery	Trauma Nurse Coordinators
Neurosurgery	Trauma PI Coordinator
Physical therapy	Nutrition services
Occupational therapy	Recreational therapy
Inpatient Warrior Family Liaison	Social work

under a trauma service that was responsible for primary management and coordination of consultative services.

As the war in Afghanistan progressed, dismounted blast injuries became the dominant injury pattern. Figure 20.1 shows how blast waves, heat, and fragmentation can simultaneously cause injuries to multiple compartments. The resulting injury pattern demonstrates how blast can truly be deemed the pan-ultimate source of polytrauma, necessitating multiple surgical services making many trips to the operating room for wound stabilization and reconstruction. Blast patients truly require hospital-wide attention.

A team of trauma surgeons, surgical residents, nurse practitioners, and physician assistants primarily managed these patients. To manage these polytrauma patients, the team held twice-weekly multidisciplinary meetings to coordinate surgical efforts, to discuss patient care, and to determine appropriate disposition (Table 20.1). These meetings were chaired by trauma surgeons, with multiple specialty representation.

As there are typically two or more surgical services required in the beginning phases of wound stabilization, every effort was made to minimize total operative time by having services operate in parallel vice series. Additionally, since DCBI patients require frequent trips to the operating room to achieve wound closure or reconstruction (as many as eight to ten), operating in parallel allowed more efficient operating room utilization [2]. To facilitate this, daily meetings were held to discuss operative planning.

Any complication or deviation from accepted practice patterns that occurred during a patient's admission to WRNMMC underwent peer review to identify potentially preventable events or opportunities for improvement. As such, the care of the complex combat-wounded patients underwent continual evolution and improvement. WRNMMC's performance improvement program also served as an integral part of the overall Joint Trauma System (JTS) performance improvement process. Participation in the weekly JTS video teleconference (VTC) connected WRNMMC to all the echelons of care from the prehospital setting to the role IV Landstuhl Regional Medical Center in Germany. It was during this conference that combat trauma cases were discussed in detail to identify system issues and to provide feedback and loop closure of open trauma issues throughout the continuum of care. All issues identified through the JTS VTC that were applicable to WRNMMC's trauma program were discussed and resolved at the WRNMMC Trauma Peer Review meeting and Systems Operations Committee with representatives from a variety of services to include orthopedic surgery, neurosurgery, emergency medicine, anesthesia, radiology, and critical care medicine. This same process continues today at both the local and Joint Trauma System level.

In 2013, WRNMMC sought and attained the American College of Surgeons' level 2 trauma center verification to ensure care provided to the high volume of combat trauma patients being managed in the National Capital Area was in keeping with accepted practices and standards. WRNMMC's process improvement program served as the backbone to successfully completing the verification process.

The following chapter provides a summary of lessons learned at WRNMMC in providing definitive care for those with DCBI.

War Consults for Blast Injury

As blast energy affects the entire body through a combination of blunt (compressive and shearing forces) and penetrating mechanisms, care must be holistic in nature. Through realizing many wounded warriors being treated at our institution had oftentimes been exposed to blast energy, whether in combat or in training exercises *before* the injury responsible for their evacuation from theater, WRNMMC instituted a policy of evaluating *all* wounded warriors with standard "blast consults" regardless of the injury mechanism. The following consultative services were routinely engaged as part of the WRNMMC blast injury protocol: physical therapy, occupational therapy, social work, audiology, dental, and the traumatic brain injury (TBI) service. By departmental policy, all blast consults were completed prior to hospital transfer or discharge. While social work, physical therapy, and occupational therapy are routine consultation requests in many trauma centers, the latter two focused on evaluating balance and gait as alterations can be physical manifestations of repeated whole-body exposure to blast energy. It must be emphasized that these consultations were obtained while under care of the trauma service, with the trauma surgeon responsible for ensuring all recommendations were coordinated, reconciled, and completed. With frequent trips to the operating room, multiple subspecialty recommendations, and multiple medications being part of the polytrauma blast injury patients' recovery, it was imperative that a single service over saw the patients.

In blast, hearing can easily be affected either by tympanic membrane disruption or by injury to the middle/inner ear. Hearing tests are part of every pre-deployment medical evaluation and provide a baseline from which to compare. Post-injury audiology evaluations provided the trauma team with additional information when developing rehabilitation plans.

Whether it's a pressure wave causing the jaw to quickly shut, penetrating fragmentation injuries, or direct trauma, the face can easily be injured. Oftentimes, in the initial phases of wound stabilization, patients do not realize they have lost a filling, chipped a tooth, or, in some cases, lost teeth. In the initial years of the war, many complained of dental issues weeks after initial injury. Therefore, post injury dental screening became part of the evaluation protocol.

The third blast-specific consultation was provided by the traumatic brain injury (TBI) team. As mentioned above, wounded warriors had oftentimes been exposed to blasts (combat or training) prior to the injury requiring medical evacuation. Knowing concussive blast effects to the brain are additive in nature, TBI screening was performed in all wounded warriors – regardless of their presenting injury pattern or mechanism of injury. There is a full chapter devoted on mild TBI screening and therapies, but here we highlight our program's specifics.

Traumatic Brain Injury Service

A wide spectrum of severity in traumatic brain injury is encountered in DCBI patients. This can be due primarily to the blast pressure itself or through direct blunt and penetrating injuries from secondary and tertiary blast effects. The TBI service consists of a physician medical director who oversees a team of neuropsychologists, psychiatrists, and physician assistants with expertise in traumatic brain injury. The initial TBI screening, even if performed at echelons prior to WRNMMC, was repeated for comparison or was initiated if it had not been previously performed. The evaluation by the TBI service was comprehensive and consisted of neuropsychological and cognitive testing, as appropriate. The TBI service combines evaluations from other consultative services to include occupational therapy, physical therapy, speech therapy, and physical medicine and rehabilitation to determine disability or impairment associated with TBI and/or acute stress syndromes.

If rehabilitation for TBI was required, the team determined whether inpatient or outpatient setting was appropriate. Inpatient rehabilitation for traumatic brain injuries were most often performed through the Veterans Affairs' Polytrauma Centers [3]. With five major VA polytrauma rehabilitation centers and numerous network sites throughout the country, the VA system for polytrauma and TBI covers the continental United States. These sites offer a continuum of rehabilitation services including specialized emerging consciousness programs for severe TBI, acute rehabilitation for complex and severe polytraumatic injuries, rehabilitation for spinal cord injuries, and residential transitional rehabilitation programs [1, 4, 5]. Outpatient therapy can occur at many military treatment facilities throughout the country.

Other Care Components

As discussed in other chapters of the text, improvised explosive devices can be associated with as many as five different injury mechanisms. The blast wave, alone, can be devastating, but when adding the other components associated with explosion – fragmentation, involuntary movement of objects/victim, biologic wound contamination, and psychological/post-traumatic stress disorders – the team and intricacies of care necessary to successfully treat DCBI patients continue to grow.

Complex Wound Care Team

The complex wound care team consisted of nurse practitioners and registered nurses certified in wound care. They were responsible for the non-operative, bedside management of open wounds. With the large volume of open wounds on the trauma service at WRNMMC, the wound care team was invaluable in their role as physician extenders responsible for both the care and monitoring of the progress of traumatic wounds. This team ensures wounds were examined regularly and alerted the primary team when wounds were not healing properly and operative debridement was required.

In addition to inpatient care, the team provided wound care continuity in outpatient clinics colocated with the trauma service and in the outpatient rehabilitation center. Through these clinics, the team provided wound care to patients with complex, chronic open wounds, e.g., soft tissue defects from the initial injury, pressure ulcers from decubiti or prosthetic limb attachments, and wounds healing by secondary intention. The team provided local wound care with the overall goal of wound healing and preventing secondary wound complications. The wound care team also identified those wounds requiring additional operative debridement or those that were ready for definitive closure.

Pain Management

Due to the high incidence of multi-system trauma in the DCBI population, multimodal analgesia became a cornerstone of inpatient acute pain management. A combination of pharmacological agents and regional anesthesia techniques were utilized to ease pain allowing for rest, recovery, and participation in rehabilitative programs. DCBI pain complexes were a direct result of their trauma and numerous surgical procedures. Blast-injured patients often developed a mixed nociceptive and neuropathic pain pattern with variable response to the different classes of pain medications. Consequently, this may have resulted in the escalation of opioid demand, thereby resulting in the uneasiness of some providers in managing these patients' multimodal pain therapy.

To complement opioid therapy, continuous peripheral nerve and/or epidural catheters were frequently utilized [6] with the goal of enhancing the analgesic therapy within a multimodal regimen to reduce the amount of oral or IV narcotics necessary for pain control. It was imperative that the provider prescribing these different classes of drugs were familiar with their interactions and side effects.

Due to the potential morbidities associated with multimodal drug prescribing, WRNMMC developed a robust acute pain service through the anesthesia department. In order to provide safe and consistent care, this service was responsible for writing all orders for pain medications in patients with in-dwelling neuraxial or peripheral nerve catheters with or without narcotic infusions and were available as consultants when the primary service requested assistance. While all medical services are trained to address various pain regimens, acute pain services can function either in a consultant role or in a primary medical pain management role until the patient is on a stable medical regimen. The model of a single service prescribing opioid or other adjunct pain medications alleviated the risk found with interservice communication errors in dosing, drug to drug interactions, and opioid titration.

Invasive Fungal Infections

Invasive fungal infections (IFI) with *Mucorales* and *Aspergillus* species became a significant source of morbidity and mortality in the DCBI patient. A March 2013 study determined risk factors for developing IFI to be:

1. Warrior on foot patrol (dismounted) in Southern Afghanistan who was injured by blast energy
2. Injury pattern involving a traumatic above-knee amputation
3. Initial resuscitation of at least 20 units of packed red blood cells within the first 24 h of injury [7]

While the mainstay of IFI treatment was aggressive surgical debridement, appropriate use of antimicrobials and topical adjuncts were also important in minimizing tissue loss and disease progression. IFI should be considered in blast patients who are tachycardic, hyperthermic, and possess a rising leukocytosis in the setting of recurring wound bed necrosis seen 5–7 days from injury [8, 9].

Recurrent wound bed necrosis was the most telling physical exam finding in blast patients that distinguished between systemic inflammatory response and IFI. If a healthy-appearing wound with good blood flow on a previous operative trip became necrotic without other explanation or does not appear to be contracting with the development of good granulation tissue by day 7 from injury, IFI should be suspected [10, 11].

Potential IFI patients were treated with high suspicion for invasive infection. Confirmatory tests involved histopathology at the border of healthy and necrotic tissue in addition to tissue culture. Tissue histopathology consisted of hematoxylin and eosin (H&E) stains, Grocott-Gomori's methenamine silver (GMS) stains, and periodic acid-Schiff (PAS) stains. By hospital protocol, histopathology results were available within 24 h. Mucormycosis grows well in culture; however, aspergillus sometimes does not. Therefore, cultures taken from suspicious wounds were checked daily for the first week and then weekly for an additional 4 weeks [11].

Secondary to the high morbidity and mortality associated with IFI infection, multimodal therapy began as soon as IFI was suspected. This multimodal therapy consisted of broad-spectrum intravenous antimicrobials, placement of wound bed antimicrobial beads, usage of negative pressure instillation topical therapy devices, and aggressive (sometimes daily) surgical debridement [11, 12].

The antimicrobial choices were liposomal amphotericin B, intravenous voriconazole, meropenem, and vancomycin. The data supportive of such broad antimicrobial use was found in the first 36 IFI patients and was reported in the Trauma Infectious Disease Outcomes Study (TIDOS) IFI Case Investigation technical report dated April 15, 2011 [7]. In this series, 47% of

IFI wounds were infected with mucormycosis species and were susceptible to amphotericin B. 41% were infected with *Aspergillus* species. However, *Aspergillus* is susceptible to voriconazole, not amphotericin. To confound matters, 28% of the wounds infected with mucormycosis were coinfected with a second (and sometimes third) species of mold. Finally, 75% of IFI wounds were coinfected (or colonized) with gram-positive and gram-negative bacteria. Antimicrobials were tailored to culture results as they returned.

Histopathology proven angioinvasive mold infections required daily trips to the operating room for debridement. Clinically, these wounds appeared healthy after a debridement, only to continually develop tissue necrosis while the infection was active. The typical duration of antifungal therapy was 2–3 weeks, and consultation with infectious disease was obtained in order to manage these patients with therapy tailored toward proven cultures as soon as possible. Serial wound debridements with cultures and tissue histopathology were performed in conjunction with systemic antimicrobial therapy until the wound was amenable for closure. This was indicated by the healthy, well-vascularized appearance of the wound with the absence of invasive infection on histopathology.

Operative Planning and Logistics

Enteral nutrition is a key aspect to recovery in critically ill patients. Numerous studies support the use of enteral feedings to promote healing, decrease wound infection rates, facilitate weaning from mechanical ventilation, and improve survival from critical illness [13, 14]. As with all patients who undergo procedures involving anesthesia, appropriate fasting guidelines are needed to minimize the risk of perioperative aspiration events [15].

However, it was not uncommon for blast patients in the early phases of wound stabilization or for those who were dealing with invasive fungal infection to be in operating room every other day for weeks. While aspiration events can be devastating, limiting caloric intake can lead to infection, delayed wound healing, reconstruction failures, and other wound complications.

Although pre-operative fasting guidelines exist for ambulatory patients, few are available for guidance in critically ill patients who are intubated or who have a tracheostomy and are being fed distal to the pylorus [15]. With the incidence of reflux decreasing proportionally to the distance from the pylorus, placing distal feeding tubes while using cuffed intraoperative airway devices should minimize aspiration risk [14]. As such, more liberal guidelines were used regarding the appropriate fasting guidelines in DCBI patients.

The following are suggested guidelines regarding nutrition:

1. All patients (intubated or extubated) receiving *gastric* or *post-pyloric* (i.e., proximal to the ligament of Treitz) feeding should be made NPO after midnight on the day of procedure, as per ASA guidelines [15].
2. Intubated/tracheostomy patients who have documented *post-pyloric* feeds may continue tube feeds up to and throughout the duration of surgery.
3. Extubated patients with documented *post-ligament of Treitz* feeds may continue tube feeds up to and throughout the duration of surgery.

These guidelines are at the discretion of the clinician caring for the patient in the operating room. As a matter of principle, tube feeds were held for intra-abdominal surgery and prone positioning regardless of airway condition or position of feeding tube.

Venous Thromboembolism Disease

With 20–30% of all DCBI patients developing venous thromboembolism disease, VTE prophylaxis and screening are of utmost importance [16]. Studies have shown decreased VTE rates in DCBI patients who received 30 mg of subcutaneous low-molecular-weight heparin twice per day [17]. As expected, those who missed fewer doses experienced less VTE. Interestingly, Caruso et al. found that usage of epidural catheters and 40 mg of once-daily low-molecular-weight heparin is protective against VTE [18]. Regardless, chemical VTE is important.

However, there may be times when chemical VTE prophylaxis is contraindicated. In these cases, the use of inferior vena cava (IVC) filters should be considered. Vena cava filters do not prevent or treat venous thrombosis [19]. The purpose of vena cava filters is to prevent clinically significant or fatal PE by trapping venous emboli. Generally, the use of vena cava filters is indicated when primary chemotherapy cannot be started, must be stopped, or is insufficient to protect the patient from a clinically significant PE [19]. The following guidelines are a stepwise approach to VTE prophylaxis one may want to consider when dealing with DCBI patients [16–20]:

1. Dosing of low-molecular-weight heparin (LMWH): Unless contraindicated, prophylactic doses of LMWH administered 30 mg twice daily should be used in patients without documented evidence of VTE.
2. Solid organ injury is not a contraindication to prophylaxis as long as the injury has been stable and prophylaxis should not be held for patients going to the operating room. Low-molecular-weight heparin 40 mg once daily should be used for those patients with neuroaxial catheters.
    (a) Dose should not be administered within 24 h of pulling catheters. For example:
        (i) Patient receives 40 mg at 0900 on a Monday. The catheter may be pulled at 0900 on Tuesday.
        (ii) Dosing at 30 mg twice daily may resume 2 h after catheter is pulled.
        (iii) In order to minimize time where patient is "uncovered" with prophylaxis LMWH, logistical coordination with the acute pain service is essential.
3. Bleeding complications on therapeutic anticoagulation: For patients with PE or DVT who develop a complication from therapeutic anticoagulation, a vena cava filter should be considered and anticoagulation stopped.
4. Patients with VTE and contraindication to medical therapy: For patients with PE or DVT who have a contraindication to therapeutic anticoagulation, a vena cava filter should be considered.
    (a) If the contraindication is anticipated to be lifelong, the filter placed should be permanent.
    (b) If the contraindication to therapeutic anticoagulation is temporary, a temporary filter should be placed.
5. Removing IVC filters: In patients with vena cava filters, therapeutic anticoagulation or prophylactic anticoagulation (whichever is indicated) should be resumed once the contraindication to its use no longer exists, and the patient should be evaluated for filter removal.

While every institution has different policies regarding preoperative chemical VTE prophylaxis utilization, unless absolutely contraindicated, its use is highly recommended. DCBI patients frequently find themselves in and out of the operating room on an every-other-day basis. In cases such as these, missing the morning dose will effectively cause them to miss three of ten (30%) of doses in a 5-day period.

As migration, fracture, and thrombosis have been reported with IVC filter placement, the decision to place an IVC filter is not one to be taken lightly, and, if utilized, IVC filters should be retrievable. A registry of IVC filters helped with tracking and served as an objective reminder to remove the filter when it was no longer necessary. While reported registry success rates have been variable, a recent retrospective review by Lucas et al. of a military IVC tracking registry showed a 95% contact rate with 60% retrieved, 15% remained in situ for ongoing indications, 10% unable to be retrieved, and 5% lost to follow-up [20].

Medication Dosing Schedules and Hand-Off Communication Tools

As we have previously mentioned, DCBI patients make frequent trips to the operating room. As such, attention must be paid to medication dosing schedules. For example, some antimicrobial medications are administered once daily. If the order to administer is written as "Q Day" vice to give at 0600, depending on the EMR, "Q Day" may default to 0900. Should the wounded warrior be in the operating room at 0900, administration of the medication may be delayed for several hours or worse, missed all together. In the case of IFI patients, liposomal amphotericin B is administered once per day. Missing a dose of this medication has disastrous consequences.

The same considerations should be made with all scheduled medications. Another example is with twice-daily low-molecular-weight heparin. If written for BID, the EMR may default to 0900 and 2100. As with liposomal amphotericin B, the 0900 dose would be due when the wounded warrior was in the operating room. Missing LMWH doses is undesirably associated with increased risk of VTE [17]. Performing daily medical reconciliation is necessary. This is especially vital when patients are returning to the floor following trips to the operating room and should be part of all post-op checks.

Conclusion

The complex dismounted blast injury patients presented many unique challenges to the care team at WRNMMC. The lessons learned presented in this chapter list the unique practices found to have the most impact in the care of these patients. In summary, the care of these patients requires a coordinated and holistic approach with a goal toward continual process improvement to ensure optimal outcomes in our combat wounded.

References

1. Dismounted Complex Blast Injury: Report of the Army Dismounted Complex Blast Injury Task Force. 18 June 2011. http://armymedicine.mil/Documents/DCBI-Task-Force-Report-Redacted-Final.pdf. Accessed 17 July 2017.
2. Lewandowski LR, Weintrob AC, Tribble DR, Rodriguez CJ, Petfield J, Lloyd BA, Murray CK, Stinner D, Aggarwal D, Shaikh F, Potter BK, The IDCRP Outcomes Study Group. Early complications and outcomes in combat injury related invasive fungal wound infections: a case-control analysis. J Orthop Trauma. 2016 March;30(3):e92–9.
3. Polytrauma/TBI System of Care. U.S. Department of Veterans Affairs. Retrieved from https://www.polytrauma.va.gov/system-of-care/index.asp. Accessed 27 Dec 2016.
4. Gironda RJ, Clark ME, Ruff RL, Chait S, Craine M, Walker R, Scholten J. Traumatic brain injury, polytrauma, and pain: challenges and treatment strategies for the polytrauma rehabilitation. Rehabil Psychol. 2009;54(3):247–58.
5. Uomoto JM, Williams RM. Post-acute polytrauma rehabilitation and integrated care of returning veterans: toward a holistic approach. Rehabil Psychol. 2009;54(3):259–69.
6. Stojadinovic A, Auton A, Peoples GE, McKnight GM, Shields C, Croll SM, Bleckner LL, Winkley J, Maniscalco-Theberge ME, Buckenmaier CC. Responding to challenges in modern combat casualty care: innovative use of advanced regional anesthesia. Pain Med. 2006;7(4):330–8.
7. Rodriguez CJ, Weintrob AC, Shah J, Malone D, Dunne JR, Weisbrod AB, Lloyd BA, Warkentien TE, Murray CK, Wilkins K, Shaikh F, Carson ML, Aggarwal D, Tribble DR, Infectious Disease Clinical Research Program Trauma Infectious Disease Outcomes Study Group. Risk factors associated with invasive fungal infections in combat trauma. Surg Infect. 2014;15(5):521–6.
8. Tribble DR, Rodriguez CJ. Combat-related invasive fungal wound infections. Curr Fungal Infect Rep. 2014;8(4):277–86.
9. Weintrob AC, Weisbrod AB, Dunne JR, Rodriguez CJ, Malone D, Lloyd BA, Warkentien TE, Wells J, Murray CK, Bradley W, Shaikh F, Shah J, Aggrawal D, Carson ML, Tribble DR, The IDCRP TIDOS Study Group. Combat trauma-associated invasive fungal wound infections: epidemiology and clinical classification. Epidemiol Infect. 2015;143(1):214–24.
10. Rodriguez CJ, Weintrob AC, Dunne JR, Weisbrod AB, Lloye B, Warkentien T, Malone D, Wells J, Murray CK, Shaikh BW, Shah J, Carson ML, Aggarwal D, Tribble DR, The IDCRP TIDOs Study Team. Clinical relevance of mold culture positivity with and without recurrent wound necrosis following combat-related injuries. J Trauma Acute Care Surg. 2014;77(5):769–73.

11. Rodriguez, Tribble, Murray, Jessie, Khan, Fleming, Potter, Gordon, Shackelford. "Invasive Fungal Infection in War Wounds". Joint Trauma System Clinical Practice Guideline. August 2016, published online. http://www.usaisr.amedd.army.mil/cpgs/Invasive_Fungal_Infection_04_Aug_2016.pdf . Accessed 6/26/2017.
12. Lewandowski L, Purcell R, Fleming M, Gordon W. The use of dilute Dakin's solution fo the treatment of Angioinvasive fungal infection in the combat wounded: a case series. Mil Med. 2013;178(4):e503–7.
13. Elke G, van Zanten A, Lemieux M, McCall M, Jeejeebhoy K, Kott M, Jiang X, Day A, Heyland D. Enteral versus parenteral nutrition in critically ill patients: an updated systematic review and meta-analysis of randomized controlled trials. Crit Care. 2016;20:117. Published online 2016 Apr 29.
14. Blumenstein I, Shastri YM, Stein J. Gastroenteric tube feedings: techniques, problems, and solutions. World J Gastroenerol. 2014;20(26):8505–24.
15. Practice Guidelines for Preoperative Fasting and the Use of Phamacologic Agents to Reduce the Risk of Pulmonary Aspiration: Application to Healthy Patients Undergoing Elective Procedures: An Updated Report by the American Society of Anesthesiologists Committee on Standards and Practice Parameters. Anesthesiology. 2011;114(3):495–511.
16. Fang R. Venous thromobembolism among military combat casualties. Current Trauma Rep. 2016;2(1):48–53.
17. Holley AB, Petteys S, Mitchell JD, Holley PR, Collen JF. Thromboprophylaxis and VTE rates in soldiers wounded in operation enduring freedom and operation Iraqi freedom. Chest. 2013;144(3):966–73.
18. Caruso JD, Elster EA, Rodriguez CJ. Epidural placement does not result in an increased incidence of venous thromboembolism in combat-wounded patients. J Trauma Acute Care Surg. 2014;77(1):61–6.
19. Grabo, Seery, Bradley, Zakaluzny, Kearns, Fernandez, Tadlock. "The Prevention of Deep Venous Thrombosis- Inferior Vena Cava Filter": Joint Clinical Practice Guidelines published online. http://www.usaisr.amedd.army/cpgs/prevent_deep_venous_thrombosis_IVC_Filter_02_Aug_2016.pdf. Accessed 3 July 2017.
20. Lucas DJ, Dunne JR, Rodriguez CJ, Curry KM, Elster E, Vicente D, Malone DL. Dedicated tracking of patients with retrievable IVC filters improves retrieval rates. Am Surg. 2012 Aug;78(8):870–4.

Infection Control and Prevention After Dismounted Complex Blast Injury

Heather C. Yun, Dana M. Blyth, and Clinton K. Murray

Background

While combat injury and subsequent infection have been common throughout history, changes in mechanisms of injury continue to necessitate changes to prevention strategies. Dismounted complex blast injuries (DCBI) by no means emerged in the past few years. Similar injuries certainly took place in prior conflicts, including WWII, Vietnam, and Korea. However, these previously often unsurvivable injuries have become much more commonly seen in follow-up due to advances in field care and forward surgical care. However, perhaps no conflict has been so uniquely defined by DCBI, with such a large proportion of severely injured survivors, as the recent conflict in Afghanistan where DCBI was caused almost exclusively by improved explosive devices (IEDs), as opposed to unexploded ordinance or landmines (as seen in previous conflicts). While IEDs were used in Iraq, many caused injuries while combat troops were in vehicles (i.e., mounted). However, in Afghanistan, the tactics and terrain of the country led to predominantly injuries sustained while on foot patrol (i.e., dismounted).

H. C. Yun (✉) · D. M. Blyth · C. K. Murray
San Antonio Military Medical Center,
JBSA-Fort Sam Houston, TX, USA

Uniformed Services University of the Health Sciences, Bethesda, MD, USA
e-mail: Heather.c.yun.mil@mail.mil

The DCBI Task Force noted in June 2011 that the number of DCBI had increased during the previous 15 months, with a doubling in the number of service members with triple limb amputations [1]. DCBI is often characterized by high above-knee amputations and genital and perineal injuries, further contributing to their complexity and predisposition to infection. The fighting season that followed the Task Force's report saw an even higher rate of amputations, with 17.4/month reported during 2011 and over 35 in the month of June, alone [2]. From 2010 to 2011, driven by DCBI, the rate of amputations in trauma patients admitted to combat support hospitals (CSHs) rose from 3.5% to 14% [3].

The risk factors for infection after these injuries are numerous. First, the degree to which DCBI wound contamination occurs has been well described in the literature and the lay media and witnessed by the author during her own 2011 Afghanistan deployment to the intensive care unit at Craig Joint Theater Hospital [4]. The variety and volume of detritus removed from these wounds is impressive and is often discovered even after several debridements. Soil, vegetation, rocks, man-made objects, parts of the boots and uniform, and even fragments of body parts of self or others may be found; the author experienced one case where the calcaneus of the soldier was discovered just inferior to his scapula after tracking through his soft tissues all the way from his amputated leg.

From the time when first entering the continuum of care, the casualty undergoes numerous operative procedures, often in austere circumstances with less-than-ideal sanitary environments. Beyond that what is associated with trauma, DCBI patients frequently sustain further immunosuppression secondary to massive blood product transfusion; are treated alongside multiple additional casualties, some of whom may be colonized with drug-resistant bacteria as a result of community or hospital acquisition; and undergo no fewer than ten transitions of care, at least two of which occur in a supine position across thousands of miles before finally arriving in the USA for definitive care. This context of care and risk for infection is incredibly unique.

Unsurprisingly, the risk for infectious complications in combat casualties after DCBI is high. The overall cohort of casualties injured and evacuated from theater has been characterized in the Trauma Infectious Disease Outcomes Study (TIDOS). This prospective observational study began enrolling subjects in 2009, the same year that injuries sustained by US personnel in Afghanistan began to outnumber those from Iraq, with a concomitant increase in risk in DCBI [1]. The initial report from the TIDOS cohort on infectious complications included 233 of 311 subjects injured in Afghanistan, with blast injuries accounting for 69% of those enrolled [5]. A total of 27% of all hospitalized patients developed at least one infectious complication; this included 50% of all those admitted to an intensive care unit. Using standardized definitions for healthcare-associated infections as defined by the National Healthcare Safety Network, wound, skin, and soft tissue infections accounted for 20%, followed by osteomyelitis at 10%, bloodstream infections at 9%, and pneumonia at 3%.

A recent analysis, including 524 wounded personnel from Iraq and 4766 from Afghanistan, found overall infection rates were higher in casualties from Afghanistan compared to those from Iraq (34% vs 28%, respectively) [6]. Independent risk factors driving this difference were large-volume blood product transfusions, high injury severity scores, and IEDs as an injury mechanism. Those injured in Afghanistan combat experienced a 47% incidence of skin/soft tissue infection, a 14% incidence of pneumonia, a 14% incidence of bloodstream infection, and a 6% incidence of osteomyelitis. In total, 36% developed >1 infection.

Microbiology

Recent infectious complications of combat casualties, with or without DCBI, have been most remarkable for the prevalence of multidrug-resistant (MDR) gram-negative rods (GNR). The most prevalent bacteria isolated either as colonizing or infecting pathogens after DCBI have less to do with the mechanism of injury and more to do with the theater in which the injury occurred, prevailing nosocomial pathogens at the time, and time after injury. During operations in Iraq, MDR *Acinetobacter baumannii-calcoaceticus* complex (ABC) emerged as a predominant pathogen among evacuated casualties, even earning the unfortunate nickname, "Iraqibacter" [7]. However, early sampling of wounds after injury revealed typical skin flora, including staphylococcal spp., and clinical cultures obtained from US casualties, while hospitalized at deployed medical facilities revealed the same [8, 9]. Colonization and infection rates with MDR ABC and other GNR including *Klebsiella pneumoniae* and *Pseudomonas aeruginosa* rose as the patient progressed through the evacuation chain and were most common (up to 70% for ABC in osteomyelitis) in initial established wound and bone infections [5, 10, 11]. By the time the patient relapsed with their osteomyelitis, however, *Staphylococcus aureus* was once again most common.

As large-scale combat operations shifted from Iraq to Afghanistan, the predominant pathogens changed. This was seen early in active surveillance cultures performed in evacuated casualties. From 2005–2009, ABC colonization rates began to decline and be replaced by other MDR GNR [12]. By 2009–2012, when most casualties were occurring in Afghanistan, the predominant colonizing pathogens were *Escherichia coli*, *P. aeruginosa*, and *Enterobacter aerogenes* [13]. *E. coli* alone (most of which produced extended-spectrum beta-lactamase [ESBL]) accounted for 67–83% of all MDR isolates recovered at US medical treatment facilities, while ABC accounted for only 7%. While E. coli was the most common colonizing pathogen, the most common GNR isolated during any evaluation for infection in casualties evacuated from Afghanistan was *P. aeruginosa*, followed by *E. coli* [6]. An evaluation of the acutely mangled extremity in Afghanistan typically revealed polymicrobial contamination with low-virulence environmental organisms and skin flora which generally did not persist on repeat sampling or appear to cause infection. Enterococci were frequently isolated from these wounds and did not often appear to be responsible for infection. Anaerobes were also isolated, although outcomes do not appear to correlate with the use of antimicrobials active against them [14]. Lastly, *Candida* spp. were isolated from about 5% of TIDOS cohort wounds, typically in polymicrobial infections, and were not associated with mortality in this context [15].

When evacuated casualties from Iraq and Afghanistan first began presenting with MDR infectious complications, the source of these organisms was not obvious. Initially, it was hypothesized that these organisms, MDR ABC in particular, were found in the local environment, heavily contaminating wounds at the time of injury, and selected for as the patient received antimicrobials and progressed through treatment. Historical data from the Vietnam era were referred to as evidence, although neither ABC taxonomy nor a mechanism for the organisms' introduction into wounds was identified, in spite of major ecological differences between Vietnam and Southwest Asia [16, 17]. Additionally, subsequent studies revealed that ABC and MDR Enterobacteriaceae were not found in fresh combat wounds shortly after the time of injury, in either Iraq or Afghanistan [8, 18], and microbiologic sampling of soil from various locations throughout Iraq and Afghanistan also failed to identify MDR GNR [19].

It was also considered that personnel may have been colonized with MDR GNR prior to injury, with gut or skin flora serving as the major contributor to endogenous infection with these organisms. However, active assessments of colonization with MDR pathogens have consistently demonstrated rising rates as patients progress through the chain of evacuation, with colonization rates increasing two to three times between admission to Landstuhl Regional Medical Center (LRMC) and US-based military treatment facilities [12, 13]. Uninjured personnel were also screened for ABC colonization prior to deployment, while serving in Iraq, and after evacuation from Iraq for non-trauma diagnoses, with no evidence of MDR ABC in any of those groups [20–22]. For ABC at least, pre-injury colonization appears to have no role in post-injury infection. For ESBL-producing Enterobacteriaceae, the data are less clear. Multiple studies of civilian travelers have demonstrated risk for ESBL acquisition over the course of international travel [23–25]. While active surveillance has continued to demonstrate rising rates of colonization in evacuated military casualties between Level IV and V facilities, this surveillance does not involve perirectal swabs which might be more likely to identify Enterobacteriaceae. One assessment of healthy deployed personnel in Afghanistan revealed an ESBL-producing *E. coli* colonization rate of 11%, about five times that seen in nondeployed military personnel [26]. These rates have been noted to be as high as 35% in French military personnel after aeromedical evacuation from Afghanistan [27]. Evaluations of serial colonizing and infecting isolates have revealed that a majority of *E. coli* isolates are related in the same patient over time, indicating a potentially greater role for endogenous infection [28]. It is worth noting, though, that the first of these isolates were recovered at LRMC, not at the time of injury or before.

The third hypothesis, and ultimately the one borne out by the literature, was that nosocomial transmission of MDR GNR was occurring during the chain of combat casualty care. An early assessment of clinical cultures performed at a CSH in Iraq demonstrated that US personnel's cultures grew predominantly *S. aureus*, coagulase-negative staphylococci, and streptococcal spp., while the cultures from local patients (who often had prolonged hospitalizations at the CSH) grew ABC, *K. pneumoniae*, and *P. aeruginosa* [9]. This suggested a potential role for cross-transmission from long-term intensive care unit patients to freshly injured casualties. Another study from Iraq demonstrated decreasing ABC colonization rates among US personnel when the hospital census, and specifically the numbers of non-US personnel admitted to the CSH, decreased [29]. A large epidemiologic assessment of ABC isolates from US military casualties, patients treated alongside casualties, and hospital environments demonstrated clonal relatedness among isolates recovered from multiple Level Vs, LRMC, the Comfort (a US military hospital ship), and a CSH in Baghdad; one strain was also recovered from British and Canadian injured personnel [22, 30]. Major outbreaks of clonally related *E. coli* isolates have not been seen in this context. However, studies performed in both Iraq and Afghanistan have demonstrated high rates of community-associated MDR GNR among local national patients treated in CSHs there and establishment of those GNR as the endemic flora of those facilities [31–33]. Taken together, the bulk of the evidence supports ongoing introduction of MDR GNR to military hospitals in the theater of operations, with cross-transmission occurring there and during higher echelons of casualty care.

Concurrent with the rise in DCBI and amputation rates in Afghanistan, invasive fungal infections (IFI) emerged as an infectious complication for which this population was uniquely at risk. Among patients evacuated to Landstuhl Regional Medical Center (LRMC), the IFI rate was 2% in the fourth quarter of 2009 and steadily rose to 5% over the following 9 months, eventually complicating 12% of intensive care unit (ICU) admissions [34, 35]. These patients presented with fever, hypotension, and tachycardia, along with recurrent myonecrosis, a median of 10 days after injury. Risk factors were identified as blast injury, being dismounted at the time of injury, above-the-knee amputations and massive transfusion (>20 units of packed red blood cells) requirements in the first 24 h [36]. Among IFI cases, 79% had lower extremity amputations, and 74% had genitalia or groin injuries; 93% were related to DCBI. Multiple amputations were also common, with bilateral lower extremity amputations seen in 68% of the original cohort and 16% involving three limbs [34]. These injuries were sustained during dismounted patrols specifically in the agricultural Kandahar and Helmand provinces of Afghanistan, which are southern, lower altitude, wetter, and better habitats for many environmental fungi [37]. Unlike MDR GNR, these pathogens are generally inoculated directly from the environment. Numerous fungi have been responsible for these infections, including Mucorales, *Aspergillus*, and *Fusarium* spp., and concurrent growth of MDR GNR has been reported in approximately one-third [38].

Outcomes

Multiple clinical outcomes have been evaluated in the setting of infection after combat-related injury, and given the nature of recent conflicts, many of these have been related to blast injuries including DCBI. Outcomes clearly are poorer than in uninfected patients. Even the presence of bacteria in uninfected appearing type III tibia fractures has been demonstrated to increase risk of amputation, with the risk increasing in the setting of more than one species of bacteria [39]. Patients without infection had a 19% rate of amputation, compared to 34% among those with osteomyelitis and 40% with deep wound infections; reoperation rates and times to fracture union were also increased. Failures of limb salvage, unplanned operative takebacks, and readmissions have all been associated with deep wound infection and osteomyelitis [40–42]. Similar to data from prior conflicts, those injured in recent conflicts who die from their wounds often do so related to sepsis or multiorgan system failure related to infection [43, 44]. IFI in general, and particularly those involving *Mucorales* spp., significantly prolonged the time to eventual wound closure compared to those without IFI, including those with bacterial infections. A recent case-control study found significant differences in outcomes between those with IFI and those without; those with IFI required a greater number of changes in amputation level, a higher number of operative procedures, and longer duration to wound closure [45]. Six percent of those with IFI died, compared to 1% of those without, although this did not reach statistical significance.

Prevention

Wound Management

The prevention of wound infection begins in the earliest stages of injury management. Wounds are to be dressed with sterile bandages at the point of injury, limiting further contamination. Debridement and irrigation should begin at the earliest opportunity, whether as part of prehospital care or in a medical setting without surgical capabilities (Level I/II). Irrigation with normal saline, sterile water, or even potable water as an alternative is recommended under low pressure [46]. Increasing volumes of irrigation fluid are recommended with increasing Gustilo grade of fracture (3 L for Type I, 6 L for Type II, and 9 L for Type III). The use of additives is not recommended, given the lack of available evidence to demonstrate improvement in outcomes and the potential risk for toxicity; recent data from the FLOW study also corroborated no improvements with the addition of castile soap [47]. The use of high-pressure delivery systems has been associated with increases in wound bacterial burden under experimental conditions and in some instances caused outbreaks of nosocomial organisms including MDR ABC [48, 49]. Soft tissue foreign bodies and fragments, commonly seen with DCBI, can typically be retained and observed if there is no evidence of infection, associated entry and exit wounds are <2 cm, and there is no vascular, pleural, peritoneal, or bony involvement. The use of negative pressure wound dressings (NWPD) has been well established in this population, including during aeromedical evacuations, although its role in infection prevention is not completely clear [50–52].

Evacuation to surgical capability is recommended at the earliest opportunity. However, combat and weather conditions can make rapid evacuation challenging. Additionally, the effect of timing of surgical debridement on infectious disease outcomes has not been well established. LEAP data and other previous studies have not demonstrated that timing of surgical debridement impacts infection rates, at least out to 24 h after injury [53]. More recent prospective data from Canadian trauma centers using similar treatment and antibiotic protocols has shown that while increasing Gustilo grade and the presence of tibia/fibula fractures increase infection risk, the time to either initial surgery or antibiotics does not [54]. It is likely that the thoroughness and adequacy of initial debridements matters more than timing. This can be particularly challenging in DCBI patients given the complexity and heavy contamination of their injuries, the frequency of multiple injuries, and physiological limitations to prolonged operative interventions in critically injured and often hemodynamically unstable patients. Daily surgical debridement is not unusual in this context, at least initially, to ensure that all wounds have been extended, directly visualized, and explored and debris and devitalized tissue have been removed. The optimal methods of fracture fixation have not been firmly established by available evidence. Internal fixation is typically delayed until after multiple debridements, evacuation, and stabilization and may be performed later than in civilian trauma settings. Internal fixation for local national patients must carefully be considered in the context of possible complications and what healthcare capacity is available to the patient in the local community. The World Health Organization cautions against implantation of orthopedic devices that may not be removable by local surgical capabilities in the event of infection [55]. In the acute setting, external fixation is the preferred US military approach; the UK often uses casting initially with good outcomes, although these may not translate in settings with longer evacuation times or increased numbers of casualties [56]. Wound cultures are recommended only when there is a clinical suspicion of wound infection.

Most wounds should undergo repeated exploration and debridement prior to closure typically 3–5 days after injury; only injuries involving the face or dura have a recommendation for primary closure. Primary repair of colonic injuries should be avoided, especially those with multiple concomitant injuries, hemodynamic instability, or massive blood transfusion, such as often seen in DCBI with rectal injuries.

Antimicrobial Use

While surgical management is the mainstay of infection prevention after DCBI, antimicrobials plan an important adjunctive role. Like wound management, their use may begin at the earliest point of care, with recommendations for initial dosing within 3 h from the time of injury. Tetanus vaccine and immunoglobulin must be considered and given when indicated. Point-of-injury (POI) antibiotics (Level I) are recommended as a single dose in the event that evacuation is delayed or expected to be delayed [57]. The currently recommended POI agent is moxifloxacin, with ertapenem given as an alternative in the event of shock, a penetrating abdominal injury, or inability to take an oral medication. These agents were chosen based on an activity against expected infecting pathogens, stability in austere field environments, and ease of dosing. Most patients do not require POI antibiotics, and high-dose cefazolin (2 g IV q6-8 h) is the backbone of recommended antimicrobial prophylaxis in combat injuries including DCBI. The 2011 guidelines also included recommendations for redosing in the event of blood transfusion totaling 1500–2000 cc. The addition of metronidazole is recommended for penetrating hollow viscus injuries or central nervous system injuries involving gross contamination with organic material. The recommended duration of antimicrobial prophylaxis is short, totaling 1–3 days for extremity injuries, 5 days for most central nervous system injuries, and typically 1 day for abdominal or thoracic injuries (Table 21.1). Longer durations are not recommended in the event of drains, external fixators, or open wounds.

The use of broader-spectrum coverage is specifically discouraged. Gas gangrene has not been seen in this population, despite the destructive injuries and the agricultural regions in which they occur, and adjunctive penicillin is not recommended. Recommendations against the use of extended-spectrum gram-negative agents, such as aminoglycosides or fluoroquinolones, were based on the absence of definitive evidence that these lower infection rates and on the concern for potentially increasing selection of MDR organisms [57]. This has been a source of controversy in civilian open fracture guidelines [58, 59]. Recent TIDOS data have indicated that antimicrobial prophylaxis is associated with increased risk of colonization by MDR GNR, with an odds ratio of 3.5 for cefazolin and 5.4 for fluoroquinolones [60]. Data recently presented at IDWeek also demonstrated that among 1043 TIDOS patients, 81% of whom had sustained blast injuries, expanded GNR coverage with a fluoroquinolone or aminoglycoside did not affect rates of osteomyelitis or MDR colonization [61]. It is also problematic to select a prophylaxis agent that would cover the resistant GNR seen in infectious complications from recent conflicts, given that these tend to be highly drug resistant. By 2007, ABC isolates had reported susceptibilities to amikacin of <40%; <10% of ICU patients' isolates were susceptible [62]. More importantly, there has been no evidence that these isolates are even present in casualties' wounds shortly after injury, at the time that prophylaxis would be given. Prophylaxis with systemic antifungals is not recommended, dilute Dakin's solution has been shown to have broad activity against a variety of molds with limited toxicity, and its application to wounds in high-risk patients has been recommended [63, 64].

Infection Prevention and Control (IPC)

Multiple sets of international, national, and combat-specific guidelines have been published and serve as excellent references to the practice of IPC, and an exhaustive reiteration of all these

Table 21.1 Antimicrobial therapeutic agents and duration for prevention of infection in combat-related trauma

Injury	Preferred agent(s)	Alternate agent(s)	Duration
Extremity wounds (includes the skin, soft tissue, bone)			
Skin, soft tissue, no open fractures	Cefazolin, 2 g IV q6-8h	Clindamycin (300–450 mg po, or 600 mg IV q8h)	1–3d
Skin, soft tissue, with open fractures, exposed bone, or open joints	Cefazolin, 2 g IV q6-8h[a]	Clindamycin 600 mg IV q8h	1–3d
Thoracic cavity			
Penetrating chest injury without esophageal disruption	Cefazolin, 2 g IV q6-8h	Clindamycin (300–450 mg po, or 600 mg IV q8h)	1d
Penetrating chest injury with esophageal disruption	Cefazolin, 2 g IV q6-8h, plus metronidazole 500 mg IV q8-12h	Ertapenem 1 g IV × 1 dose or moxifloxacin 400 mg IV × 1 dose	1d after definitive washout
Abdomen			
Penetrating abdominal injury with suspected/known hollow viscus injury and soilage; may apply to rectal/perineal injuries as well	Cefazolin, 2 g IV q6-8h, plus metronidazole 500 mg IV q8-12h	Ertapenem 1 g IV × 1 dose or moxifloxacin 400 mg IV × 1 dose	1d after definitive washout
Maxillofacial			
Open maxillofacial fractures or maxillofacial fractures with foreign body or fixation device	Cefazolin, 2 g IV q6-8h	Clindamycin 600 mg IV q8h	1d
Central nervous system			
Penetrating brain injury	Cefazolin 2 g IV q6-8 h. Consider adding metronidazole 500 mg IV q8-12 h if gross contamination with organic debris	Ceftriaxone 2 g IV q24h. Consider adding metronidazole 500 mg IV q8-12h if gross contamination with organic debris. For penicillin allergic patients, vancomycin 1 g IV q12h plus ciprofloxacin 400 mg IV q8-12h	5 days or until CSF leak is closed, whichever is longer
Penetrating spinal cord injury	Cefazolin 2 g IV q6-8h. Add metronidazole 500 mg IV q8-12h if abdominal cavity is involved	As above. Add metronidazole 500 mg IV q8-12h if abdominal cavity is involved	5 days or until CSF leak is closed, whichever is longer
Eye wounds			
Eye injury, burn, or abrasion	Topical: Erythromycin or bacitracin ophthalmic ointment QID and PRN for symptomatic relief. Systemic: No systemic treatment required	Fluoroquinolone one drop QID	Until epithelium healed (no fluorescein staining)
Eye injury, penetrating	Levofloxacin 500 mg IV/PO once daily. Before primary repair, no topical agents should be used unless directed by ophthalmology		7d or until evaluated by a retinal specialist

(continued)

Table 21.1 (continued)

Injury	Preferred agent(s)	Alternate agent(s)	Duration
Burns			
Superficial burns	Topical antimicrobials with twice daily dressing changes (include mafenide acetate or silver sulfadiazine; may alternate between the two), silver-impregnated dressing changed q3–5 d, or Biobrane	Silver nitrate solution applied to dressings	Until healed
Deep partial-thickness burns	Topical antimicrobials with twice daily dressing changes or silver-impregnated dressing changed q3–5d, plus excision and grafting	Silver nitrate solution applied to dressings plus excision and grafting	Until healed or grafted
Full-thickness burns	Topical antimicrobials with twice daily dressing changes plus excision and grafting	Silver nitrate solution applied to dressings plus excision and grafting	Until healed or grafted

From Ref. [77]
[a]These guidelines do not advocate adding enhanced gram-negative bacterial coverage (i.e., addition of aminoglycoside or fluoroquinolone) in type III fractures

is outside the scope of this chapter. However, it is worth noting that attention to these practices is often an afterthought or, at worst, may be considered pointless or unattainable in austere environments. This is clearly not the case. For all the reasons outlined in the paragraphs above, infection prevention is of paramount importance to prevent unnecessary suffering. However, prioritization of focus areas is necessary in deployed military treatment facilities, based on the overall risk, the evidence base, and the feasibility of the proposed interventions; these are summarized in Table 21.2.

Command Support and Administrative Controls

Throughout the history of military preventive medicine efforts, a strategic vision and the support of the command have been the key to the efforts' eventual success or failure. Our main recommendation for IPC in combat casualties, including DCBI, is the establishment of a structured, systematic process for conducting and studying IPC, with an individual leader responsible. Frequently, successful interventions have been sporadic, limited in scope, and spearheaded by a deployed clinician with a particular interest on a several-month rotation. While on-the-ground efforts can often only be executed by deployed individuals to specific facilities, without an overarching strategic vision, these efforts will result in only piecemeal successes. Ideally, a joint, theater-level consultant with IPC expertise, operational experience, and ability to assist with development and conduction of multicenter research protocols to address knowledge gaps would be appointed in order to continuously improve processes and respond to evolving issues [46, 65]. This individual should also be responsible for ongoing development and deployment of theater-level standard operating procedures with regard to IPC. Deployments of IPC experts to assess in-theater practices took place in 2008, 2009, and 2012 and revealed a number of ongoing areas for improvement, including training of IPC practitioners, microbiology capabilities, policies for IPC and blood-borne pathogen exposures, and policies and procedures for both IPC and hospital disinfection [66]. Support for development and maintenance of clinical practice guidelines should also be provided; these were developed in 2008 with a substantial revision in 2011 [57, 67]. These will require updating as both risks and available evidence evolve.

Diagnostic Microbiology Capabilities

In order to ensure appropriate empiric therapy for infected patients, a reliable hospital antibiogram

Table 21.2 Specific infection prevention areas for prioritization in deployed military treatment facilities

Focus area	Recommendation
Command support/ administrative controls	Establish joint, theater-level expert infection prevention consultant responsible for directing IPC activities from levels I–IV, including annual risk assessments and plans Establish theater-level IPC SOPs Commit to deployed expert microbiology support and integrated surveillance for HAIs and MDROs Commit to ongoing education for deploying and deployed infection preventionists and clinicians Commit to resourcing clinically relevant IPC/HAI research in theater Commit to resourcing updated clinical practice guidelines
Essential IPC tactical priorities	Follow national and international guidelines for prevention and treatment of HAI Implement robust hand hygiene programs and monitor adherence Implement VAP bundles and monitor adherence Implement evidence-based SSI prevention measures Ensure cohorting of short-term vs long-term patients Standardize environmental disinfection, including both low- and high-level disinfection, and processing of sterile supplies Implement antimicrobial stewardship programs and monitor adherence with published guidelines

IPC Infection prevention and control, *SOP* Standard operating procedure, *HAI* Healthcare-associated infection, *MDRO* Multidrug-resistant organism, *VAP* Ventilator-associated pneumonia, *SSI* Surgical site infection, *BBP* Blood-borne pathogen

is required, and in order to deescalate therapy, rapid and accurate culture results must be obtained. Both of these are dependent upon a capable, adequately supported microbiology laboratory, which has not always been available downrange. Both expertise and appropriate automated systems must be in place to accurately identify MDR pathogens, including ESBL-producing organisms; this in particular has been a challenge in recent conflicts. Future IPC strategies must include a focus on establishment and maintenance of appropriate diagnostic microbiology capabilities, with flexibility to adjust as pathogens of concern change.

Education and Training

Ideally, every deployed hospital would be equipped with an IPC officer with knowledge and experience in the field. This is not currently attainable, as only a small number of active duty personnel have such experience. In order to provide predeployment training to personnel tasked with performing IPC officer roles, the Infection Control in the Deployed Environment Course was developed in 2008. This was initiated at Brooke Army Medical Center through the AMEDD Center and School in San Antonio, Texas. Uptake by Army and Air Force personnel deploying in this role has become regular, with >100 (most deploying to Afghanistan) having attended the course to date [66].

Systems for Research and Surveillance

Research and surveillance gaps can quickly become apparent as new infectious disease problems surface in the context of combat casualty care. However, multiple barriers exist toward addressing these gaps, such that many research efforts have been single-center, retrospective studies. Gradually, programmatic improvements in this have been implemented. The Army orchestrated some deployments specifically for infectious disease research. The Department of Defense Trauma Registry had infectious disease modules added in an effort to capture these complications. TIDOS was initiated and began enrolling subjects in 2009, concurrently with the multidrug-resistant organisms repository and surveillance network's collection of isolates for characterization and assessment of global epidemiology. These were admirable efforts which ultimately led to dissemination of robust, multicenter scientific knowledge nearly a decade into combat operations. Development of such capabilities obviously requires considerable time and resources, and they must not be left to founder during times of relative peace.

Tactical IPC Priorities

Guideline-Driven Care

As previously stated, numerous national and international guidelines exist with recommendations for prevention and treatment of healthcare-associated infections. In general, these can be applied to any context of care, and the guidelines for prevention of infections in combat casualties specifically address more austere environments of care [46]. Given the high prevalence of MDR pathogens in deployed hospitals, questions frequently arise about universal contact precautions (gowns and gloves). In general standard precautions should always be applied, with the transmission-based precautions reserved for their typical applications. Cohorting is recommended in order to reduce the risk of cross-transmission from long-term inpatients to patients who will undergo short-term evacuation.

Hand Hygiene

It would be challenging to design an IPC intervention more ideally suited for the deployed (or any other) healthcare environment than hand hygiene. Besides being practically universally applicable to the prevention of infection or transmission of any healthcare-associated infection organism, it is inexpensive, highly evidence based, not highly dependent on context of care or supply chains, and easy to implement and monitor adherence. Alcohol-based handrub (ABHR) is usually preferable to soap and water due to ease of use, lack of required infrastructure, and general acceptance by healthcare workers. It must be easily accessible; if personnel have to go out of their way, they will not use it readily. One intervention at a deployed hospital in Afghanistan involved installing ABHR dispensers on every bedside table in the ICU, after which hand hygiene adherence saw a sustained increase from 28% to 80% [66]. Previously there had been a single sink in each open bay, with dispensers mounted on the walls outside the ICU. Soap and water is still preferred when hands are grossly contaminated. Surveillance for adherence should be performed by trained observers in a standardized fashion and may lead to both on-the-spot feedback and trend determination for reporting to unit and hospital leadership.

Ventilator-Associated Pneumonia Prevention

DCBI patients and other combat casualties are at considerable risk for healthcare-associated, predominantly ventilator-associated pneumonia (VAP). One assessment from the TIDOS cohort during 2009–2010, when DCBI was a predominant mechanism of injury, found that 18% of evacuated ICU patients developed this complication [68]. Implementation of VAP bundles and surveillance for VAP are practical at Level IIIs and are specifically recommended by Joint Theater Trauma System clinical practice guidelines [69]. Application of these guidelines has been demonstrated to significantly reduce VAP rates in both Iraq and Afghanistan Level IIIs. In Iraq, the VAP rate fell from 60 to 11 per 1000 ventilator days, and in Afghanistan this was reduced from 40 to 13 per 1000 ventilator days [66, 70].

Surgical Site Infection Prevention

Surveillance for surgical site infections is clearly recommended in US-based hospitals; however, this is challenging to perform in forward echelons of care given the long durations of follow-up required to ascertain cases, especially when orthopedic hardware is involved. Broad-based interventions designed at lowering risks of operative complications, including the use of operative checklists, can be used in any environment of care. These interventions include the use of alcoholic chlorhexidine for skin preparation, avoidance of shaving when hair removal is necessary, avoidance of hypothermia and hyperglycemia, maintenance of normal oxygenation, and use of appropriate preoperative antimicrobials with adherence to redosing schedules [71–74].

Environmental Disinfection, Sterile Supply, and Endoscope Processing

Housekeeping in deployed environments is often provided by local contractors, but disinfection of equipment used in patient care is typically the purview of nurses and technicians. This equipment, including ventilators, monitors, bedside tables, and hospital beds, can present high risks for indirect transmission of organisms. As an additional, nonclinical duty, disinfection of these items can suffer from lack of standardization. We suggest maintaining a schedule of cleaning patient care equipment, including not only terminal disinfection but regularly during the care of longer-term inpatients, with a checklist to ensure completion by assigned staff. Processing sterile supplies and endoscopes requires specific training and expertise that may be limited in the deployed environment. This duty may fall to inexperienced personnel with on the job training. As such, careful attention should be paid to development of straightforward SOPs and checklists to ensure that quality control procedures have been completed according to standards. A monitoring program should be developed calling for frequent audits to ensure that correct procedures are being used for disinfection.

Antimicrobial Stewardship

Widespread use of antimicrobials in settings treating combat casualties is inevitable. For all the reasons articulated earlier, these casualties, and DCBI patients in particular, are at high risk for infection, and prophylaxis is generally warranted. Unfortunately, adherence to guideline-recommended therapy is variable—both in terms of choice of agent and duration. In 2009, the use of an antibiotic consistent with guidelines was 76% in Iraq and 58% in Afghanistan [75]. Follow-up data showed improvement to 75% compliance overall, but guideline-directed use of antimicrobials in penetrating abdominal injuries still lagged at 68% [76]. These suggest ongoing need for both surveillance and education, particularly in the light of more recent data supporting increasing risk of MDR colonization with the use of fluoroquinolones [60]. It is worth noting that antimicrobial stewardship, in addition to other locally implemented IPC practices, can have a perceptible, rapid impact on antimicrobial susceptibilities of commonly isolated organisms. One evaluation out of Balad, Iraq, assessed ABC susceptibilities after focusing on decreasing carbapenem use, in addition to implementing ventilator-associated pneumonia (VAP) bundles and improving hand hygiene and environmental disinfection. Over a 4-month period, there were statistically significant improvements in ABC susceptibilities to both meropenem (46–64%) and amikacin (41–68%) [70]. Local review of guideline adherence, utilizing pharmacy records, is easy to implement in the deployed setting and can focus attention on problematic patterns of use. Admission order sets should prespecify antibiotics recommended for prophylaxis, with durations for use selected up front. Treatment of established infections in patients admitted to deployed hospitals must involve broader-spectrum empiric agents when MDR pathogens are suspected, but these should be deescalated as quickly as possible based on culture results.

Conclusions

Patients affected by combat wounds in general, and DCBI in particular, frequently suffer infectious complications. These affect 34% of those injured in and evacuated from Afghanistan and 50% if only ICU patients are considered. The destructive nature of their injuries, heavy contamination, frequent need for massive blood transfusions, and complex and austere environments and transitions of care all contribute to risk. These infections are often made more challenging to treat due to the presence of MDR pathogens transmitted in the healthcare environment. While MDR infection varies based upon the context of injury, in recent years ESBL-producing *E. coli* has been the predominant MDR pathogen among DCBI patients. Those injured in Afghanistan, particularly those with severe injuries, amputations, and massive blood transfusion requirements, have shown unique risk for IFI. Preventing these infectious complications involves careful, context-appropriate surgical management of wounds, judicious antimicrobial prophylaxis, and deliberate attention to IPC practices both on the strategic and tactical levels.

Conflicts of Interest The authors declare no conflicts of interest and no funding source used in the preparation of this manuscript.

Disclaimer The views expressed herein are those of the authors and do not reflect the official policy or position of Brooke Army Medical Center, the US Army Medical Department, the US Army Office of the Surgeon General, the Department of the Air Force, the Department of the Army, the Department of Defense, or the US Government.

References

1. Dismounted complex blast injury: report of the army dismounted complex blast injury task force. 2011.
2. Center AFHS. Deployment-related conditions of special surveillance interest. Med Surveill Mon Rep. 2012;19(4):25.
3. Krueger CA, Wenke JC, Ficke JR. Ten years at war: comprehensive analysis of amputation trends. J Trauma Acute Care Surg. 2012;73(6 Suppl 5):S438–44.
4. Reilly C. A chance in hell, part 3: blood and grit. The Virginian-Pilot, 2011, 2.
5. Tribble DR, Conger NG, Fraser S, Gleeson TD, Wilkins K, Antonille T, et al. Infection-associated clinical outcomes in hospitalized medical evacuees after traumatic injury: trauma infectious disease outcome study. J Trauma. 2011;71(1 Suppl):S33–42.
6. Tribble DR, Li P, Warkentien TE, Lloyd BA, Schnaubelt ER, Ganesan A, et al. Impact of operational theater on combat and noncombat trauma-related infections. Mil Med. 2016;181(10):1258–68.
7. Centers for Disease C, Prevention. Acinetobacter Baumannii infections among patients at military medical facilities treating injured U.S. service members, 2002-2004. MMWR Morb Mortal Wkly Rep. 2004;53(45):1063–6.
8. Murray CK, Roop SA, Hospenthal DR, Dooley DP, Wenner K, Hammock J, et al. Bacteriology of war wounds at the time of injury. Mil Med. 2006;171(9):826–9.
9. Yun HC, Murray CK, Roop SA, Hospenthal DR, Gourdine E, Dooley DP. Bacteria recovered from patients admitted to a deployed U.S. military hospital in Baghdad, Iraq. Mil Med. 2006;171(9):821–5.
10. Johnson EN, Burns TC, Hayda RA, Hospenthal DR, Murray CK. Infectious complications of open type III tibial fractures among combat casualties. Clin Infect Dis Off Publ Infect Dis Soc Am. 2007;45(4):409–15.
11. Yun HC, Branstetter JG, Murray CK. Osteomyelitis in military personnel wounded in Iraq and Afghanistan. J Trauma. 2008;64(2 Suppl):S163–8. discussion S8.
12. Hospenthal DR, Crouch HK, English JF, Leach F, Pool J, Conger NG, et al. Multidrug-resistant bacterial colonization of combat-injured personnel at admission to medical centers after evacuation from Afghanistan and Iraq. J Trauma. 2011;71(1 Suppl):S52–7.
13. Weintrob AC, Murray CK, Lloyd B, Li P, Lu D, Miao Z, et al. Active surveillance for asymptomatic colonization with multidrug-resistant gram negative bacilli among injured service members--a three year evaluation. Msmr. 2013;20(8):17–22.
14. White BK, Mende K, Weintrob AC, Beckius ML, Zera WC, Lu D, et al. Epidemiology and antimicrobial susceptibilities of wound isolates of obligate anaerobes from combat casualties. Diagn Microbiol Infect Dis. 2016;84(2):144–50.
15. Blyth DM, Mende K, Weintrob AC, Beckius ML, Zera WC, Bradley W, et al. Resistance patterns and clinical significance of Candida colonization and infection in combat-related injured patients from iraq and afghanistan. Open Forum Infect Dis. 2014;1(3):ofu109.
16. Tong MJ. Septic complications of war wounds. JAMA. 1972;219(8):1044–7.
17. Murray CK, Yun HC, Griffith ME, Hospenthal DR, Tong MJ. Acinetobacter infection: what was the true impact during the Vietnam conflict? Clin Infect Dis Off Publ Infect Dis Soc Am. 2006;43(3):383–4.
18. Wallum TE, Yun HC, Rini EA, Carter K, Guymon CH, Akers KS, et al. Pathogens present in acute mangled extremities from Afghanistan and subsequent pathogen recovery. Mil Med. 2015;180(1):97–103.
19. Keen EF, Mende K, Yun HC, Aldous WK, Wallum TE, Guymon CH, et al. Evaluation of potential environmental contamination sources for the presence of multidrug-resistant bacteria linked to wound infections in combat casualties. Infect Control Hosp Epidemiol Off J Soc Hosp Epidemiol Am. 2012;33(9):905–11.

20. Griffith ME, Ceremuga JM, Ellis MW, Guymon CH, Hospenthal DR, Murray CK. Acinetobacter skin colonization of US Army soldiers. Infect Control Hosp Epidemiol Off J Soc Hosp Epidemiol Am. 2006;27(7):659–61.
21. Griffith ME, Lazarus DR, Mann PB, Boger JA, Hospenthal DR, Murray CK. Acinetobacter skin carriage among US army soldiers deployed in Iraq. Infect Control Hosp Epidemiol Off J Soc Hosp Epidemiol Am. 2007;28(6):720–2.
22. Scott P, Deye G, Srinivasan A, Murray C, Moran K, Hulten E, et al. An outbreak of multidrug-resistant Acinetobacter Baumannii-Calcoaceticus Complex infection in the US military health care system associated with military operations in Iraq. Clin Infect Dis Off Publ Infect Dis Soc Am. 2007;44(12):1577–84.
23. Tangden T, Cars O, Melhus A, Lowdin E. Foreign travel is a major risk factor for colonization with Escherichia Coli producing CTX-M-type extended-spectrum beta-lactamases: a prospective study with Swedish volunteers. Antimicrob Agents Chemother. 2010;54(9):3564–8.
24. Ostholm-Balkhed A, Tarnberg M, Nilsson M, Nilsson LE, Hanberger H, Hallgren A, et al. Travel-associated faecal colonization with ESBL-producing Enterobacteriaceae: incidence and risk factors. J Antimicrob Chemother. 2013;68(9):2144–53.
25. Laupland KB, Church DL, Vidakovich J, Mucenski M, Pitout JD. Community-onset extended-spectrum beta-lactamase (ESBL) producing Escherichia Coli: importance of international travel. J Infect. 2008;57(6):441–8.
26. Vento TJ, Cole DW, Mende K, Calvano TP, Rini EA, Tully CC, et al. Multidrug-resistant gram-negative bacteria colonization of healthy US military personnel in the US and Afghanistan. BMC Infect Dis. 2013;13:68.
27. Janvier F, Delacour H, Tesse S, Larreche S, Sanmartin N, Ollat D, et al. Faecal carriage of extended-spectrum beta-lactamase-producing enterobacteria among soldiers at admission in a French military hospital after aeromedical evacuation from overseas. Eur J Clin Microbiol Infect Dis Off Publ Eur Soc Clin Microbiol. 2014;33:1719.
28. Mende K, Beckius ML, Zera WC, Yu X, Cheatle KA, Aggarwal D, et al. Phenotypic and genotypic changes over time and across facilities of serial colonizing and infecting Escherichia Coli isolates recovered from injured service members. J Clin Microbiol. 2014;52(11):3869–77.
29. Griffith ME, Gonzalez RS, Holcomb JB, Hospenthal DR, Wortmann GW, Murray CK. Factors associated with recovery of Acinetobacter Baumannii in a combat support hospital. Infect Control Hosp Epidemiol Off J Soc Hosp Epidemiol Am. 2008;29(7):664–6.
30. Turton JF, Kaufmann ME, Gill MJ, Pike R, Scott PT, Fishbain J, et al. Comparison of Acinetobacter Baumannii isolates from the United Kingdom and the United States that were associated with repatriated casualties of the Iraq conflict. J Clin Microbiol. 2006;44(7):2630–4.
31. Ake J, Scott P, Wortmann G, Huang XZ, Barber M, Wang Z, et al. Gram-negative multidrug-resistant organism colonization in a US military healthcare facility in Iraq. Infect Control Hosp Epidemiol Off J Soc Hosp Epidemiol Am. 2011;32(6):545–52.
32. Huang XZ, Frye JG, Chahine MA, Glenn LM, Ake JA, Su W, et al. Characteristics of plasmids in multi-drug-resistant Enterobacteriaceae isolated during prospective surveillance of a newly opened hospital in Iraq. PLoS One. 2012;7(7):e40360.
33. Sutter DE, Bradshaw LU, Simkins LH, Summers AM, Atha M, Elwood RL, et al. High incidence of multidrug-resistant gram-negative bacteria recovered from Afghan patients at a deployed US military hospital. Infect Control Hosp Epidemiol Off J Soc Hosp Epidemiol Am. 2011;32(9):854–60.
34. Warkentien T, Rodriguez C, Lloyd B, Wells J, Weintrob A, Dunne JR, et al. Invasive mold infections following combat-related injuries. Clin Infect Dis Off Publ Infect Dis Soc Am. 2012;55(11):1441–9.
35. Weintrob AC, Weisbrod AB, Dunne JR, Rodriguez CJ, Malone D, Lloyd BA, et al. Combat trauma-associated invasive fungal wound infections: epidemiology and clinical classification. Epidemiol Infect. 2015:143(1):214–24.
36. Rodriguez CJ, Weintrob AC, Shah J, Malone D, Dunne JR, Weisbrod AB, et al. Risk factors associated with invasive fungal infections in combat trauma. Surg Infect. 2014;15:521.
37. Tribble DR, Rodriguez CJ, Weintrob AC, Shaikh F, Aggarwal D, Carson ML, et al. Environmental factors related to fungal wound contamination after combat trauma in Afghanistan, 2009-2011. Emerg Infect Dis. 2015;21(10):1759–69.
38. Warkentien TE, Shaikh F, Weintrob AC, Rodriguez CJ, Murray CK, Lloyd BA, et al. Impact of Mucorales and other invasive molds on clinical outcomes of Polymicrobial traumatic wound infections. J Clin Microbiol. 2015;53(7):2262–70.
39. Burns TC, Stinner DJ, Mack AW, Potter BK, Beer R, Eckel TT, et al. Microbiology and injury characteristics in severe open tibia fractures from combat. J Trauma Acute Care Surgery. 2012;72(4):1062–7.
40. Napierala MA, Rivera JC, Burns TC, Murray CK, Wenke JC, Hsu JR, et al. Infection reduces return-to-duty rates for soldiers with type III open tibia fractures. J Trauma Acute Care Surgery. 2014;77(3 Suppl 2):S194–7.
41. Huh J, Stinner DJ, Burns TC, Hsu JR, Late Amputation Study T. Infectious complications and soft tissue injury contribute to late amputation after severe lower extremity trauma. J Trauma. 2011;71(1 Suppl):S47–51.
42. Masini BD, Owens BD, Hsu JR, Wenke JC. Rehospitalization after combat injury. J Trauma. 2011;71(1 Suppl):S98–102.
43. Kelly JF, Ritenour AE, McLaughlin DF, Bagg KA, Apodaca AN, Mallak CT, et al. Injury severity and

causes of death from operation Iraqi freedom and operation enduring freedom: 2003-2004 versus 2006. J Trauma. 2008;64(2 Suppl):S21–6. discussion S6-7.
44. Holcomb JB, McMullin NR, Pearse L, Caruso J, Wade CE, Oetjen-Gerdes L, et al. Causes of death in U.S. special operations forces in the global war on terrorism: 2001-2004. Ann Surg. 2007;245(6):986–91.
45. Lewandowski LR, Weintrob AC, Tribble DR, Rodriguez CJ, Petfield J, Lloyd BA, et al. Early complications and outcomes in combat injury-related invasive fungal wound infections: a case-control analysis. J Orthop Trauma. 2016;30(3):e93–9.
46. Hospenthal DR, Green AD, Crouch HK, English JF, Pool J, Yun HC, et al. Infection prevention and control in deployed military medical treatment facilities. J Trauma. 2011;71(2 Suppl 2):S290–8.
47. Investigators F, Bhandari M, Jeray KJ, Petrisor BA, Devereaux PJ, Heels-Ansdell D, et al. A trial of wound irrigation in the initial management of open fracture wounds. N Engl J Med. 2015;373(27):2629–41.
48. Owens BD, White DW, Wenke JC. Comparison of irrigation solutions and devices in a contaminated musculoskeletal wound survival model. J Bone Joint Surg Am. 2009;91(1):92–8.
49. Maragakis LL, Cosgrove SE, Song X, Kim D, Rosenbaum P, Ciesla N, et al. An outbreak of multidrug-resistant Acinetobacter Baumannii associated with pulsatile lavage wound treatment. JAMA. 2004;292(24):3006–11.
50. Lalliss SJ, Stinner DJ, Waterman SM, Branstetter JG, Masini BD, Wenke JC. Negative pressure wound therapy reduces pseudomonas wound contamination more than Staphylococcus Aureus. J Orthop Trauma. 2010;24(9):598–602.
51. Murray CK, Obremskey WT, Hsu JR, Andersen RC, Calhoun JH, Clasper JC, et al. Prevention of infections associated with combat-related extremity injuries. J Trauma Inj Infect Crit Care. 2011;71:S235–S57.
52. Moues CM, Vos MC, van den Bemd GJ, Stijnen T, Hovius SE. Bacterial load in relation to vacuum-assisted closure wound therapy: a prospective randomized trial. Wound Repair Regen. 2004;12(1):11–7.
53. Pollak AN. Timing of debridement of open fractures. J Am Acad Orthop Surg. 2006;14(10 Spec No.):S48–51.
54. Weber D, Dulai SK, Bergman J, Buckley R, Beaupre LA. Time to initial operative treatment following open fracture does not impact development of deep infection: a prospective cohort study of 736 subjects. J Orthop Trauma. 2014;28(11):613–9.
55. Giannou C, Baldan M, for the International Committee of the Red Cross. War surgery: working with limited resources in armed conflict and other situations of violence, vol. 1; 2010. p. Geneva–ICRC.
56. Dharm-Datta S, McLenaghan J. Medical lessons learnt from the US and Canadian experience of treating combat casualties from Afghanistan and Iraq. J R Army Med Corps. 2013;159(2):102–9.
57. Hospenthal DR, Murray CK, Andersen RC, Bell RB, Calhoun JH, Cancio LC, et al. Guidelines for the prevention of infections associated with combat-related injuries: 2011 update: endorsed by the Infectious Diseases Society of America and the Surgical Infection Society. J Trauma. 2011;71(2 Suppl 2):S210–34.
58. Hauser CJ, Adams CA Jr, Eachempati SR, Council of the Surgical Infection S. Surgical Infection Society guideline: prophylactic antibiotic use in open fractures: an evidence-based guideline. Surg Infect. 2006;7(4):379–405.
59. Hoff WS, Bonadies JA, Cachecho R, Dorlac WC. East practice management guidelines work group: update to practice management guidelines for prophylactic antibiotic use in open fractures. J Trauma. 2011;70(3):751–4.
60. Gilbert LJ, Li P, Murray CK, Yun HC, Aggarwal D, Weintrob AC, et al. Multidrug-resistant gram-negative bacilli colonization risk factors among trauma patients. Diagn Microbiol Infect Dis. 2016;84(4):358–60.
61. Lloyd B, Murray CK, Shaikh F, Schnaubelt E, Whitman T, Blyth DM, Carson L, Tribble DR. Addition of fluoroquinolones or aminoglycosides to post-trauma antibiotic prophylaxis does not decrease risk of early osteomyelitis. IDWeek; 28 October 2016; New Orleans, LA, 2016.
62. Murray CK, Yun HC, Griffith ME, Thompson B, Crouch HK, Monson LS, et al. Recovery of multidrug-resistant bacteria from combat personnel evacuated from Iraq and Afghanistan at a single military treatment facility. Mil Med. 2009;174(6):598–604.
63. Barsoumian A, Sanchez CJ, Mende K, Tully CC, Beckius ML, Akers KS, et al. In vitro toxicity and activity of Dakin's solution, mafenide acetate, and amphotericin B on filamentous fungi and human cells. J Orthop Trauma. 2013;27(8):428–36.
64. Joint Theater Trauma System Clinical Practice Guideline: Invasive Fungal Infection in War Wounds. 2016.
65. Hospenthal DR, Crouch HK, English JF, Leach F, Pool J, Conger NG, et al. Response to infection control challenges in the deployed setting: operations Iraqi and enduring freedom. J Trauma. 2010;69(Suppl 1):S94–101.
66. Yun HC, Murray CK. Infection prevention in the deployed environment. US Army Med Dep J. 2016;(2–16):114–8.
67. Hospenthal DR, Murray CK, Andersen RC, Blice JP, Calhoun JH, Cancio LC, et al. Guidelines for the prevention of infection after combat-related injuries. J Trauma. 2008;64(3 Suppl):S211–20.
68. Yun HC, Weintrob AC, Conger NG, Li P, Lu D, Tribble DR, et al. Healthcare-associated pneumonia among U.S. combat casualties, 2009 to 2010. Mil Med. 2015;180(1):104–10.
69. Joint Theater Trauma System Clinical Practice Guideline: Ventilator Associated Pneumonia 2012 [Available from: http://www.usaisr.amedd.army.mil/assets/cpgs/Ventilator_Associated_Pneumonia_17_Jul_12.pdf.
70. Landrum ML, Murray CK. Ventilator associated pneumonia in a military deployed setting: the impact of an aggressive infection control program. J Trauma. 2008;64(2 Suppl):S123–7. discussion S7-8.

71. Anderson DJ, Kaye KS, Classen D, Arias KM, Podgorny K, Burstin H, et al. Strategies to prevent surgical site infections in acute care hospitals. Infect Control Hosp Epidemiol Off J Soc Hosp Epidemiol Am. 2008;29(Suppl 1):S51–61.
72. Bratzler DW, Hunt DR. The surgical infection prevention and surgical care improvement projects: national initiatives to improve outcomes for patients having surgery. Clin Infect Dis Off Publ Infect Dis Soc Am. 2006;43(3):322–30.
73. de Vries EN, Prins HA, Crolla RM, den Outer AJ, van Andel G, van Helden SH, et al. Effect of a comprehensive surgical safety system on patient outcomes. N Engl J Med. 2010;363(20):1928–37.
74. Darouiche RO, Wall MJ Jr, Itani KM, Otterson MF, Webb AL, Carrick MM, et al. Chlorhexidine-alcohol versus Povidone-iodine for surgical-site antisepsis. N Engl J Med. 2010;362(1):18–26.
75. Tribble DR, Lloyd B, Weintrob A, Ganesan A, Murray CK, Li P, et al. Antimicrobial prescribing practices following publication of guidelines for the prevention of infections associated with combat-related injuries. J Trauma. 2011;71(2 Suppl 2):S299–306.
76. Lloyd BA, Weintrob AC, Hinkle MK, Fortuna GR, Murray CK, Bradley W, et al. Adherence to published antimicrobial prophylaxis guidelines for wounded service members in the ongoing conflicts in Southwest Asia. Mil Med. 2014;179(3):324–8.
77. Yun HC, Murray CK. Practical approach to combat-related infections and antibiotics. In: Martin M, Beekley A, Eckert M, editors. Front Line Surgery: Switzerland: Springer International Publishing; 2017.

Organizing the Trauma Team in the Military and Civilian Settings

Michael B. Yaffe, Alok Gupta, Allison Weisbrod, and James R. Dunne

Military Setting

Walter Reed National Military Medical Center (WRNMMC) functioned as the primary medical evacuation site for patients who were injured on the Operation Iraqi Freedom (OIF) and Operation Enduring Freedom (OEF) battlefields. This required a transformation from a 250-bed university-affiliated teaching hospital into an American College of Surgeons (ACS) Committee on Trauma (COT)-verified trauma center [1]. Continuous monitoring of outcomes and process improvement drove the evolution of new practice guidelines and emphasized the importance of multidisciplinary teamwork in order to optimize care for the nation's wounded warriors.

M. B. Yaffe
Acute Care Surgery, Trauma and Surgical Critical Care, Beth Israel Deaconess Medical Center, Boston, MA, USA

A. Gupta
Division of Acute Care Surgery, Trauma, and Critical Care, Beth Israel Deaconess Medical Center, Harvard Medical School, Boston, MA, USA

A. Weisbrod
Department of Surgery, Naval Hospital Camp Lejeune, Camp Lejeune, NC, USA

J. R. Dunne (✉)
Department of Trauma/Surgical Critical Care, Memorial Health University Medical Center, Savannah, GA, USA
e-mail: dunneja1@memorialhealth.com

Medevac Preparation

Communication was a cornerstone for efficient and effective medical care. Specialists at each level of treatment can minimize wasted resources and logistics by working as a team. Afterward, care plans must be appropriately communicated in transition to the new team.

Once a military member was injured on the battlefield, provider-to-provider handoff was continued as the patient proceeded through each progressive echelon of care. Weekly video teleconferences occurred between Landstuhl Regional Medical Center (LRMC) and WRNMMC in order to discuss patients who were expected to transfer in the near future as well as to augment supporting details about prior transported patients. This was enhanced by reports given by flight physicians and nurses who accompanied the patients in-transit.

Thirty-six hours prior to transport, a manifest was published that listed each patient expected to make the transatlantic flight. This, in turn, triggered admission planning at WRNMMC. Each expected patient had an electronic medical record in the Theater Medical Data Store (TMDS) that included all uploaded medical documentation from each level of care. This repository held paper charts from initial battlefield assessments, in-flight documentation, progress notes, operative reports, and both plain film and axial imaging. The day prior to arrival, each patient's chart was reviewed and a problem list was generated.

An early consult was placed to each medical specialty expected to be involved in a patient's care. This allowed the consulted specialty to review the existing chart and imaging in order to identify additional specialty-specific orders to be placed to streamline the admission process.

At WRNMMC, medical evacuations occurred on Sundays, Tuesdays, and Fridays and were expected to be large-scale, high-resource, simultaneous admission processes. Admission orders were placed the morning of arrival to optimize personnel and logistic efficiency for later that day. Orders included admission labs: complete blood count (CBC), electrolyte panel, coagulation factors, blood cultures, urinalysis and culture, screening cultures for multidrug-resistant organisms (MDROs), type and cross, and prealbumin level. At that time, the patient's medications and antibiotics were also ordered, so that the nursing staff could reconcile dosing times within the medical record prior to arrival and have necessary medications available as the transport staff brought the patient through the door. Imaging studies were preordered, including an admission chest X-ray, an abdominal film to confirm feeding tube placement, immediate computed tomography of the head for patients who sustained a brain injury, as well as any injury-specific films recommended by specialists, thus allowing for an organized and comprehensive visit to the radiology suite.

When each patient was admitted, an admission care team was waiting in his room. This included nursing staff and medical technicians. A trauma, orthopedic, and neurosurgical resident, as a team, evaluated each new patient in order of descending acuity. If a consulted specialty had identified a concern through their earlier chart review, a representative provider joined the admission team assessment. Simultaneous evaluation allowed for minimized discomfort to the patient and initiated early discussion and implementation of coordinated multidisciplinary care. This team of providers also functioned to create a unified message of the patient's care plan to family members.

All wounded warriors had consults placed on admission to the following services: physical therapy, occupational therapy, audiology, dental, social work, psychology/traumatic brain injury, recreational therapy, and speech pathology.

Streamlining Care

Daily Rounds

The trauma team functioned as the primary care team for each polytrauma patient and rounded on each patient twice daily. The patient, his family, and his nurse were all considered important members of each rounding encounter as each provided input into care plans. Due to the collaboration of numerous specialists for each patient, accurate daily documentation was stressed to ensure appropriate written communication was available when verbal communication was not. The trauma team then used this information to reconcile the competing needs of all involved care team members.

Multidisciplinary Conference

WRNMMC held multidisciplinary rounds twice a week to facilitate longitudinal care plans and to address inter-specialty concerns. A large core staff was involved, including a trauma attending, who facilitated the meeting; representatives from the surgical teams taking care of the patients (trauma, neurosurgery, orthopedic surgery, oral maxillary facial surgery/otolaryngology); a provider each from the acute pain service, neurology, and psychology; rehabilitation specialists from physical therapy, occupational therapy, speech therapy, and nutrition, as well as a physical rehabilitation physician; involved social workers and case managers; and representatives from the administration and nursing staff.

Each patient was announced and then his active problem list was reviewed. Concerns about the current care priorities or barriers were addressed. An estimate was given regarding the patient's expected hospital course with an opportunity for discussion from involved specialties. Finally, the expected disposition location and level of care were addressed.

At the end of the rounds, each participant was given a chance to discuss any concerns unique to their specialty in order to ensure that all wounded warrior caretakers were functioning as an effective team. An example included the failure to communicate changes in weight-bearing status in a timely manner to rehabilitation services. Representatives from different services were able to solve problems quickly right then or decide to collaborate outside the meeting in order to find an appropriate solution. In these meetings, a large amount of information was covered efficiently. All participants walked away from the meeting with a global sense of the patient, the patient's priorities, and expected timeline and were therefore able to incorporate their provider plans accordingly.

Operating Room Management

Patients injured in Iraq and Afghanistan had significant operative requirements. Injury patterns commonly included one or more limb amputations and multiple orthopedic injuries in the setting of contaminated soft tissue wounds. This necessitated repetitive debridement prior to definitive orthopedic care.

On patient arrival at WRNMMC, each patient was evaluated for need of immediate operative intervention. Any patient with an open abdomen or who was acutely toxic was brought to the OR on the night of admission. Additionally, if the trauma census was high and a patient needed only minimal operative care or could be definitively treated that night, the patient was brought to the OR in order to facilitate logistics.

In general, all patients were scheduled for operative debridement three times a week on a Monday, Wednesday, and Friday schedule. Three ORs were dedicated to the wounded warriors in order to facilitate care and to minimize the potential for cross contamination of *Acinetobacter* or invasive fungal infections. Acutely ill and recently arrived patients had precedent for first case. Intraoperative care was a multidisciplinary effort with surgeons from each necessary specialty working simultaneously, often within the same wound, in support of each other. This approach streamlined operative time, maximized resources, minimized nothing per os (NPO) status, and encouraged provider teamwork. Prior to the end of the procedure, the logistics of each patient's subsequent case were decided, including necessary team members, operative timing, and instrument requirements.

Conclusion

WRNMMC successfully transitioned from a medium-sized university-affiliated teaching hospital that did not see active trauma into an ACS COT-verified trauma center by focusing on multidisciplinary teamwork and continuous process improvement. The creation of practice guidelines and standard operating protocols was imperative to maintain an optimized care level in a setting of constant personnel turnover – a logistic that was expected in a facility staffed by deploying military members and rotating graduate medical education house staff. The resultant care received high satisfaction ratings from treated patients.

Civilian Setting

Management of a mass casualty incident in the civilian sector presents a variety of unique challenges, including logistics, personnel, and operations management in a setting where at least some degree of routine hospital operations and patient flow needs to be maintained [2].

Disaster Planning

Similar to the military planning process, management of a mass casualty event begins long before the mass casualty itself ever occurs. At a minimum, every civilian Level I trauma center, and ideally every hospital regardless of its trauma designation, should have a clear, well-defined disaster plan. The disaster plan should be an "all-hazards plan," designed to address a wide variety of scenarios and contingencies including active shooter incidents, explosions and building collapses, floods, earthquakes, tornadoes, hurricanes, chemical spills and chemical weapons attacks, radiological accidents, and possibly even widespread dissemination of an infectious disease including bubonic plague or Ebola [3, 4]. Contingencies that should be addressed in the plan include the possibility of failure of the commercial electrical grid, loss of the municipal water supply, flooding of the hospital, lack of critical personnel, communications failure involving the telephone system and cell phone networks, and structural damage to the hospital as a direct result of the mass casualty event. Consequently, a chain of succession of command for hospital-wide management, and within each department, needs to be developed and widely disseminated long before any mass casualty event occurs [5]. In addition, a mechanism for rapidly establishing security at the hospital and preventing secondary casualty-producing events from transpiring there remains a critical component of the MCI plan.

Even the best developed plan will prove to be useless unless the plan is repeatedly put into practice by regular mock mass casualty drills [6]. Our experience is that, for maximum effectiveness, these drills need to be conducted twice a year at a minimum and must involve key personnel/representatives from all stakeholders to include the emergency department, general/trauma surgery, orthopedics, neurosurgery, cardiothoracic surgery, medicine, infectious disease, opthalmology and anesthesiology. In addition, leaders from the intensive care units, operating room, recovery area, blood bank, laboratroy, admissions, medical records, information technology and the morgue will also be needed. Quarterly mock mass casualty drills, with at least one of those each year taking place at off-hours when the hospital is at its lowest staffing level, are ideal. A particularly useful exercise is to incorporate one or more of the contingencies mentioned above into the mock mass casualty drills. Our hospital has developed a series of magnetic whiteboards and scenario exercises for mass casualty planning, and we have successfully exported these to other medical centers across the country. Similar scenario boards can be developed locally or imported from other hospitals such as ours in which correct and incorrect practices have been identified, refined, and improved through real-world application during mass casualty events [7].

In our experience both locally and nationally with conducting disaster drills, we have come to learn that the most effective planning exercises are ones that drill deep into the system to expose vulnerabilities. The debrief to follow – or after-actions review – should aim to identify errors made by personnel, challenges encountered by participants, and system-wide deficiencies. These are then used to create an action plan for future benefit. A disaster planning drill that identifies no opportunities for improvement is a lost opportunity. This can also create a false sense of security.

Patient Management During Disasters

Once mass casualty victims arrive at the medical center, their management occurs in four distinct phases: (1) initial evaluation and triage, (2) immediate resuscitation, (3) initiation of definitive care, and (4) the extended recovery phase. Our management strategy to accomplish these phases reflects the authors' collective experience during the 9/11 terrorist attack in New York City in 2001 [8], the catastrophic Haitian earthquake in 2010 [9, 10], the Boston Marathon bombing in 2013 [11, 12], and the Taliban attack on the US Army Special Forces Camp Integrity in Kabul, Afghanistan, in 2015 [13]. Several key aspects of civilian disaster management strategy differ from those used in the military sector, while other aspects are shared. For example, in both civilian and military disaster management, there is a need for rapid secondary triage of casualties upon arrival at the medical treatment center, in addition to the field triage that occurred at the location of the disaster. The status of the casualties can rapidly change en route, and injuries that were not immediately apparent in the commotion of the initial response often become apparent and/or better defined in a more resource-rich environment. We have found it very expedient to have pre-prepared colored triage tags and mass casualty patient "packets" containing a standard trauma H&P form, a set of standing orders and nursing notes, and a template sheet on which to write lab results and blood product infusions [14]. Triage classifications are relatively uniform across the civilian and military sectors and include "urgent" (green tag), "urgent surgical" (red tag), delayed (yellow tag), and expectant (black tag) categories. The specific time requirements for treatment of each triage category are not absolute in the civilian sector, in contrast to the military response. Following secondary triage, immediate resuscitation typically is continued/performed in the emergency department, including previously designated overflow locations, which typically include the adjacent parking lot abutting the ED in fair weather and/or the family waiting areas outside the ED during periods of inclement weather. In civilian mass casualty events, resource limitations for the resuscitation phase (IVs, fluids, bandages, personnel capable of monitoring vital signs) are rarely the limiting factor, in contrast to the situation in forward-deployed military mass casualty events. Unstable patients who do not need immediate surgical intervention should be rapidly transferred to the intensive care unit. The early involvement of anesthesiology, psychiatry, and social work during this phase of care may help reduce the subsequent incidence of post-traumatic stress disorder [15–17].

The initial bottleneck in civilian mass casualty events is typically the availability of ICU beds, operating rooms, and availability of appropriate surgical providers. Operations that are already in progress at the medical center prior to arrival of the MCI patients need to be concluded as rapidly as possible, and pending cases need to be canceled. ORs and associated staff are then re-prioritized, trying to maintain at least one circulator or scrub nurse who has experience with the specific case type (orthopedics, vascular, thoracic, neurosurgery, trauma/general surgery) in the room. Surgeons may be asked to perform emergency cases in areas outside their typical civilian practice and comfort zone, including amputations, vascular repair, fasciotomies, burn debridement, and escharotomies. Surgeon extenders, including PAs and surgical residents, can play key roles by accompanying and monitoring unstable patients during the resuscitation and initial operative treatment phases. Senior and chief surgical residents may function as the senior surgeon in appropriate cases should the demand require it. Specific types of equipment, medications, and dressings such as burn supplies may be limited during the first 24–48 h after the MCI, compromising patient care. During the Boston Marathon bombing, a system of interhospital sharing and exchange proved critical for distribution of certain key orthopedic, plastic surgery, and burn supplies [12]. In addition, several major medical suppliers immediately volunteered to provide urgently needed supplies outside of the traditional requisition and payment systems. Ideally, such arrangements could be incorporated in the pre-disaster planning phase.

Options for Extended Clinical Service Care of MCI Victims

Management of care of these patients during the ensuing days and weeks after the mass casualty event presents another distinct challenge. Many of these patients will require repeated trips to the operating room as their wounds evolve or if the initial operation was limited to damage control. Depending on the size of the injured patient population, a fixed number of operating rooms needs to be set aside and removed from the regular scheduling process as the medical center transitions back to its daily routine that was in place prior to the MCI. This may also require a temporary increase in the staffing of anesthesiologists, operating room nurses, attendants, and other OR staff. This requires support from the highest levels of leadership in clinical departments and hospital administration. Exactly how the mass casualty patients themselves should be followed and managed during the extended recovery phase is equally challenging. We present three distinct models for the extended care phase and describe each briefly below.

The most traditional model for mass casualty event patient flow during the recovery phase is to utilize the standard trauma model in use at most Level I trauma centers. In this model, patients with single-system injuries (orthopedics, vascular, thoracic) are cared for on separate services devoted to these specialties, while those with multisystem injuries (i.e., a vascular injury in the setting of a fracture) are cared for on the trauma service, usually managed by a general surgeon with fellowship training in trauma and critical care. The advantage of this model is that it utilizes the ingrained patient flow mechanism that is already well established and functional in the medical center.

An alternative model involves placing all of the mass casualty patients on the existing trauma service, regardless of whether their injuries are multisystem or single system. This expansion of the existing trauma service allows integration of these patients into a trauma-focused primary clinical service and maintains a single provider (the attending trauma surgeon) as the overseer of care for all patients from a single event. The sudden surge in patient numbers, however, will likely necessitate additional clinical staffing, including attending surgeons, fellows, residents, and mid-level providers. Furthermore, increased ancillary care staffing needs should be anticipated, including nursing, respiratory therapy, physical therapy, occupational therapy, and social work. Every attempt is made to maintain business as usual for the non-MCI patients, although resources must be shared, based on patient acuity – i.e., ordering of the daily OR case sequence, patient priority during rounds, etc. A major advantage of this existing trauma service model is that it allows a direct line of communication between one trauma-skilled designated provider, the attending trauma surgeon, with hospital leadership in order to secure all needed resources such as an ICU and ward beds, OR block time, and related administrative issues.

The third model involves the spontaneous creation of a dedicated Mass Casualty Service (MCS) as an entirely separate, independent clinical service. This obviously creates separate staffing needs such as an MCS attending surgeon and a cadre of resident and mid-level providers whose clinical efforts are dedicated to this unique patient population. The central advantage of this approach is that it allows all of the patients who shared the same physical and emotional trauma to be cared for under a single distinct "umbrella of care," even if the patients are geographically distributed across the hospital. Furthermore, it facilitates the integration of multidisciplinary rounds under the direction of the MCS attending (a trauma/general surgeon) in which one or more representatives from each of the other key services (orthopedics, neurosurgery, vascular surgery, plastic surgery, anesthesiology, infectious disease, psychiatry, nursing, social work, OT/PT) are present. This insures a well-coordinated plan for patient care in which all critical areas are adequately covered during daily or twice daily rounds. In addition, the identification of a specific cohort of ancillary staff required for only MCI patients makes it easier to disseminate clinical information in real time and markedly enhances the efficiency with which these personnel can be trained and updated with regard to security issues, HIPAA concerns, and emerging clinical priorities. The MCS approach also minimizes the total number of ancillary staff that are "exposed" to MCI patients, enhancing the comfort of the MCS patients and likely reducing secondary PTSD events among the staff. Communication with hospital leadership is *very* streamlined in this model, and it specifically allows the needs of the MCS patients to be addressed separately from those of other trauma patients. Furthermore, the MCS concept can then be extended into the outpatient arena, facilitating further care following discharge. Additional details of the MCS concept will be presented elsewhere, but the concept should be considered during disaster planning scenarios.

Other Considerations

Specific issues that require high prioritization during mass casualty events include media management, security management, and manpower management. There is an intense media presence at the medical center following an MCI which needs to be controlled and coordinated in order to provide information to both the local government and general public, calm fears and limit rumors, and simultaneously protect patient confidentiality [18]. We have found that this is best accomplished by having a single point person act as the media representative, typically a senior official from the department of media relations and communication. If necessary, this person should be accompanied by a single knowledgeable physician, typically a trauma surgeon or ER provider to provide appropriate clinical details.

It is imperative that individual providers do not speak directly with the media without specific designation and approval from the hospital administration in order to limit the chaos that inevitably flows in such events.

Following an MCI, the medical center itself becomes a secondary target for additional attacks. A security plan that limits visitors and nonmedical personnel and screens packages, including those marked as "medical supplies" upon arrival, is paramount. Following the Boston Marathon bombing, our medical center cared for both the victims and the two people identified as the bombers responsible for the event. Maintaining separation between these two groups was paramount to prevent additional episodes of violence.

Finally, it must be remembered that MCI management, even in the acute phases, requires prolonged efforts in manpower [3]. It is important not to deploy all of your resources and personnel immediately. Instead, a cohort of clinical and nonclinical staff will be needed for later shifts and should be held in reserve, if possible. If traffic conditions and road closures limit access to and from the medical area, it may be necessary to provide this group of people with lodging and food and maintain them on site until the time of their duty shift. Ideally all of these contingencies including media, security, and manpower issues should be contained in a well-constructed MCI disaster plan.

References

1. Elster EA, Pearl JP, DeNobile JW, Perdue PW, Stojadinovic A, Liston WA, et al. Transforming an academic military treatment facility into a trauma center: lessons learned from operation Iraqi freedom. Eplasty. 2009;9:e31.
2. Adini B, Goldberg A, Laor D, Cohen R, Zadok R, Bar-Dayan Y. Assessing levels of hospital emergency preparedness. Prehosp Disaster Med. 2006;21:451–7.
3. Klein JS, Weigelt JA. Disaster management. Lessons learned. Surg Clin North Am. 1991;71:257–66.
4. Biddinger PD, Savoia E, Massin-Short SB, Preston J, Stoto MA. Public health emergency preparedness exercises: lessons learned. Public Health Rep. 2010;125(Suppl 5):100–6.
5. Schmalzried HFallon LF Jr. Succession planning for local health department top executives: reducing risk to communities. J Community Health. 2007;32:169–80.
6. Jenckes MW, Catlett CL, Hsu EB, Kohri K, Green GB, Robinson KA, Bass EB, Cosgrove SE. Development of evaluation modules for use in hospital disaster drills. Am J Disaster Med. 2007;2:87–95.
7. Dausey DJ, Buehler JW, Lurie N. Designing and conducting tabletop exercises to assess public health preparedness for manmade and naturally occurring biological threats. BMC Public Health. 2007;7:92.
8. Reibman J, Levy-Carrick N, Miles T, Flynn K, Hughes C, Crane M, Lucchini RG. Destruction of the world trade center towers. Lessons learned from an environmental health disaster. Ann Am Thorac Soc. 2016;13:577–83.
9. Auerbach PS, Norris RL, Menon AS, Brown IP, Kuah S, Schwieger J, Kinyon J, Helderman TN, Lawry L. Civil-military collaboration in the initial medical response to the earthquake in Haiti. N Engl J Med. 2010;362:e32.
10. Merin O, Miskin IN, Lin G, Wiser I, Kreiss Y. Triage in mass-casualty events: the Haitian experience. Prehosp Disaster Med. 2011;26:386–90.
11. Boston Trauma Center Chiefs C. Boston marathon bombings: an after-action review. J Trauma Acute Care Surg. 2014;77:501–3.
12. Gates JD, Arabian S, Biddinger P, Blansfield J, Burke P, Chung S, Fischer J, Friedman F, Gervasini A, Goralnick E, Gupta A, Larentzakis A, McMahon M, Mella J, Michaud Y, Mooney D, Rabinovici R, Sweet D, Ulrich A, Velmahos G, Weber C, Yaffe MB. The initial response to the Boston marathon bombing: lessons learned to prepare for the next disaster. Ann Surg. 2014;260:960–6.
13. Schauer SG, April MD, Simon E, Maddry JK, Carter R, Delorenzo RA. Prehospital interventions during mass-casualty events in Afghanistan: a case analysis. Prehosp Disaster Med. 2017;32(4):465–468.
14. Hong R, Sexton R, Sweet B, Carroll G, Tambussi C, Baumann BM. Comparison of START triage categories to emergency department triage levels to determine need for urgent care and to predict hospitalization. Am J Disaster Med. 2015;10:13–21.
15. Hobfoll SE, Watson P, Bell CC, Bryant RA, Brymer MJ, Friedman MJ, Friedman M, Gersons BP, de Jong JT, Layne CM, Maguen S, Neria Y, Norwood AE, Pynoos RS, Reissman D, Ruzek JI, Shalev AY, Solomon Z, Steinberg AM, Ursano RJ. Five essential elements of immediate and mid-term mass trauma intervention: empirical evidence. Psychiatry. 2007;70:283–315. discussion 316-269.
16. Watson PJ, Friedman MJ, Ruzek JI, Norris F. Managing acute stress response to major trauma. Curr Psychiatry Rep. 2002;4:247–53.
17. Ruzek JI, Kuhn E, Jaworski BK, Owen JE, Ramsey KM. Mobile mental health interventions following war and disaster. Mhealth. 2016;2:37.
18. Lowrey W, Evans W, Gower KK, Robinson JA, Ginter PM, McCormick LC, Abdolrasulnia M. Effective media communication of disasters: pressing problems and recommendations. BMC Public Health. 2007;7:97.

Index

A

Abdomen
  CONUS, 130
  DCBI, 66, 130, 131
  laparotomy, 66
  solid organ injury, 66
Abdominal trauma
  assessment and initial evaluation, 123–124
  blast injury, 122
  catastrophic intra-abdominal hemorrhage, 121
  damage control laparotomy, 127
  DCBI, 121, 124
  demographics, 122–123
  fecal diversion, combat trauma, 128
  historical perspective, 121–122
  IEDs, 121
  intra-abdominal injuries, 131
  IR—interventional radiology, 125
  prehospital care, 131
  research, 131
  surgical management
    complications, 130
    damage control, 124–126
    fecal diversion, 128–130
    second-look operations and definitive treatment, 126–128
Abdominoperineal resection (APR), 129
Abnormal penile curvature, 156
ACell® products, 191
Acinetobacter baumannii-calcoaceticus complex (ABC), 182, 270–274, 279, 287
Activities of daily living (ADLs), 234
Acute Lung Injury Rescue Team (ALIRT), 117
Acute respiratory distress syndrome (ARDS), 53, 114, 116, 117
Acute traumatic coagulopathy (ATC), 46
Adjacent tissue transfer (ATT), 214
Advanced Surgical Skills for Exposure in Trauma (ASSET), 79
Advanced Trauma Life Support (ATLS), 30
Advanced Trauma Operative Management (ATOM), 79
Alcohol-based handrub (ABHR), 278
AlloDerm®, 130

American Association for the Surgery of Trauma (AAST), 152, 154, 156
Amputation
  blast trauma casualties, 226, 232, 237
  complications, 171–174
  DCBI, 166
  defense-funded study, 175
  definitive management, 168–170
  early complications, 170–171
  IEDs, 166
  individuals, 226, 234, 236, 237
  initial management, 166–168
  lower limb, 225, 227, 236
  MTFs, 225
  osseointegration, 175
  outcomes, 174–175
  pain, 234
  peripheral nerves, 235
  proximal transfemoral, 229
  surgical techniques, 175, 235
  transhumeral osseointegrated implants, 175
  transtibial, 237
  traumatic, 226, 228, 236
  upper limb, 225, 226, 231
Analgesia, 17
Ankle-brachial index (ABI), 136, 137
Anterolateral thoracotomy incision, 87
Antimicrobial therapeutic agents, 275–276
Aorta
  abdominal aorta, 90–93
  infrarenal aorta, 91
  intermittent occlusion, 94–95
  partial occlusion, 95
  thoracic aorta, 87
  visceral segment, 90
Arterial
  access, 93
  concomitant, 139
  subclavian artery injuries, 145
  venous injuries, 138, 143
  wounds, 65
Arteriovenous fistulae, 137, 141
Automated Neuropsychological Assessment Metrics (ANAM), 243

© Springer International Publishing AG, part of Springer Nature 2018
J. M. Galante et al. (eds.), *Managing Dismounted Complex Blast Injuries in Military & Civilian Settings*, https://doi.org/10.1007/978-3-319-74672-2

Axillary artery, 81
Axillosubclavian artery injury, 145–147

B
Balanced resuscitation, 47
Barotrauma, 10
Bladder injuries, 68, 153
Blast injury, 9–11, 13, 100, 103–105
    DCBI, 121
    DRTs, 217
    free tissue transfer, 216
    hybrid reconstructive ladder, 218–219
    ISS, 209
    lower extremity, 210
    pathophysiology, 122
    primary (*see* Primary blast injuries)
    quaternary (*see* Quaternary blast injuries)
    reconstructive ladder, 214–215
    secondary (*see* secondary blast injuries)
    severe soft tissue injury, 211–212
    tertiary (*see* Tertiary blast injuries)
    upper extremity, 211, 215
Blast lung injury (BLI)
    air emboli and bronchopulmonary fistula, 113
    ARDS and BLI, 114
    clinical features, 113
    description, 112
    hypoxia, 117
    incidence, 111
    prognosis, 114
Bleeding Control for the Injured (B-Con), 26
Body-powered arm, 232
Borg's Rate of Perceived Exertion (RPE), 247
Boston Marathon bombing, 44, 78
Brachial artery, 81, 146
Bronchopleural fistula, 114
Bronchoscopy, 116
Burn
    airway, 197
    dermis, 205
    dressing, 204, 206, 207
    inhalation, 198
    intubation, 198
    patients, 205, 207
    resuscitation, 199–203
    TBSA, 198–202, 204
    wound, 204

C
Care under fire, 16
Case fatality rate (CFR), 159
Certified registered nurse anesthetists (CRNA), 37
Chest and pelvic films, 62
Civilian disaster, 197
Civilian setting, 287
Clinical practice guidelines (CPG), 183
Coalition forces, 203, 204
Coda catheter, 93
Cognitive disorders
    arousal, 254
    memory impairment, 254
    pharmacologic treatment, 254
Cognitive therapy, 254
Colonic reanastomosis, 67
Colostomy, 121, 128, 129
Combat
    bowel injuries, 66
    casualties, 270, 271, 276, 278, 279
    CSHs, 269
    injury, 269
    trauma, 128–130, 275–276
    and weather conditions, 273
    wounded, 259, 266
Combat application tourniquet (CAT), 1, 167
Combat-related extremity wound infection (CEWI)
    analysis, 193
Combat-related wounds
    abdominal cavity, 187, 188
    agricultural debris, 184
    amputation wound, 191
    bacterial and fungal pathogens, 194
    bowel and mesentary, 188
    CEWI analysis, 193
    diagnosis, 184–185
    dismounted blast wounds, 182
    higher-level amputations, 186
    immunosuppression, 192–193
    infection, 181–184, 193
    invasive fungal infection (*see* Invasive fungal infection)
    ischemia, 192
    liver, 187
    local nonoperative wound care, 188–190
    necrotic fibroadipose tissue, 189
    pain control, 193
    pathogens, 181
    proximal vascular control, 184
    reconstruction, 190–191
    recurrent necrosis, 185
    soft tissue sheen, 187
    systemic therapy, 191–192
    timing, wound closure, 190
    treatment
        debridement, 185–187
        operative exploration, 185–187
        surgical and medical, 185
Committee for Tactical Emergency Casualty Care, 26
Common femoral artery (CFA), 84, 144
Complete blood count (CBC), 286
Complex wound care, 211, 215, 217
Complications, TBI
    autonomic storming, 255
    heterotopic ossification (HO), 256
    hydrocephalus, 256
    pituitary gland, 256
    spasticity, 256
    VTE prophylaxis, 256
Component therapy, 49
Comprehensive care, 226

Index

Computed tomographic angiography (CTA), 137
Computed tomography (CT), 252
Concussion
    chronic cognitive sequelae, 244
    intracranial abnormalities, 242
    MACE, 243
    mTBI, 241
    SCAT, 243
    sleep disturbances, 245
    vestibular dysfunction, 245
Continental United States (CONUS), 124
Cosmetic cover, 233
Crystalloid, 44, 45, 51
Cystostomy tube, 69

D

Damage control laparotomy, 66
Damage control orthopedics (DCO), 163
Damage control principles, 57–60
Damage control resuscitation (DCR), 60
    multiorgan failure, 48
    plasma and RBCs, 47
    PRBCs, 48
    tenants, 47
Damage control surgery, 124–126, 128–131
DCBI patients
    blast energy affects, 261
    care components, 262
    challenges, WRNMMC, 266
    enteral nutrition, 264
    guidelines, nutrition, 264
    hand-off communication tools, 266
    IFI, 263, 264
    multidisciplinary trauma team, 260
    pain management, 262–263
    polytrauma, 260
    TBI service, 261, 262
    VTE, 264, 265
    wound care team, 262
    WRNMMC, 259–261
Debridement, 204, 207
Defense and Veteran Brain Injury Center (DVBIC), 247
Definitive resuscitation
    blast-injured patients, 52
    empiric therapy and TEG-guided therapy, 52
    PBLI, 53
    PROPPR trial, 51
    TEG/ROTEM, 52
Definitive socket, 228
Deflagration, 7
Department of Defense Trauma Registry (DoDTR), 154, 156
Department of Veterans Affairs/Department of Defense (VA/DoD), 241
Deputy commander for clinical services (DCCS), 40
Dermal regeneration template (DRT), 163, 215
Dermanet®, 207
Dermis, 205
Detonation, 7–9, 12

Diffuse axonal injury (DAI)
    classification grading scale, 252
    intracranial bleeding, 252–253
    neuroimaging, 252–253
    tensile strain and disruption, 252
Disasters
    patient management, 288–289
    planning, 287–288
Dismounted complex blast injuries (DCBI)
    administrative controls, 276
    in Afghanistan, 270
    antimicrobial stewardship, 274, 279
    airway management, 62
    description, 225
    diagnostic microbiology capabilities, 276–277
    drug-resistant bacteria, 270
    education and training, 277
    endoscope processing, 279
    environmental wound contamination, 63
    evaluation and management, 61
    guideline-driven care, 278
    hand hygiene, 278
    healthcare-associated infections, 270
    IEDs, 269
    IFI, 63
    IPC, 274
    MDR infection, 280
    microbiology, 270–272
    outcomes, 272–273
    patients, 279
    perineal soft tissue injuries, 13
    research and surveillance, 277–278
    risk factors, 269
    surgical site infection, 278
    TIDOS, 270
    traumatic amputations, 13
    triple limb amputations, 269
    unsurvivable injuries, 269
    VAP, 278
    wound management, 273–274
Disorders of consciousness (DOC), 254
Dressing, 2, 204, 206, 207
Duplex ultrasound (DUS), 137

E

Electrocautery, 161, 168
Emergency department, 251
Empiric therapy, 52
Endotracheal tubes, 197–199
Endovascular
    aortic occlusion, 93
    REBOA, 141, 147
    trauma, 146–147
Energy return feet, 231
Enterobacteriaceae, 271
Epicenter, 8, 9
Epidural hematomas, 252
ER thoracotomy, 41
Ertapenem, 274

Escharotomy, 201, 202
ET tube, 198
Evacuation care phase, 23
Excessive fluid administration, 43
Expanded polytetrafluoroethylene (ePTFE) grafts, 143
Explosive blasts
   artillery shell, 11, 12
   blunt, 8
   casualties, 7, 9, 10, 13
   devices, 7, 8, 11, 13
   high-order explosives
      blast wave, 8
      blast wind, 8
      brisance, 8
      detonation, 7
   low-order explosives, 7
   multidimensional injuries, 9
   penetrating injuries, 8
   personal protective equipment, 9, 12, 13
Extended-spectrum beta-lactamase (ESBL), 182, 271
External genital injury, 153, 158
External hemorrhage control, 21
Extracellular matrices (ECM), 215
Extremity
   DCBI, 161, 167, 173
   dysvascular, 167
   heterotopic ossification, 159
   LEAP study, 174
   limb prostheses, 174
   METALS study, 174
   in multi-trauma patients, 163
   myoelectric prosthetics/upper, 173, 175
   traumatic, 160

F
Fasciotomies, 65, 140
Femoral artery injuries, 144
Fibronectin, 219
Fluid resuscitation, 17
Fluoroquinolones, 274, 279
Focused abdominal sonography for trauma (FAST), 102, 124
Fogarty balloon catheter, 142

G
Gastroenterology, 3
Genitourinary injuries, 69, 70
Genitourinary trauma
   abdominal trauma secondary, 151
   bladder injuries, 153
   expeditious management, 158
   external genitals and urethra, 158
   flap-based renorrhaphy, 152
   Gerota fascia, 151
   IED blast, 151, 155
   OEF and OIF, 151, 152
   penile and testicular laceration, 157
   penile injuries, 153–155
   renal and ureteral trauma, 152–153
   scrotal and testicular injuries, 156–157
   scrotal skin avulsion, 156
   testis injury scale, 156
   tunica albuginea, 157
   urethral injuries, 155–156
Glasgow Coma Scale (GCS), 105, 251, 254
Glycosaminoglycans, 217, 219
Grafting, 200, 203–208
Gram-negative rods (GNR), 270
Grocott-Gomori's methenamine silver (GMS) stains, 263
Guillotine amputations, 68, 167

H
Head injury, 23
Hematochezia, 124
Hematomas
   epidural, 252
   subdural, 252, 253, 256
Hematoxylin and eosin (H&E) stains, 263
Hemipelvectomy, 3, 4, 174
Hemorrhage control
   axillary artery, 81
   blast-injured casualty, 78
   brachial artery, 81
   CFA, 84, 85
   expedient exposure, 79
   extremity vascular injury, 138
   iliac vessels, 83–84
   inguinal ligament, 84
   noncompressible torso, 141
   popliteal artery, 85
   prehospital care, 77
   SCA, 79
   traumatic amputation, 77
   tourniquets, 144
Hemorrhagic shock, 197, 201
Hemostatic resuscitation, 60
Heterotopic ossification (HO), 164, 172, 174, 175, 236
Hibiclens solution, 199, 203–205
Host nationals, 199, 203, 204
Hybrid reconstructive ladder, 215, 217–220
Hyperinsulinemia, 173
Hypocoagulability, 160
Hypotensive resuscitation
   DCR, 47
   rebleeding systolic blood pressure, 46
   theory of rebleeding, 46
Hypothermia, 17, 23

I
Iliac vessels, 83–84
Implantable myoelectric electrode systems (IMES), 221
Improved explosive devices (IEDs), 1, 115, 151, 153, 156, 209, 210, 222, 225, 269, 270
Infection prevention and control (IPC), 274–276
Inferior vena cava (IVC) filters, 265
Infrarenal aorta, 91

Index

Inguinal ligament, 84
Initial damage control resuscitation, 61
Injury
    bleeding, 1, 2
    dressings, 2, 3
    examination, 2
    hemorrhage, 1, 2
    Wounded Warrior, 1–5
Innominate artery injury, 147
Internal skeletal fixation, 104
Intracranial pressure (ICP), 253
Intraparenchymal airspace, 113
Intrapelvic hemorrhage, 100
Intrepid Dynamic Exoskeletal Orthosis (IDEO), 165
Intubation, 22, 198
Invasive fungal infection (IFI), 63, 161, 164, 171, 183, 184
    antimicrobial, 263
    blast patients, 263
    debridement, 264
    geographical differences, 183
    morbidity and mortality, 263
    Mucorales and *Aspergillus* species, 263
    surgical doctrine, 186
    tissue histopathology, 263

J
Joint Theater Trauma Registry (JTTR), 111, 135
Joint Trauma System (JTS), 260

L
Lactated Ringer's (LR) solution, 44
Landstuhl Regional Medical Center (LRMC), 272, 285
Laparotomy, 121, 123–127, 129, 130
Large-volume resuscitation, 45
Legacy Emanuel DOR capability, 71
Length of coma (LOC), 251
Leukocytosis, 3
Lidocaine, 236
Liner, 227
Low back pain (LBP), 236
Lower Extremity Assessment Project (LEAP) study, 174
Lower limb prosthetics, 229–231
Low-molecular-weight heparin (LMWH), 265

M
Major exsanguinating external hemorrhage, 22
Mangled extremity, 77
MASCAL, *see* Mass casualty incidents
Mass casualty incidents
    anesthesia, 31
    communication, 42
    CRNA, 37
    CSH, 38
    DCN and DCCS, 40
    dead, 39
    emergent, 36
    EMT section, 32, 35
    expectant patient, 39
    ICU and operating room, 32
    leadership position, 34
    management, 31
    minimal category, 38
    narcotic administration, 41–42
    NCOs, 30
    operating room, 40, 41
    patient movement, 31
    principle, 29, 41
    traditional/garrison model, 31
    trauma experience, 30
    triage category system, 35
    triage officer, 32, 34, 42
    workup and treatment, 38
Mass Casualty Service (MCS), 290
Mechanical knees, 230
Medevac preparation, 285–286
Median sternotomy, 89
Medical care and medical evacuation (MEDEVAC), 225
Memory impairment, 254
Microprocessor knees, 230
Mild traumatic brain injury (mTBI)
    acute assessment, 242–243
    cognitive deficits, 244
    definition, 241
    demographics, 241–242
    DVBIC guidelines, 246, 247
    mechanisms, 242
    natural course, 247
    PCS, 243, 244
    post-traumatic headache, 245
    PTHA, 244
    recovery patterns, 243
    SIS, 246
    sleep disturbances, 245–246
    vestibular dysfunction, 245
    Zurich guidelines, 246–247
Military
    deployed military treatment facilities, 277
    echelons of care, 212
    nondeployed military personnel, 271
    setting, 285
    the US military casualties, 272
    wounding studies, 15
Military Acute Concussion Evaluation (MACE), 11
Military Extremity Trauma Amputation versus Limb Salvage (METALS) study, 174
Minimally conscious state (MCS), 254
Modern casualties, 39
Moral, welfare, and recreation (MWR), 40
Moxifloxacin, 274
Mucormycosis, 171
Multidrug-resistant (MDR), 270
Multidrug-resistant organisms (MDROs), 286
Myodesis, 169, 173
Myoelectric arm, 232

N

National Trauma Data Bank (NTDB), 73, 136
Necrosis, 3
  consecutive debridements, 191
  effects, 182
  operating room, 187
Needle thoracostomy, 22
Negative pressure wound therapy (NPWT), 213
Neurobehavioral dysfunction
  agitation, 255
  environmental stimuli, 255
  hypoarousal and sleep disturbances, 255
  pharmacologic treatment, 255
  posttraumatic agitation, 255
  rehabilitation team and family, 255
Neurobehavioral symptom inventory (NSI), 247
Non-compressible torso hemorrhage (NCTH), 64
Non-wartime civilian trauma, 151
Normal saline (NS), 188

O

Obstructive sleep apnea (OSA), 245
Open aortic occlusion, 86
Open chest wound, 115
Open pelvic fracture, 99, 101, 105
Operating room management, 287
Operation enduring freedom (OEF), 209, 285
Operation Iraqi Freedom (OIF), 209, 285
Orchiectomy, 107
Orthopedic surgeons, 2
Ostomy, 124, 128–130
Overseas contingency operations (OCOs), 156
Ovine forestomach matrix, 219

P

Palovarotene, 172
Pelvic blast injuries, 99
Pelvic fracture, 62, 63, 67, 68
  acute surgical care, 101–104
  cavity, 101
  colostomy, 104
  emergent management, 101
  hemipelves, 99
  hemorrhage control, 103
  NPWT, 104
  pelvic ring disruptions, 100
  prehospital care, 100–101
  reconstructive care, 104–106
  soft tissue management, 103
  treatment, 106–107
  viscus rupture, 100
Pelvic packing and direct control methods, 102
Penetrating cardiac wounds, 65
Penile injuries, 153–155
Perineal blast injuries, 153
Periodic acid-Schiff (PAS) stains, 263
Permissive hypotension, 46
Persistently symptomatic residual limbs (PSRLs), 172, 174
Personal protective equipment, 9, 12, 13
Phantom pain, 234, 235
Plastic ThermoLyn material, 227
Pleural airspace, 113
Pneumothorax, 113–117
Point-of-care management
  LR and NS, 51
  prehospital environment, 51
  shock, 51
  TCCC guidelines, 51
Polytrauma
  blast injuries, 260
  Veterans Affairs' Polytrauma Centers, 262
  WRNMMC, 260
Polytrauma system of care (PSC), 256
Popliteal artery, 85–86, 144–145
Posaconazole, 192
Post-concussive syndrome (PCS), 243
Posterior tibial artery (PTA), 145
Posterolateral thoracotomy, 88–89
Posttraumatic amnesia (PTA), 251
Post-traumatic headaches (PTHA), 244
Posttraumatic seizures (PTS), 256
Post-traumatic stress disorder (PTSD), 228, 237
Pragmatic Randomized Optimal Platelet and Plasma Ratios (PROPPR) trial, 47
Preventable death, 15, 19, 27
Primary blast injuries
  delayed injuries, 10
  devastating, 10
  gastrointestinal injuries, 10
  implosion, 9
  tympanic membrane, 9, 10
Primary blast lung injury (PBLI), 53
Profunda femoris artery (PFA), 144
Prosthetic device, 226–229, 231, 232, 234–237
Prosthetists, 229
Proteoglycans, 219
Pseudoaneurysm, 87, 94, 137, 141, 147
Pulmonary barotrauma, 253

Q

Quadratus lumborum, 151
Quaternary blast injuries, 13, 116

R

Radial artery injuries, 146
Radiographic images, 2, 3
Recurrent tissue necrosis, 63
Regenerative medicine, 210, 215, 221
Rehabilitation
  ACRM, 241
  blast trauma casualties, 226
  mTBI, 244
  phases of, 232–234
  PM&R specialist, 226

residential transitional, 262
TBI service, 262
vestibular, 245
WRAMC, 259
Repair
arterial and venous injury, 143
axillary and subclavian arteries, 146
blunt aortic injury, 147
femoral vein injury, 139
vascular, 144
vein, 139–140
venous injuries, 143
Resuscitation
ATC, 46
blast-injured patients, 43
crystalloid, 45
crystalloids/colloids, 44
goals, 43
primary injury, 43
Resuscitation fluids, 44, 45
Resuscitative endovascular balloon for occlusion of the aorta (REBOA), 64, 93, 126
Retroperitoneal approach, 92–93
Right iliac artery, 83
Rotational thromboelastometry (ROTEM), 52
Ruptured testes, 70

S
Scrotal injuries, 156–157
Second impact syndrome (SIS), 246
Secondary blast injuries, 11, 13
Secondary thoracic blast injury, 115–116
Short Musculoskeletal Function Assessment (SMFA), 174
Shrapnel, 11
Shrinker socks, 226, 227, 229
Sigmoid colon, 2, 3, 67
Skin grafting, 204, 205, 207
Small intestinal submucosa (SIS), 219
Soft tissue injury
amputations (*see* Amputations)
buttocks and bilateral lower extremity, 165
complications, 164–166
contaminated extremity wound, 160
definitive management, 161–162
early echelon care, 160–161
fracture management, 163–164
guillotine amputation, 168
HO morbidity, 159
in Iraq and Afghanistan, 159
JTTR, 159
left transfemoral amputation, 169
left transhumeral amputation, 172
left upper extremity, DCBI patient, 167
military health-care system, 175
musculoskeletal extremity wounds, 159
pelvic fracture, 164
pelvis and lower abdomen, DCBI patient, 164
perineal and pelvic injury, 159
principles, DCBI, 160
reconstructive ladder, 162–163
symptomatic limbs, 175
Somatic pain, 234
Sphincteroplasty, 130
Split-thickness skin graft (STSG), 163, 165, 170
Sport Concussion Assessment Tool (SCAT), 243
Staffing
ancillary care, 290
anesthesiologists, 289
MCS, 290
Sternotomy, 65, 115
Streamlining care
multidisciplinary conference, 286–287
polytrauma patient, 286
Subarachnoid hemorrhage, 252, 253
Subclavian artery (SCA), 79
Subdural hematomas, 253
Superficial femoral artery (SFA), 144, 145
Supraceliac aorta, 90, 91
Suprapubic tube (SPT), 155, 156
Surgeon-centric technique, 2, 5, 33
Symptoms
non-pharmacologic treatment, 255
pharmacologic treatment, 255

T
Tactical combat casualty care (TCCC)
care under fire, 16
concept, 15
guidelines, 17
principles, 15, 18
tactical field care, 17
tenets, 16–18
Tactical emergency casualty care (TECC)
circulation, 22
evacuation care phase, 23
guidelines, 18, 19
hot zone, 20
implementation, 24–27
MARCHE, 21
prehospital environments, 19
respiration, 22
TECC, 19
tenets, 20–24
warm zone, 21
Tactical Evacuation Care, 18
Tactical Field Care phase, 17
Targeted muscle reinnervation (TMR), 175, 221, 236
Temporary check socket, 228
Temporary thoracic closure, 66
Temporary vascular shunts (TVS), 138, 139
Terminal devices, 233
Tertiary blast injuries, 13
Tertiary thoracic blast injury, 116
Testicular injuries, 156–157
The Committee on Tactical Combat Casualty Care (TCCC), 101
Theater Medical Data Store (TMDS), 285
Theoretical maximum heart rate (TMHR), 247

Thermoplastic socket, 229
Thoracic aortic pseudoaneurysms, 86, 87
Thoracic damage control, 65
Thoracic incision exposures, 88
Thoracic injuries
    blast lung perihilar contusion, 112
    classification, 114
    clinical presentation, 113
    demographics, 111
    ECMO initiation, 117
    ICU management, 116–118
    medical care, 114
    military and civilian settings, 111
    pathophysiology, 112–113
    PBI, 112
    primary, 118
    prognosis and injury prevention, 114–116
    quaternary, 116
    secondary, 115–116
    tertiary, 116
    timeline, 113
Thoracic stent grafts, 146
Thoracic trauma, 111, 116, 117
Thoracoabdominal incision, 89
Thoracostomy, 62, 65, 115
Thromboelastography (TEG), 52
Tibial artery injuries, 145
Tibial injuries, 145
Total body surface area (TBSA), 198–202, 204
Tourniquets, 138
Traditional patient movement, 31
Traditional US army training, 32
Trans-clavicular exposure, 80
Transcutaneous electrical nerve stimulation (TENS), 235
Transfemoral amputation, 229, 231, 237
Transperitoneal approach, 90
Trauma
    civilian settings, 273
    Department of Defense Trauma Registry, 277
    Joint Theater Trauma System clinical practice, 278
    non-trauma diagnoses, 271
    WRAMC and NNMC, 259
Trauma Infectious Disease Outcomes Study (TIDOS), 183, 263, 270, 271, 274, 277, 278
Traumatic brain injury (TBI), 10, 225
    acute medical management, 254
    blast injury (*see* Blast injury)
    blast-specific consultation, 261
    cognitive disorders (*see* Cognitive disorders)
    complications (*see* Complications, TBI)
    consciousness (DOC), 254
    DAI, 252
    DCBI patients, 261
    description, 252
    epidemiology, 251
    grading, 251
    intracranial bleeding, 252
    mental health disorders (*see* Symptoms)
    morbidity and mortality, 251
    neurobehavioral dysfunction (*see* Neurobehavioral dysfunction)
    neuroimaging, 252
    neuropsychological and cognitive testing, 255, 262
    pathophysiology, 253
    polytrauma, 262
    rehabilitation, 262
    severity classification, 252, 261
    VA-DoD (*see* VA-DoD continuum)
Traumatic limb amputation, 186
Triage category system, 35
Triamcinolone, 236
Trinitrotoluene (TNT), 8
Tube thoracostomy, 111, 115
Tympanic membrane, 9, 10

U

Ulnar artery injuries, 146
Upper limb prosthetics, 231–232
Ureteropelvic junction (UPJ), 152
Urethral injuries, 68, 155–156
US Army Medical Department, 29
US military system, 30

V

Vacuum-assisted closure (VAC), 126
VA-DoD continuum
    PSC, 256
    rehabilitation, 257
Vascular injuries
    arterial and venous injury, 138
    axillary artery, 147
    axillosubclavian artery, 145–146
    blast injury, 135
    brachial artery, 146
    diagnosis, 136–137
    endovascular therapies, 146–147
    epidemiology, 135–136
    femoral artery, 144
    femoral vein injury, 139
    interposition graft repair, 143
    in Iraq and Afghanistan, 135
    management
        collateral damage, 137
        fasciotomy, 140
        nonoperative, 141
        operative, 141–146
        tourniquets, 138
        TVS, 138, 139
        vein repair, 139–140
    popliteal artery, 144, 145
    radial and ulnar artery, 146
    tibial artery, 145
Vascularized composite allotransplantation (VCA), 221
Vasodilated ischemic tissue, 95
Vehicle-borne IEDs (VBIEDs), 159

Vein repair, 139–140
Venovenous extracorporeal membrane oxygenation (vvECMO) cannulation, 117
Ventilation, 198, 203
Verrucous hyperplasia, 237
Volumetric muscle loss (VML), 165
Voriconazole, 192

W

Walter Reed National Military Medical Center (WRNMMC)
 admission processes, 286
 and NNMC, 259
 blast injury protocol, 261
 combat trauma patients, 261
 complication, 260
 DCBI patients, 259
 in Afghanistan, 260
 JTS VTC, 260
 military Role V hospitals, 259
 OIF and OEF battlefields, 285
 patient, 287
 polytrauma patients, 260
 surgical services, 260
Warm, fresh, whole blood (WFWB), 49
Wound, management, 273–274
Wrap, 199, 204, 205, 207

Z

Zurich guidelines, 246–247

Printed by Printforce, the Netherlands